NEUROLOGY - LABORATORY AND CLINICAL RESEARCH DEVELOPMENTS

CONTEMPORARY ISSUES IN PERIPHERAL NEUROPATHY

NEUROLOGY - LABORATORY AND CLINICAL RESEARCH DEVELOPMENTS

Additional books in this series can be found on Nova's website
under the Series tab.

Additional e-books in this series can be found on Nova's website
under the e-book tab.

NEUROLOGY - LABORATORY AND CLINICAL RESEARCH DEVELOPMENTS

CONTEMPORARY ISSUES IN PERIPHERAL NEUROPATHY

DANIEL L. MENKES
EDITOR

NOVA BIOMEDICAL

New York

Library of Congress Cataloging-in-Publication Data

ISBN: 978-1-62948-681-9

Library of Congress Control Number: 2013955178

Published by Nova Science Publishers, Inc. † New York

Contents

Preface

The challenge of any editor is to insure that any publication provides value added benefit for the reader. There are numerous publications that address the subject of peripheral neuropathy from short articles intended for continuing medical education to weighty tomes designed to be encyclopedic in nature. This book attempted to focus on issues that confront the clinician, both novice and expert, who routinely treats patients with peripheral neuropathies. I have learned that most editors assign the chapter topics to be written such that the book is an outgrowth of the editor's vision. This book took an entirely novel approach. Rather than assign the topics, the author allowed the publisher to request clinicians who were passionate about a particular subject to write about topics that were encountered in their usual clinical practice. My role as editor was to insure that these diverse topics were amalgamated into a coherent publication. I am of the opinion that the work speaks for itself in that it addresses subjects that are hardly ever contained in one text. These include the introductory chapters on hereditary neuropathies, genetic testing and the use of electrodiagnostic methodologies. This is followed by a discussion of the acquired demyelinating neuropathies, as noted in the Guillain Barre syndrome. Subsequently, there are two chapters devoted to chronic inflammatory demyelinating polyneuropathy; one in children, the other in adults. This is followed by a discussion of acquired neuropathies from diverse conditions such as the monoclonal gammopathies, familial amyloidosis and neuropathies associated with HIV. This book concludes with a discussion of pelvic floor neuropathies and a surgical approach to the treatment of compressive and traumatic neuropathies. The goal was to provide a textbook that would address the most current topics in the field of peripheral neuropathy authored by other specialists in addition to neurologists.

Acknowledgment

In addition to the chapter authors, the editor would like to thank all of his patients for educating him on the subtleties of diagnosing and treating these disorders.

In: Contemporary Issues in Peripheral Neuropathy
Editor: Daniel L. Menkes
ISBN: 978-1-62948-681-9

Chapter I

The Role of Clinical Neurophysiology in the Diagnosis of Peripheral Neuropathies

Elisabeth Chroni*
Department of Neurology, University of Patras, Greece

Abstract

Peripheral nerve disorders manifest with symptoms attributable to dysfunction of one or more of the following peripheral nervous system's functions; sensory, motor and autonomic. While clinical neurophysiological testing provides useful information beyond what is obtainable by physical examination, one cannot underestimate the importance of a detailed history and examination.

Nerve conduction studies (NCS) assess the function of the largest diameter, most heavily myelinated nerve fibers. These fibers include the motor fibers and the sensory fibers that subserve vibration and position. As such, NCS does not concernthe thinly myelinated (e.g. autonomic) or unmyelinated (e.g. nociceptive) fibers. NCS may provide information about the extent and severity of nerve pathology, differentiate between primary axonal and demyelinating processes, establish the pattern of nerve involvement (e.g., symmetric, length dependent, multiple mononeuropathics) and narrow the differential diagnosis regarding the underlying cause. Advanced techniques such as transcranial magnetic stimulation and autonomic nervous system testing may provide additional salient information. Needle electromyography [EMG] may provide additional data regarding the duration of nerve injury (acute or chronic) the degree of reinnervation on subsequent studies follow-up studies), evaluate the possibility of a coexisting myopathic process and may occasionally disclose an abnormality suggestive of a particular condition (e.g. neuromyotonia in Isaac syndrome or myokymia in radiation plexopathies).

* Correspondance: Elisabeth Chroni, M.D, Ph. D., Department of Neurology, School of Medicine, University of Patras, Rio-Patras 26504, Greece. Tel. : +30.2610.994 485, Fax : +30.2610.993949, E-mail: echroni@yahoo.com.

In conclusion, clinical neurophysiological examinations assist in confirming the clinical diagnosis of a peripheral neuropathy and help delimit the range of diagnostic possibilities

Keywords: Neurophysiology, motor and sensory conduction, F-waves, conduction block, axonal and demyelinating neuropathies, electromyography

Introduction

This review outlines the basic neurophysiological tests employed for the diagnosis and management of peripheral neuropathies. A specific emphasis is placed on the various aspects of these nerves diseases as characterized by clinical neurophysiology testing. In addition, these tests' limitations and potential pitfalls that should be avoided will also be discussed. Given the frequency and diversity of peripheral nerve diseases encountered in clinical practice, this review focuses on well-established nerve conduction study techniques, especially those involving large diameter motor and sensory fibers. Before any clinical neurophysiology examinations are performed, it is imperative that the physician obtain all relevant clinical information and perform an appropriate physical examination. This allows the physician to narrow the differential diagnosis to a maximum of two or three potential diagnoses that will be evaluated. By focusing on a narrower range of diagnostic possibilities, fewer electrodiagnostic tests are required resulting in minimal patient discomfort while obtaining a maximum amount of information in a limited period of time. [1-3] As there are different techniques that evaluate sensory, motor and autonomic functions, it is important to have an understanding of these techniques.

1. Routine Electrodiagnostic Studies

1.1. Motor Nerve Conduction Studies

Electrical stimulation of a motor nerve through intact the skin induces an evoked response from one or more muscles innervated by that nerve, which is designated the compound muscle action potential (CMAP). This represents the summation of all of the evoked responses from the group of muscles that respond to supramaximal motor nerve stimulation. It should be recalled that when the motor fibers of the median nerve are supramaximally stimulated, the resulting CMAP response is from a group of median nerve innervated thenar muscles and not just from the abductor pollicis brevis (APB). Therefore, when the report reads that a median motor nerve conduction study was performed to the APB, this indicates that the median motor fibers were supramaximally stimulated and the results were obtained from the thenar muscles supplied by the median nerve in the region, primarily the APB. Useful CMAP measurements include the distal motor latency, its amplitude, its area and its duration. While motor nerve conduction velocities are useful, it is necessary to stimulate the same nerve at a proximal site in order to calculate the motor nerve conduction velocity for this intervening segment. It is also useful to examine the CMAP's configuration as dispersion of this waveform may indicate the presence of myelin sheath dysfunction. Localization of a focal lesion requires a comparison of the amplitude, area and duration of CMAP obtained from proximal stimulation to that obtained from distal stimulation. Motor nerve conduction studies should be performed such that the segments across the common sites of compression are evaluated. These include the median nerve across the wrist, the ulnar nerve across the elbow and the fibular nerve (previously known as peroneal nerve) across the fibular head.

1.2. Sensory Nerve Conduction Studies

These are somewhat similar to motor nerve conduction studies with some minor differences. First, the supramaximal stimulation may be performed in the usual direction of sensory nerve conduction (orthodromic) or in the opposite direction of sensory nerve conduction (antidromic). As an example, orthodromic median nerve stimulation would be performed by supramaximal over the index finger. The response, known as a sensory nerve action potential (SNAP), would be recorded at the wrist. If an antidromic technique were to be used, the stimulating and recording sites would be reversed. There are different ranges of normal for SNAP amplitudes obtained from orthodromic and antidromic stimulation. The SNAP amplitudes derived from antidromic stimulation are greater in amplitude because the SNAP is recorded at a site much closer to the signal generator. Thus, it is important to know the manner in which the recordings were obtained and the ranges of normal for that laboratory. The most useful SNAP measurements include its amplitude and latency. Unlike motor nerve conduction velocities, sensory nerve conduction velocities can be obtained directly without the need to stimulate a second time at a more proximal site. The sensory nerve conduction velocity is calculated by measuring the distance over which the nerve was conducted in millimeters and dividing this by the latency in milliseconds. Most clinicians prefer to use conduction velocities because this value remains the same over differing distances. SNAP morphology is less useful than CMAP morphology because fewer sensory fibers contribute to the SNAP. Furthermore, SNAP amplitudes are measured in microvolts whereas CMAP amplitudes are measured in millivolts. Therefore, the motor responses are three orders of magnitude larger than the sensory responses. Therefore, desynchronization of a SNAP is hardly ever observed given that phase cancellation usually results when the sensory segment is affected by a demyelinating process. Nonetheless, the SNAP may manifest an increased duration when it is measured across a site of compression such as the median nerve at the wrist or in the earlier stages of an inherited myelinopathy.

1.3. F-Waves

These are evoked responses of the muscles that result after the CMAP has occurred such that F-waves are commonly referred to as "late responses." Electrical impulses applied to a peripheral nerve propagate proximally as well as distally. Some of the largest and most heavily myelinated motor fibers have enough capacitance to generate a second action potential after the refractory period has ended. These largest motor fibers, which comprise 1-3% of the total number of motor fibers, discharge a second time and emit a response that may be recorded from certain distal limb muscles. However, it should be recalled that sufficient time must elapse between the last contracting muscle fibers contributing to the CMAP and the arrival of the F-wave for this finding to be observed on the oscilloscope. With few exceptions, F-waves are most easily recorded from the intrinsic hand and foot muscles. While F-waves do not occur after every stimulus, a series of consecutive stimuli usually evokes F-waves varied in shape, latency, and amplitude. Characteristics of F-waves such as latency and persistence (i.e. number of F-waves in a series of stimuli) vary between nerves. [4, 5] The most useful F-wave parameter is the F-wave minimum latency, which is defined as the shortest latency obtained from a series of consecutive stimuli. In addition, the range of latencies designated "F-chronodispersion", has been reported to be a sensitive and early marker of motor fiber dysfunction. [4, 6, 7]. An adequate number of stimuli are needed in order to obtain reliable measurements. Many authorities recommend that a sample of 40 F-waves should be obtained in order to make an accurate assessment of all F-wave parameters. [8] However, 20 stimuli should be sufficient for an accurate measurement of F-wave minimum" or mean latency. [9]

1.4. Electromyography (EMG)

Electromyography or needle EMG is recorded by placing either a concentric or a monopolar needle electrode into a muscle for evaluation. In most instances, needle EMG must be performed in order to provide an accurate assessment of peripheral nervous system function. However, EMG examination is not obligatory in all cases as it may not provide much value added benefit in the evaluation of carpal tunnel syndrome with normal CMAP amplitudes. Similarly, it may not provide additional information on those follow-up examinations performed to monitor the status of a previously diagnosed entrapment neuropathy or acquired demyelinating neuropathy.

Approximately 0.5 seconds after a needle is inserted into a region area outside the end-plate zone of a healthy muscle, no EMG activity is expected. Restated, the muscle should be quiet. Any activity, other than end-plate noise, that is observed thereafter is designated spontaneous activity. Spontaneous activity is an abnormal finding and often indicates that pathology is present. Spontaneous activity of varied morphology and pathophysiology is always abnormal but is hardly ever specific (Figure 1). Fibrillation potentials are biphasic (initially negative) action potentials of single muscle fibers that are of low amplitude (<1000 μV) and short (5ms) duration. Their appearance usually follows muscle membrane or axonal damage after an initial lag time of 7 to 14 days with a peak at 1-2 months after disease onset. Positive sharp waves (PSWs) differ in morphology from fibrillation potentials. PSWs manifest an initial sharp positive phase, are of lesser amplitude but of longer duration than fibrillation potentials and usually appear within 1-2 weeks after disease onset. Both fibrillation and PSWs should be interpreted similarly in that they indicate that the motor axon has been disconnected from the muscle membrane. Many authors refer to these as "denervation potentials," but it should be recalled that they may be observed in necrotizing myopathies as well as in neuropathic processes. Fasciculation potentials, which should not be confused with fibrillation potentials, represent isolated spontaneous discharges of motor units. Unlike fibrillation potentials, fasciculation potentials may be observed through the skin, tend to be of much higher amplitude, have a more complex morphology and a distinctive "popping" sound on EMG. Complex repetitive discharges (CRDs) are also a non-specific spontaneous EMG abnormality. They consist of runs of rapidly discharging motor fibres with an abrupt onset and a uniform amplitude and configuration (Figure 2). [10] They have a distinctive sound likened to a motorcycle revving its engine. Spontaneous activity of any type should be quantified by its frequency. Two main classifications are used. One qualitative system classifies its presence as abundant, moderate or sparse. Another system semi-quantifies this by the number of muscle sites in which it is present using a scale of zero to 4+. Nonetheless, the amount of spontaneous activity does not necessarily reflect the amount of underlying pathology given that the muscle is sampled at random. Once the muscle has been evaluated at rest, the physician asks the patient to contract the muscle gently in order to assess the motor unit action potentials (MUAPs). MUAPs represent the action potentials of a group of muscles fibers belonging to the same histochemical type and innervated by the same motor neuron. However, it should be recalled that Type II or "white" muscle is not evaluated at low levels of contraction. MUAP parameters that may be useful diagnostically include the amplitude, duration, the number of phases, number of turns, the firing rate and the recruitment ratio. These may be assessed visually or with a specially designed software program. [10-13]

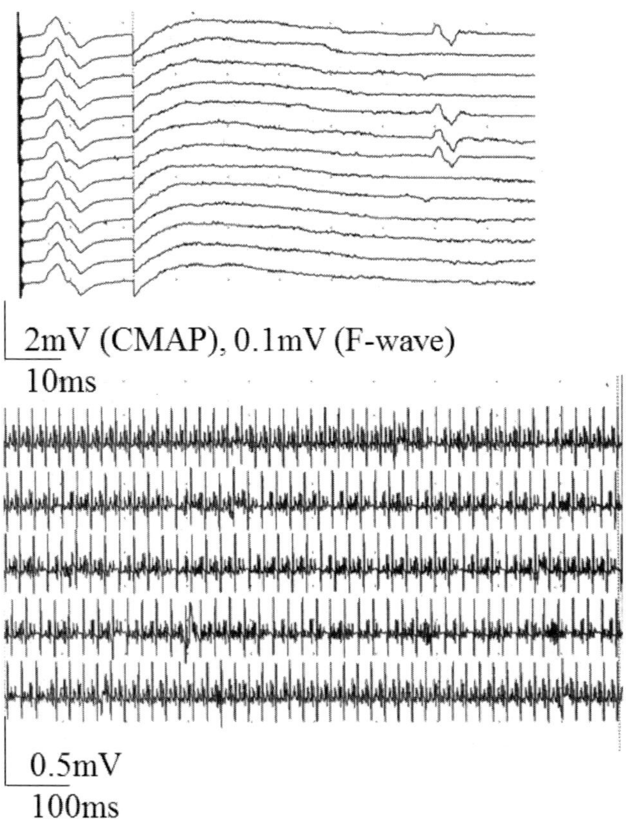

Figurc 1. A 56 year-old male patient presented with muscle stiffness, cramps and myalgias. Nerve conduction studies were indicative of an undefined asymmetric polyneuropathy. Upper tracing: Stimulation of the fibular nerve evoked a CMAP from the extensor digitorum communis muscle of low amplitude, followed by infrequently occurring F-waves with a very prolonged latency (79 ms). Lower tracing: Needle electromyography from tibialis anterior muscle demonstrated a neuromyotonic discharge consisting of a prolonged series of multiple motor unit action potentials firing at a high (50Hz) intraburst frequency.

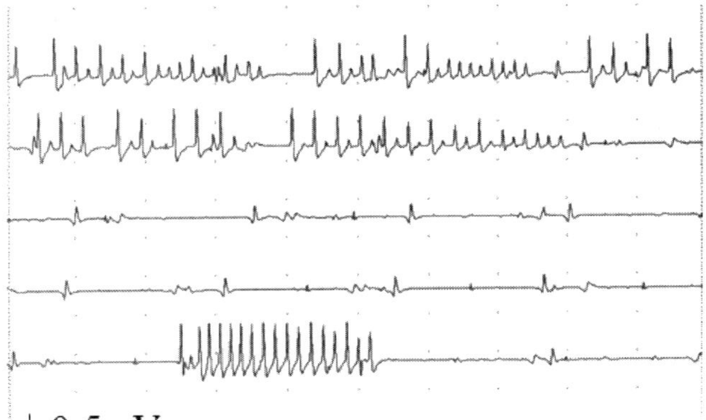

Figure 2. Isolated fibrillation potentials associated with bursts of abrupt onset and equally abrupt cessation of complex repetitive discharges in a patient with an idiopathic plexopathy.

1.5. Autonomic Tests

These tests are not routinely performed as part of an electrodiagnostic evaluation unless dysautonomia is a prominent presenting symptom. The most commonly utilized tests evaluate cardiovascular function. These include the Valsalva maneuver, R-R variability during deep breathing and the tilt test. [14, 15] Signal analysis that includes estimation of time and frequency domain measurements provides a reasonable assessment of the sympathetic-parasympathetic balance. [16] Sweating function may be assessed by recording of the sympathetic skin responses, an easily performed study with low sensitivity, or by the quantitative sudomotor axon-reflex test (QSART). [17-20] QSART and more labor intensive investigations such as thermoregulatory sweat testing are techniques that are usually performed at centers that specialize in autonomic nervous system testing.

1.6. Transcranial Magnetic Stimulation (TMS)

Magnetic stimulation of an appropriate area of the motor cortex may induce an evoked response from a limb muscle. This technique measures the time required for the cortex to generate a muscle response. The conduction time along the peripheral motor nerve, the neuromuscular junction and muscle may be calculated using the F-wave minimum latency. The peripheral motor conduction time is calculated by measuring the F wave minimum latency and subtracting 1 ms as the estimate of the "turn-around time" for the F wave to be generated. The distal motor latency is added to this figure and then divided by two. When this peripheral motor conduction time is subtracted from the latency obtained by cortical stimulation, a central conduction time within the corticospinal tract may be derived. This technique allows for the assessment of central nervous system motor function subserved by the corticospinal tract. A less common use of TMS is the confirmation of a proximal conduction block by stimulating the anterior motor roots at their exit zone while recording from a distal target muscle. [21, 22]

2. Methodology

2.1. Test Selection

Although the American Association of Neuromuscular and Electrodiagnostic Medicine has published guidelines on the maximum number of nerve conduction studies (NCS) that should be performed in over 90% of cases, this refers to routine clinical practice. [23] Nonetheless, the purpose of the study must be kept in mind. For example, it is not uncommon to detect an underlying polyneuropathy in a patient with carpal tunnel syndrome, especially when the patient has a known risk factor for peripheral neuropathy such as diabetes mellitus. This is the reason that others support the view that a more extensive examination may be required to exclude the possibility of an underlying polyneuropathy. [24, 25] Over the recent years when practice medicine shifted from expert opinion to evidence based medicine, neurophysiological criteria have been proposed for several groups of peripheral nerve disorders. [26] Nonetheless, most authors would agree that it is useful to obtain at least one normal sensory study, one normal motor study, and one normal late response (F-wave or H reflex) before proceeding to needle EMG. Needle EMG should be performed to such an extent that the distribution of the abnormalities has been conclusively determined.

2.2. Selection of Nerves / Muscles

The nerves that are most commonly studied include the median, ulnar and radial nerves in the upper limbs and the fibular, superficial fibular, tibial and sural nerves in the lower limbs. Depending on the referring diagnosis, other nerves may be of additional utility (e.g. antebrachial cutaneous nerves, phrenic nerve). There is a difference of opinion between electrodiagnostic medicine consultants as to which nerves are most useful for specific disease processes. As an example, some authors opine that the plantar nerves in the foot are more sensitive than the sural nerve for detecting length-dependent neuropathies. [27]

As previously stated, the number of muscles that should be examined depends on the referring diagnosis and the results of the nerve conduction studies. In a person referred for median neuropathy at the wrist (carpal tunnel syndrome) with normal nerve conduction studies, needle EMG is not obligatory. Contrast this with a person referred for a diagnosis of motor neuron disease who may require needle EMG of three limbs, cranial nerve innervated muscles and the thoracic paraspinal muscles. Therefore, the author recommends that a sufficient number of muscles be examined to answer the referring provider's question, determine the distribution of the needle EMG abnormalities, and to account for all abnormalities noted on nerve conduction studies.

2.3. Planning and Executing the Procedures

The first step in any EMG/NCS is to identify any abnormalities in the antecedent history and physical examination that might be indicative of peripheral nerve dysfunction. This is not always straightforward, particularly when more than one condition is present in the same individual. For example, restricted shoulder movements might be due to tendonitis, arthritis or a brachial plexus lesion. In the earliest stages of these disorders, it may be difficult to differentiate anterior horn cell disease from multifocal motor neuropathy (MMN), or motor predominant chronic inflammatory demyelinating polyneuropathy (CIDP). The second step is the documentation of nerve involvement in one or more limbs such that the pattern of abnormality may be characterized. This allows the clinician to distinguish those neuropathies that may be amenable to treatment from those for which there is little or no treatment.

The initial electrodiagnostic evaluation plan should be flexible and subject to modification during the procedure depending on the individual findings. Examination of two muscles innervated by the same root but different nerves should be performed to differentiate radiculopathies from mononeuropathies. With respect to compression neuropathies, it is important to sample muscles along the length of the involved nerve in order to localize the pathological site. At the very least, the most proximal and most distal muscle innervated by that nerve should be examined. It is also important to comment on whether or not MUAPs were observed in every muscle. The presence of even just one recruitable MUAP would indicate that there is functional continuity of the nerve to all muscles sampled, which assists the clinician in developing a treatment strategy. It should be recalled that only the largest, most heavily myelinated fibers can be examined by these techniques. Lesser myelinated autonomic nerve fibers, as well as small-diameter unmyelinated fibers cannot be evaluated by standard nerve conduction studies and require specific tests. [28] Thus, patients with pain and dysautonomia may have completely normal EMG/NCS. Such patients should be informed that they may have a "small fiber neuropathy."

Despite these limitations, EMG/NCS have proven useful in that they often help to differentiate pathology affecting the large myelinated nerve fibers as either primary myelinopathies for primary axonopathies. Since these structures coexist in peripheral nerves, injury to one component often results in secondary or collateral damage to the other component. As such, it is not useful to state that a neuropathy affecting these large fibers is a "mixed axonal and demyelinating polyneuropathy" given that this is almost always true but is rarely helpful. It is essential that primary myelinopathies be distinguished from primary axonopathies. This is because acquired myelinopathies tend to be more amenable to treatment. In general, segmental myelin dysfunction may be detected by significantly prolonged distal motor latencies, slow motor nerve conduction velocities and markedly prolonged late responses. Nonetheless, these findings in and of themselves cannot differentiate inherited myelinopathies or dysmyelinating neuropathies (e.g. Charcot Marie Tooth Type I or CMT-I) from acquired demyelinating polyneuropathies (e.g. CIDP). In contrast, there are certain findings that strongly favor an acquired demyelinating polyneuropathy diagnosis over that of an inherited dysmyelinating neuropathy. These findings include conduction block (CB) and temporal dispersion (TD). Various criteria have been proposed to define these entities that have different sensitivities and specificities. Nonetheless, all criteria exclude data obtained across common sites of compression such as the ulnar nerve across the elbow and the fibular nerve across the fibular head. The author assesses for CB by comparing a CMAP derived from supramaximal stimulation of a motor nerve at a proximal site to the CMAP obtained in the same manner from supramaximal stimulation at a distal site. CB requires that the proximal CMAP amplitude and area decrease by more than 50% and that the CMAP duration increases by no more than 30%. In contrast, the author diagnoses TD when the proximal CMAP amplitude is reduced by more than 50%, the area is unchanged or reduced by no more than 50% and the duration is increased by more than 30% as compared to the distal CMAP. When the proximal CMAP demonstrates an amplitude and area reduction of more than 50% and the duration is increased by more than 30% as compared to the distal CMAP, then the author indicates that both CB and TD are present (Figure 3). Irrespective of the definition of CB or TD, their presence usually indicates that presence of acquired demyelinating pathology. It should be recalled that amplitude, area and duration measurements are made in the CMAP waveforms' initial negative phase and confirmation of CB or TD should be demonstrated over short nerve distances (e.g. 2.5cm). [29-32]

Another characteristic CMAP finding in myelinopathies is that there is poor synchronization of the waveform giving it a "wavy" or "ragged" appearance. Primary axonopathies are usually accompanied by a reduction in the amplitude and area of both SNAPs and CMAPs with minimal slowing of the conduction velocity. [3] However, it should be recalled that disorders such as the acute motor axonal neuropathy (AMAN) variant of the Guillain-Barré syndrome (GBS) may manifest these findings due to inexcitability of some of the distal motor axons. As such, this change may not result from actual axon loss but may be due to the intrinsic electrical properties of the myelin sheaths or axons themselves. Numerous criteria have been proposed to differentiate primary myelinopathies from primary axonopathies that have varying degrees of specificity and sensitivity.

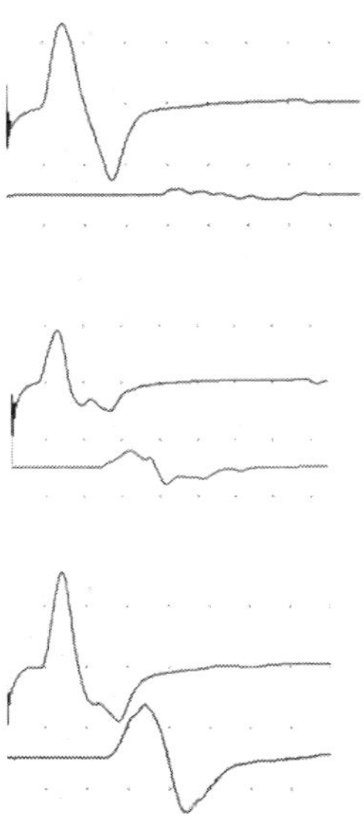

Date	St. Site	Lat (ms)	Amp (mV*ms)	Area (mV)	Dur (ms)
2007	W	4.1	2.0	8.8	6.2
	El	18.0	0.2 (-94%)	0.7 (-92%)	9.2 (49%)
2008	W	3.9	4.7	11.1	4.4
	El	12.3	1.4 (-71%)	5.5 (-51%)	7.0 (58%)
2009	W	4.3	7.8	18.7	4.6
	El	12.2	4.4 (-44%)	18.2 (-3%)	7.6 (6%)

2mV(1st), 5mV(2nd,3rd study)
5ms

Figure 3. Serial nerve conduction studies of the median nerve in a 60 year-old male patient with classical CIDP. Upper two traces: The first study showed CB and TD with distortion of the CMAP on stimulation at the elbow (El) as compared to the wrist (W). Middle two traces: This second study, conducted 8 months later, demonstrates persistence of the focal demyelinating signs, CB and TD. Lower two traces: The third study showed improvement. Note that the CMAP amplitude increased with both wrist and elbow stimulation as compared to the previous study. Moreover, only TD was detected on elbow stimulation.

In order to preserve specificity for acquired demyelination, the author recommends that motor nerve conduction study abnormalities suggestive of demyelination should be identified in at least two nerves. Nonetheless, several caveats ought to be kept in mind. Amplitude drop may result from either axonal loss or distal CB.

Inexcitability of the largest diameter, fastest conducting fibers may result in a reduced conduction velocity, which results from the excitation of a subpopulation of lesser myelinated fibers. [33] When no CMAP or SNAP is obtainable, then the underlying pathological process cannot be determined as this may be due to either axon loss or nerve inexcitability. When the abnormalities do not fit into either a primary demyelinating or a primary axonal process then the author tends to classify the neuropathy as undefined or intermediate. This tends to be the most common type of neuropathy that the author encounters in clinical practice.

F-waves are also included in various sets of criteria for the diagnosis of demyelination. However, they can offer additional information, depending on the abnormality observed. The F-wave minimum latency is the most common parameter used for neuropathy classification. A significant prolongation, after adjustment for height and age, is a clear sign of demyelination. A normal F-wave minimum latency but increased F-chronodispersion implies a non-homogeneous involvement of motor nerve fibers, as some fibers are more severely affected than others (Figure 4). A. normal F-wave minimum latency with normal F-chronodispersion but reduced F-wave persistence implies either that either some neurons are unable to generate F-waves or that there is some process that is preventing the impulse from traveling along the nerve. An increased number of F-waves identical in shape, latency and amplitude are designated F-wave repeaters, [34] (Figure 5). This is a non-specific sign of a neuronopathy or a neuropathy. Of note, high amplitude F-waves have been associated with upper motor neuron diseases and other disorders of the central nervous system. [35]

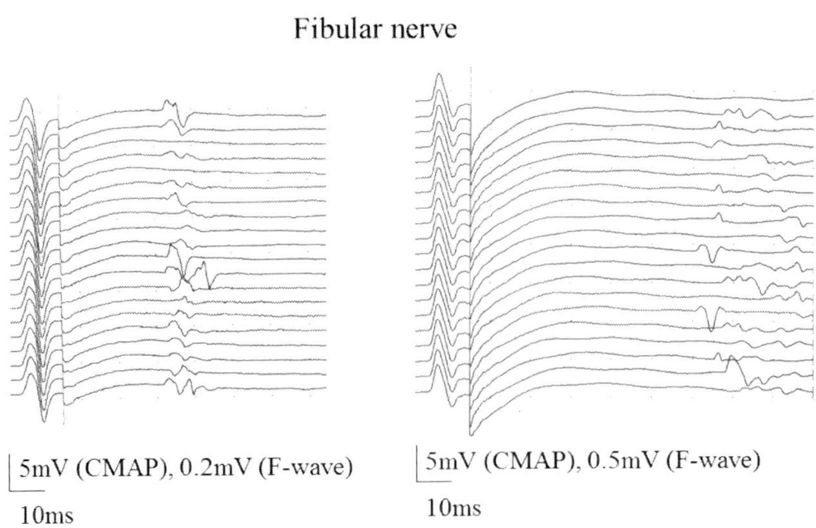

Figure 4. Standard F-waves recordings from the fibular nerve. Left side: This is a normal study with an F-wave minimum latency of 43.2 ms, F-chronodispersion of 6ms and a persistence of 95%. Contrast this with the right side: The right fibular nerve demonstrates a very prolonged F-wave minimum latency (70.1ms), increased F-chronodispersion (21.2ms) and normal persistence in a 55 year-old male patient with asymmetric CIDP.

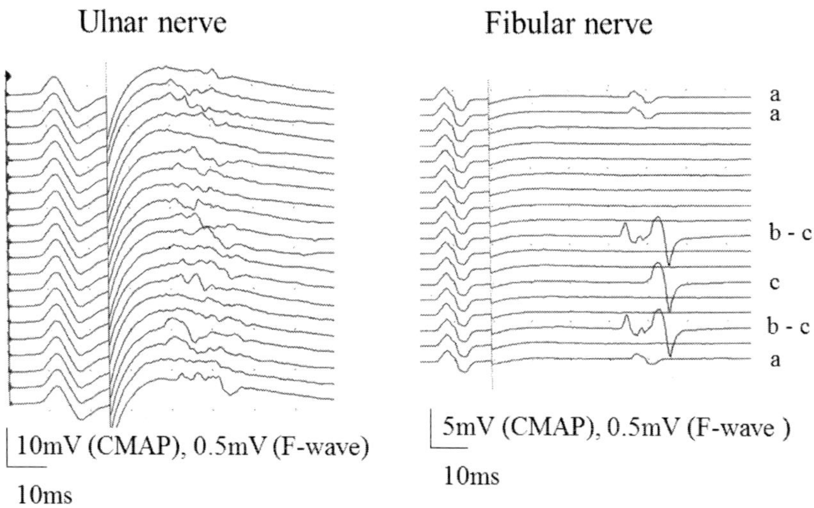

Figure 5. F-waves studies that recorded 20 consecutive traces. Left side of screen (ulnar nerve): There is a prolonged F-wave minimum latency (37.2ms), increased F-chronodispersion (8ms), and normal persistence in the ulnar nerve of a 35 year-old female patient with CIDP. Right side of screen (fibular nerve): There is low persistence and an increased number of F-wave repeaters in the fibular nerve of a 65 year-old female patient with MMN. Note that three different F-wave repeaters were recorded; two repeated three times and another one twice.

Needle EMG provides additional information on disease chronicity and its progress. In the context of a neuropathy, the presence of fibrillation potentials and positive sharp waves indicates ongoing axonal degeneration. This would not be observed in a primary myelinopathy in the absence of axon loss nor would this be observed in the recovery phase of a neuropathy (i.e. re-innervation). Spontaneous activity may also appear in patients with a severe acquired demyelinating polyneuropathy approximately two to three weeks after initial secondary axon loss. Fasciculation potentials are non-specific. When associated with objective clinical weakness or other spontaneous activity, they may be indicative of anterior horn disease. Nonetheless, they have also been reported in multifocal motor neuropathy and neuropathy associated with thyrotoxicosis. [10] Complex repetitive discharges are generally observed with chronic denervation and reinnervation, particularly in radiculopathies or other proximal motor lesions. [36] Early stages of motor axon loss are often associated with a reduced interference pattern at maximal voluntary effort along with spontaneous activity. In contrast, chronic denervation with reinnervation is characterized by MUAPs of prolonged duration. Other findings in this stage may include increased MUAP amplitudes and satellites potentials as a result of collateral sprouting. [10, 11] Consecutive discharges of these MUAPs may also demonstrate a variation in shape, known as "jiggle". The recognition of such MUAP morphological changes assists in identifying the chronicity of the neuropathic process. [37] At the chronic stage of an axonal neuropathy, MUAPs are often polyphasic, increased in amplitude and duration but stable; the maximal recruitment pattern remains reduced whereas the MUAPs demonstrate an increased firing rate. When severe muscle atrophy exists, a "pseudomyopathic" pattern with low amplitude polyphasic MUAPs may be observed. Therefore, it is better to refrain from using the terms "neuropathic" or "myopathic" when describing recruitment and interference patterns on needle EMG. Briefly, NCS and needle EMG results often allow for the neuropathy to be characterized for the following features:

- *Spatial pattern:* mononeuropathy // mononeuropathy multiple // symmetric polyneuropathy // asymmetric polyneuropathy // length dependent
- *Intra-nerve spatial pattern*: uniform // segmental // homogeneous
- *Fiber type involved*: motor // sensory // small diameter-autonomic fibers (note: special testing is required) // mixed (varied combinations)
- *Pathologic pattern*: primary axonal // primary demyelinating // undefined (intermediate)
- *Temporal pattern*: active denervation // chronic regenerative process

It is imperative that the electrodiagnostic physician have a thorough knowledge of peripheral nerve anatomy including the brachial plexus, lumbosacral plexus, and common anatomical anomalies such as the Martin-Gruber anastomosis. The electrodiagnostic physician should not have a stereotypical approach to any diagnosis such that maximum flexibility is maintained when unexpected results are encountered. Common pitfalls leading to erroneous diagnoses are listed below:

Points responsible for false positive neurophysiological results

- Busy laboratories may have insufficient time to conduct the examinations according to established methodological guidelines. Prolonged distal latencies or mild reduction of conduction may occur from low temperature or suboptimal skin contact (Figure 6). SNAPs may be affected by lower extremity edema due to higher skin resistance or increased distance from the action potential generated.

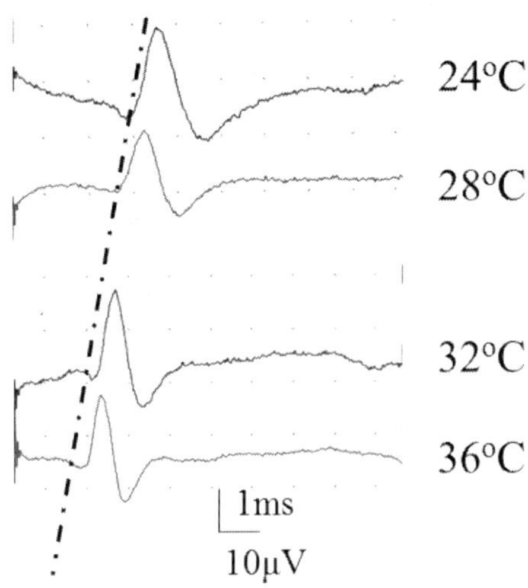

Figure 6. Sensory nerve action potentials (SNAPs) obtained from the ulnar nerve at different palm surface temperatures. The optimal skin temperature for SNAP recordings in the upper extremity is 32-34 degrees Celsius (°C). Note that with decreasing temperature, the latency, amplitude and duration all increase. With increasing temperature, the opposite is observed.

- Control data are not universal. It is recommended that each laboratory should establish its normative values. Alternatively, published data can be used, providing that the exact same techniques are employed.
- Mild abnormalities do not specifically identify the underlying pathology. For example, consider a patient in whom the upper limit of normal for an F-wave minimum latency is 29ms. An F-wave minimum latency of 30ms should not be construed as evidence of primary demyelination. Sural SNAP amplitudes in elderly people or in those swollen legs may be reduced or absent.
- Neurophysiologists often show a tendency to make the study conform to a clinical diagnosis or render a diagnosis in the absence of definitive neurophysiological data. Ideally, the EMG interpretation should be based solely on the neurophysiological findings.

Points responsible for false negative neurophysiological results

- If an examination is limited, sporadic pathology may be overlooked.
- Incorrect timing: Any study performed less than 10 days after an acute lesion is too early to establish a diagnosis with any degree of certainty. When studies are performed late in the course of the illness, the absence of evoked responses may not allow the primary pathological process to be discerned.
- Examinations that only evaluate large fibers will not detect disorders of the thinly myelinated or unmyelinated fibers (e.g. small fiber neuropathies).
- Some practitioners are reluctant to perform more extensive needle EMG such that additional diagnostic information goes undetected. [38]
- Inexperienced neurophysiologists tend to be inflexible in their approach. For example, a request for CTS turns out to be radiculopathy, mononeuropathy multiplex or even motor neuron disease.
- Failure to consider a second pathological condition. For example, consider a patient with a known inherited polyneuropathy such as CMT-I. An unexpected finding of a definite conduction block should not be attributed to the patient's condition. Instead, it should raise the suspicion of a superimposed acquired demyelinating polyneuropathy. [39]

3. Neurophysiological Findings in the Typical or Most Common Types of Neuropathy

3.1. Acquired Demyelinating Polyneuropathies

With respect to polyneuropathies, the clinical neurophysiologist is implicitly tasked with differentiating neuropathies that are potentially treatable with immunomodulating therapies from idiopathic distal symmetric axonal polyneuropathies that tend not to respond to such treatments. On general principles, the treatable neuropathies tend to be either the vasculitides (presenting in a typical "mononeuritis multiplex" pattern) or the acquired demyelinating polyneuropathies. Since vasculitides are rare, the electrodiagnostic consultant is primarily tasked with identifying acquired demyelination that may manifest as some combination of CB, TD, late response prolongation or profound conduction velocity slowing on NCS. Such significant slowing of nerve conduction studies usually fall into one of two distinct patterns; uniform slowing that is characteristic of hereditary myelinopathies and segmental demyelination often accompanied with focal conduction block, which is characteristic of acquired demyelinating neuropathies such as the inflammatory form of the GBS and CIDP. GBS is the most frequent worldwide acquired, acute, immune-mediated disorder of the peripheral nervous system. Acute inflammatory demyelinating polyneuropathy (AIDP) was the first type to be recognized, which emphasized the role of primary demyelination in GBS pathology. Subsequently, other subtypes of GBS such as AMAN with distinctive electrophysiological patterns have been acknowledged. Early electrophysiological confirmation of GBS diagnosis is of outmost clinical importance as early treatment tends to improve prognosis, which has been attributed to minimizing the degree of secondary axon loss. Several large studies have proposed single or combinations of electrophysiological parameters as more sensitive and reliable markers that would support the diagnosis during the first 5 days from the onset of clinical manifestations. Absence of H-reflex from gastrocnemius muscle, abnormalities of F-waves, proximal conduction block alone or in combination with distal lesion are few of these markers. [40-42] For practical and research reasons, the electrodiagnosis of GBS has been based on defined criteria. These various criteria have different specificity and sensitivity regarding differentiating acquired demyelinating from axonal neuropathies. [43, 44] The typical GBS abnormalities on routine motor nerve conduction studies include segmental conduction slowing with or without conduction block. In the proximal parts of the nerves that are infrequently examined, demyelination may be inferred on the basis of a significantly prolonged F-wave minimum latency and reduction of F-wave persistence. In the distal segments, prolongation of the distal motor latency, or TD of the CMAPs with the loss of their smooth configuration may be observed. Significant CMAP amplitude reduction in response to distal stimulation may be observed either on the basis of distal demyelination, axonal loss or both. [40] A significant CMAP amplitude reduction when proximal stimulation is compared to distal stimulation meeting the criteria for a CB also implies a demyelinating process. When distal CMAP amplitudes are reduced, AIDP should be differentiated from acute motor axonal neuropathy (AMAN) and a related disorder acute motor and sensory axonal neuropathy (AMSAN) in which the SNAP amplitudes are also abnormal. The additional finding of TD, as indicated by a CMAP of increased duration obtained from proximal stimulation when compared to distal stimulation, favors the diagnosis of AIDP. [3, 45, 46] Reversible conduction failure presenting as transient conduction slowing and CB at the intermediate segments without TD that may later progress to axonal degeneration, was systematically studied by Uncini and Kuwabara. [47] These authors emphasized the need for serial neurophysiological examinations in order to differentiate between temporary and persistent CB. A gradual reduction of the distal CMAP amplitude that eventually matches the amplitude of proximal stimulation, the so-called length-dependent CMAP amplitude reduction, has been attributed to Wallerian degeneration and favors an axonal process such as AMAN or AMSAN. [47] Other F-wave parameters, particularly F-chronodisperson, may demonstrate abnormalities even before other signs of acquired demyelination are noted. This reflects the underlying patchy and uneven involvement of motor nerve fibers in GBS. [48] Reduced persistence of F-waves in the median and ulnar nerves is a definite sign of conduction failure but it does not differentiate between the demyelinating and axonal variants of GBS. Sensory conduction studies in GBS are less important than motor ones but should be performed nonetheless. However, unlike the majority of neuropathies, sensory abnormalities of the ulnar and median nerve associated with a relatively preserved sural SNAP is often observed in GBS. [49] Amplitude changes of the SNAPs are more common than conduction slowing or reversible conduction failure often observed in the motor nerve conduction studies. [47] This is because there are fewer subcomponent fibers in a sensory nerve as compared to a motor nerve. Needle electromyography (EMG) has a secondary role in the diagnosis of GBS. In the earliest disease stages, needle EMG may demonstrate a reduced recruitment and interference pattern in the absence of spontaneous activity. The presence of spontaneous activity such as fibrillation potentials and positive waves suggests secondary axon loss and may portend a worse prognosis.

CIDP is the prototype of acquired, chronically relapsing or continuously progressive autoimmune neuropathy that is amenable to treatment. Since the first descriptions, an ever increasing number of CIDP variants appeared in the literature, including axonal or pure motor forms with or without conduction block, asymmetric and distal preponderance patterns. As with acquired demyelination in the AIDP variant of GBS, and the electromyographer should search for evidence of acquired demyelination such as profound segmental conduction slowing, partial CB, TD, prolonged latencies and F-waves abnormalities. [32] Electrophysiological abnormalities were employed by Kuwabara et al. to classify CIDP cases into distal, intermediate (forearm segments) and diffuse pattern groups. [50] Each electrophysiological category appears to be related to a particular disease subtype's severity and evolution, response to treatment and prognosis. As noted in the AIDP form of GBS, sensory nerve conduction studies tend to demonstrate a significant reduction in SNAP amplitude. [51] The pathophysiology of this finding is debated as to whether this represents axon loss or conduction failure. The distinctive pattern of abnormal median/ulnar with a normal sural SNAP may be observed in CIDP as well. [50]

Several authors have attempted to find electrophysiological abnormalities that are more representative of particular CIDP variants. For instance, neuropathy with antibodies against myelin-associated glycoprotein and sulfated glucuronyl paragloboside (anti-MAG/SGPG) tend to demonstrate greater involvement of the distal segments in the lower limbs in a length-dependent matter than is observed in typical cases of CIDP without these antibodies. [52, 53] In the subtype known as multifocal acquired demyelinating sensory and motor neuropathy (MADSAM), the intermediate nerve segments tend to have greater degrees of pathology than other segments. Nonetheless, none of these electrodiagnostic findings should be considered pathognomonic or unique for a certain clinical profile. Another acquired demyelinating neuropathy in which motor fibers are predominantly affected is multifocal motor neuropathy (MMN). In the later stages of MMN, the neurophysiological examination may be the only means by which one can distinguish this disorder from pure lower motor neuron variants of motor neuron disease. In the case of MMN, NCS reveal persistent partial CB that affects motor nerve but not sensory nerve conduction studies over a short segment outside common sites of compression whereas other features of demyelination tend to be less prominent. [29, 54, 55] These conduction abnormalities appear in the distribution of individual nerves or their branches such as the ulnar and median nerves in the upper extremities. [56] The identification of MMN without CB is even more difficult but needle EMG may be helpful as fasciculations occur less frequently in MMN than in motor neuronopathies. [31]

3.2. Diabetic Neuropathy

Diabetic mellitus (DM) is the cause of several clinically and pathophysiologically different neuropathy subtypes. [57, 58] A distal symmetric, sensory predominant polyneuropathy is the most frequent type of neuropathy induced by DM. [59] As this subtype of diabetic neuropathy is a typically length-dependent, the NCS reflect this process. Common findings include low amplitude or absent SNAPs with correspondingly reduced conduction velocities. The first sensory nerves affected are the sural and superficial fibular nerve, followed at a later stage by ulnar and median nerves, whereas the radial nerve is hardly ever involved. [60] Some authors opine that the median plantar and medial peroneal cutaneous nerve, being distal to the sural nerve, may be more sensitive to detecting the presence of a sensory neuropathy. [27] F-wave latency prolongation, increased F-chronodispersion, or increased F-wave repeaters in the fibular or tibial nerve constitute an early physiological sign of motor fiber involvement. [4, 34] When the diagnostic sensitivity of different neurophysiological parameters was examined, the ratio of the sural SNAP amplitude to that of the radial SNAP and the F-wave wave minimum latency in the fibular received the highest score. [61-63] With respect to the upper extremity, the ulnar is more frequently abnormal in this subtype of diabetic neuropathy than the median nerve unless a carpal tunnel syndrome coexists. When a median F-wave minimum latency is prolonged, the electromyographer should perform additional studies in order to evaluate for a superimposed median neuropathy at the wrist. While some neurophysiological abnormalities should be observed in diabetic patients, any electrodiagnostic study with complete absence of all SNAPs and reduced CMAP amplitudes in the hand muscles should raise the suspicion of another cause for the neuropathy. The electrodiagnostic physician should extend the testing in order to determine if a second pathological process such as acquired demyelination coexists.

Finally, apart from of the large diameter myelinated fibers, which are evaluated by standard nerve conduction studies, thinly myelinated and unmyelinated fibers are often affected in diabetic neuropathy. [64] Impaired autonomic nervous system function may be detected with specific tests such as the thermoregulatory sweat test, the Valsalva maneuver and laser Doppler flowmetry [64]. The absence of the sympathetic skin response from the sole of the foot, and less often, from the palm of the hand, indicates a cholinergic abnormality that may be observed in isolation or in addition to abnormalities on standard NCS. [65]

3.3. Neuropathies Related to Neoplasia

Malignancies may affect the peripheral nervous system directly by compression or neural tissue invasion or indirectly from an immune mediated response observed in paraneoplastic syndromes. Treatments directed at the neoplastic process such as radiation or chemotherapy may also have adverse effects on the peripheral nervous system. [66] Numerous chemotherapeutic agents such as platinum compounds, taxanes, and thalidomide have associated neurotoxicity. As a rule, a chemotherapy induced neuropathy manifests as a length-dependent sensory or predominately sensory neuropathy with minimum motor involvement save for some mild F-wave abnormalities. [67-69] While most chemotherapy associated neuropathies are axonal, some agents like suramin may result in a demyelinating neuropathy. [66]

Paraneoplastic neuropathies, which are defined as remote effects of cancer, are not directly related to the tumor, its metastases, its treatment or nutritional deficiency states. [66] Small cell lung cancer is the neoplastic process that is most commonly associated with a paraneoplastic syndrome. It may produce numerous subtypes of neuropathies including GBS, subacute or chronic sensorimotor polyneuropathy, autonomic neuropathy and sensory neuronopathy with or without motor involvement. [70] A sensory neuronopathy, which is characterized by low or absent SNAPs in both upper and lower extremities, even in the absence of other findings, should raise the index of suspicion for an occult tumor, especially a small cell lung carcinoma. [66]

3.4. Vasculitic Neuropathies

Connective tissue diseases may also cause a polyneuropathy. Occlusion of nutrient blood vessels resulting in hypoxic-ischemic injuries of large nerve trunks is considered the basic pathophysiologic mechanism. [71, 72] Vasculitic neuropathy is characterized by acute or subacute onset of multifocal axonal degeneration, with or without secondary myelin loss, in a pattern other than a typical distal symmetric axonal neuropathy. Therefore, the typical clinical pattern is that of "mononeuropathy multiplex," although overlapping of nerve lesions could result in asymmetric or even a symmetric sensorimotor polyneuropathy. The most frequent affected nerves are the fibular nerve at the level of the mid-thigh and the ulnar nerve in the arm. Such focal axonal lesions can be differentiated from nerve entrapment lesions by the absence of conduction slowing across common sites of compression, such as the elbow and the fibular head, and by the involvement of proximal muscles. [71] Sural, tibial, median and radial nerves are also affected in this descending order of frequency.

In addition to the typical reduction of amplitude of CMAPs and SNAPs, a finding known as "pseudoconduction block" may occur in the early phases of Wallerian degeneration. Of note, Sjögren syndrome is associated with a wide variety of neuropathic patterns, including trigeminal, autonomic and pure sensory neuropathies such that any electrodiagnostic investigation of this disorder requires specific neurophysiological testing. [73] Unlike acquired demyelinating polyneuropathies in which few needle EMG changes are noted early in the course of the illness, needle electromyography is of paramount importance in vasculitic neuropathies.

Abundant spontaneous activity, fibrillations and positive waves, is a prominent and early feature that occurs in a multifocal manner in both proximal and distal muscles. This feature helps to distinguish between idiopathic distal symmetric axonal neuropathies in which proximal spontaneous activity should not be identified and acquired demyelinating neuropathies in which spontaneous activity is usually absent early in the course of the illness. It is important to recall that re-innervation by collateral sprouting during the recovery phase will result in low amplitude polyphasic potentials on needle EMG. These findings should not be mistaken for a myopathic process.

3.5. Hereditary Neuropathies

Hereditary motor and sensory neuropathies (HMSN) constitute a large group of genetic conditions. In the past, eponyms were used to characterize a specific phenotype such as Charcot-Marie-Tooth. [74] Currently they are categorized by the specific genetic defect arising from different genetic mutations. [75, 76] HMSN may be subdivided on the basis of clinical neurophysiology into primary axonopathies and primary myelinopathies. The neurophysiological features that favor a hereditary origin are a uniform slowing along the entire length of a peripheral nerve, [77] the absence of CB and TD of the CMAPs and the normal F-chronodispersion due to the homogeneity of myelin pathology. Conduction velocities in the primary myelopathy subtypes may demonstrate severe conduction slowing to 15-20 m/s in the distal nerve segments. [78] The axonal subtype manifests length-dependent finds that occur first in the feet and then later in the hands. [77] If the first neurophysiological examination is performed later in the patient's life, secondary changes of myelin dysfunction or axonopathy may be present such that this may result in some difficulties in identifying the primary type of pathology. This is because CMAPs and SNAPs may be unobtainable in the distal limb segments. In such cases, recording from a more proximal muscle or nerve (e.g. tibialis anterior muscle or the radial nerve), may be useful. Two important exceptions to the pattern of "uniform conduction slowing" in primary myelinopathies include hereditary neuropathy with liability to palsies (HNPP) and the leukodystrophies. [79] HNPP is characterized by mild conduction slowing which becomes prominent or accompanied by CB across common sites of compression such as the fibular head for the fibular nerve and the elbow for the ulnar nerve. [80, 81] These additional conduction abnormalities can be short lasting or chronic, in which case EMG signs of denervation and reinnervation may be detected.

Conclusion

Clinical neurophysiology studies, most of which are non-invasive, provide objective data that provide significant value added benefit in the evaluation of peripheral nerve diseases. In order to maximize the diagnostic utility of these studies, several aspects must be kept in mind.

All patients who have signs or symptoms of a peripheral neuropathy should undergo appropriate neurophysiological studies. Each neurophysiological examination should be specifically tailored to address all of the clinical manifestations. Electrodiagnostic studies should be used to confirm a neuropathy, exclude other pathologies, estimate the severity of neuropathy and predict its prognosis. A normal neurophysiological examination cannot exclude a neuropathy as most conventional studies only examine the largest most heavily myelinated fibers. While neuropathies can often be classified as primary myelinopathies or axonopathies, electrodiagnostic studies do not confirm the pathological process. The tests should be performed in a timely manner, neither too early nor too late. There are very few "pathognomonic neurophysiological findings" indicative of particular processes. Finally, the interpretation of neurophysiological data and final conclusions should be strictly based on the actual neurophysiological data although the final diagnosis should be the purview of the clinician.

References

[1] Gooch CL, Weimer LH. The electrodiagnosis of neuropathy: basic principles and common pitfalls. *Neurol. Clin.* 2007; 25: 1-28.

[2] Kimura J. Kugelberg lecture: principles and pitfalls of nerve conduction studies. *Electroencephalogr. Clin. Neurophysiol.* 1998; 106: 470-476.

[3] Donofrio PD, Albers JW. AAEM minimonograph #34: polyneuropathy: classification by nerve conduction studies and electromyography. *Muscle Nerve* 1990; 13: 889-903.

[4] Panayiotopoulos CP, Chroni E. F-waves in clinical neurophysiology: a review, methodological issues and overall value in peripheral neuropathies. *Electroencephalogr. Clin. Neurophysiol.* 1996; 101: 365-374.

[5] Fisher MA. F-waves--physiology and clinical uses. *ScientificWorld Journal* 2007; 7: 144-160.

[6] Panayiotopoulos CP. F chronodispersion: a new electrophysiologic method. *Muscle Nerve* 1979; 2: 68-72.

[7] Chroni E, Panayiotopoulos CP. F tacheodispersion: quantitative analysis of motor fiber conduction velocities in patients with polyneuropathy. *Muscle Nerve* 1993; 16: 1302-1309.

[8] Chroni E, Taub N, Panayiotopoulos CP. The importance of sample size for the estimation of F wave latency parameters in the ulnar nerve. *Muscle Nerve* 1994; 17: 1480-1483.

[9] Fisher MA, Hoffen B, Hultman C. Normative F wave values and the number of recorded F waves. *Muscle Nerve* 1994; 17: 1185-1189.

[10] Kimura J. Electrodiagnosis in diseases of nerve and muscle: pricinples and practice. (edit 2) 1989; F/A. Davis company, Philaldelphia.

[11] Stalberg E. Invited review: electrodiagnostic assessment and monitoring of motor unit changes in disease. *Muscle Nerve* 1991; 14: 293-303.

[12] Stalberg E, Erdem H. Quantitative motor unit potential analysis in routine. *Electromyogr. Clin. Neurophysiol.* 2002; 42: 433-442.

[13] Stalberg E, Fuglsang-Frederiksen A, Bischoff C. Quantitation and standardization in EMG and neurography. *Suppl. Clin. Neurophysiol.* 2000; 53: 101-111.

[14] Stalberg EV, Nogues MA. Automatic analysis of heart rate variation: I. Method and reference values in healthy controls. *Muscle Nerve* 1989; 12: 993-1000.

[15] Looga R. The Valsalva manoeuvre--cardiovascular effects and performance technique: a critical review. *Respir. Physiol. Neurobiol.* 2005; 147: 39-49.

[16] Sztajzel J. Heart rate variability: a noninvasive electrocardiographic method to measure the autonomic nervous system. *Swiss Med. Wkly* 2004; 134: 514-522.

[17] Low PA, Caskey PE, Tuck RR et al. Quantitative sudomotor axon reflex test in normal and neuropathic subjects. *Ann. Neurol.* 1983; 14: 573-580.

[18] Low PA, Vernino S, Suarez G. Autonomic dysfunction in peripheral nerve disease. *Muscle Nerve* 2003; 27: 646-661.

[19] Shahani BT, Halperin JJ, Boulu P, Cohen J. Sympathetic skin response--a method of assessing unmyelinated axon dysfunction in peripheral neuropathies. *J. Neurol. Neurosurg. Psychiatry* 1984; 47: 536-542.

[20] Low PA, Denq JC, Opfer-Gehrking TL et al. Effect of age and gender on sudomotor and cardiovagal function and blood pressure response to tilt in normal subjects. *Muscle Nerve* 1997; 20: 1561-1568.
[21] Inaba A, Yokota T, Saito Y et al. Proximal motor conduction evaluated by transcranial magnetic stimulation in acquired inflammatory demyelinating neuropathies. *Clin. Neurophysiol.* 2001; 112: 1936-1945.
[22] Attarian S, Azulay JP, Verschueren A, Pouget J. Magnetic stimulation using a triple-stimulation technique in patients with multifocal neuropathy without conduction block. *Muscle Nerve* 2005; 32: 710-714.
[23] Proper performance and interpretation of electrodiagnostic studies. *Muscle Nerve* 2006; 33: 436-439.
[24] Kaul MP, Pagel KJ, Dryden JD. When to use the combined sensory index. *Muscle Nerve* 2001; 24: 1078-1082.
[25] Chang MH, Liu LH, Lee YC et al. Comparison of sensitivity of transcarpal median motor conduction velocity and conventional conduction techniques in electrodiagnosis of carpal tunnel syndrome. *Clin. Neurophysiol.* 2006; 117: 984-991.
[26] Fuglsang-Frederiksen A, Pugdahl K. Current status on electrodiagnostic standards and guidelines in neuromuscular disorders. *Clin. Neurophysiol.* 2011; 122: 440-455.
[27] Altun Y, Demirkol A, Tumay Y et al. The medial plantar and medial peroneal cutaneous nerve conduction studies for diabetic polyneuropathy. *Neurol. Sci.* 2011; 32: 849-854.
[28] Santiago S, Ferrer T, Espinosa ML. Neurophysiological studies of thin myelinated (A delta) and unmyelinated (C) fibers: application to peripheral neuropathies. *Neurophysiol. Clin.* 2000; 30: 27-42.
[29] Nobile-Orazio E, Cappellari A, Priori A. Multifocal motor neuropathy: current concepts and controversies. *Muscle Nerve* 2005; 31: 663-680.
[30] Lange DJ, Trojaborg W, McDonald TD, Blake DM. Persistent and transient "conduction block" in motor neuron diseases. *Muscle Nerve* 1993; 16: 896-903.
[31] Katz JS, Barohn RJ, Kojan S et al. Axonal multifocal motor neuropathy without conduction block or other features of demyelination. *Neurology* 2002; 58: 615-620.
[32] Sander HW, Latov N. Research criteria for defining patients with CIDP. *Neurology* 2003; 60: S8-15.
[33] Tankisi H, Pugdahl K, Johnsen B, Fuglsang-Frederiksen A. Correlations of nerve conduction measures in axonal and demyelinating polyneuropathies. *Clin. Neurophysiol.* 2007; 118: 2383-2392.
[34] Chroni E, Tendero IS, Punga AR, Stalberg E. Usefulness of assessing repeater F-waves in routine studies. *Muscle Nerve* 2012; 45: 477-485.
[35] Argyriou AA, Polychronopoulos P, Talelli P, Chroni E. F wave study in amyotrophic lateral sclerosis: assessment of balance between upper and lower motor neuron involvement. *Clin. Neurophysiol.* 2006; 117: 1260-1265.
[36] Meyer BU, Benecke R, Frank B, Conrad B. Complex repetitive discharges in the iliopsoas muscle. *J. Neurol.* 1988; 235: 411-414.
[37] Stalberg EV, Sonoo M. Assessment of variability in the shape of the motor unit action potential, the "jiggle," at consecutive discharges. *Muscle Nerve* 1994; 17: 1135-1144.
[38] Sohn MW, Whittle J, Pezzin LE et al. Electrodiagnostic consultation and identification of neuromuscular conditions in persons with diabetes. *Muscle Nerve* 2011; 43: 812-817.

[39] Marques W, Jr., Funayama CA, Secchin JB et al. Coexistence of two chronic neuropathies in a young child: Charcot-Marie-Tooth disease type 1A and chronic inflammatory demyelinating polyneuropathy. *Muscle Nerve* 2010; 42: 598-600.
[40] Gordon PH, Wilbourn AJ. Early electrodiagnostic findings in Guillain-Barre syndrome. *Arch. Neurol.* 2001; 58: 913-917.
[41] Clouston PD, Kiers L, Zuniga G, Cros D. Quantitative analysis of the compound muscle action potential in early acute inflammatory demyelinating polyneuropathy. *Electroencephalogr. Clin. Neurophysiol.* 1994; 93: 245-254.
[42] Ropper AH, Wijdicks EF, Shahani BT. Electrodiagnostic abnormalities in 113 consecutive patients with Guillain-Barre syndrome. *Arch. Neurol.* 1990; 47: 881-887.
[43] Albers JW, Donofrio PD, McGonagle TK. Sequential electrodiagnostic abnormalities in acute inflammatory demyelinating polyradiculoneuropathy. *Muscle Nerve* 1985; 8: 528-539.
[44] Asbury AK, Cornblath DR. Assessment of current diagnostic criteria for Guillain-Barre syndrome. *Ann. Neurol.* 1990; 27 Suppl: S21-24.
[45] Ho TW, Mishu B, Li CY et al. Guillain-Barre syndrome in northern China. Relationship to Campylobacter jejuni infection and anti-glycolipid antibodies. *Brain* 1995; 118 (Pt 3): 597-605.
[46] Kalita J, Misra UK, Das M. Neurophysiological criteria in the diagnosis of different clinical types of Guillain-Barre syndrome. *J. Neurol. Neurosurg. Psychiatry* 2008; 79: 289-293.
[47] Uncini A, Kuwabara S. Electrodiagnostic criteria for Guillain-Barre syndrome: A critical revision and the need for an update. *Clin. Neurophysiol.* 2012.
[48] Panayiotopoulos CP, Chroni E, Daskalopoulos C. The significance of F-chronodispersion in the electrodiagnosis of Guillain-Barre syndrome and other motor neuropathies. *Arch. Neurol.* 1992; 49: 217-218.
[49] Murray NM, Wade DT. The sural sensory action potential in Guillain-Barre syndrome. *Muscle Nerve* 1980; 3: 444.
[50] Kuwabara S, Ogawara K, Misawa S et al. Distribution patterns of demyelination correlate with clinical profiles in chronic inflammatory demyelinating polyneuropathy. *J. Neurol. Neurosurg. Psychiatry* 2002; 72: 37-42.
[51] Krarup C, Trojaborg W. Sensory pathophysiology in chronic acquired demyelinating neuropathy. *Brain* 1996; 119 (Pt 1): 257-270.
[52] Capasso M, Torrieri F, Di Muzio A et al. Can electrophysiology differentiate polyneuropathy with anti-MAG/SGPG antibodies from chronic inflammatory demyelinating polyneuropathy? *Clin. Neurophysiol.* 2002; 113: 346-353.
[53] Franssen H, Notermans NC. Length dependence in polyneuropathy associated with IgM gammopathy. *Ann. Neurol.* 2006; 59: 365-371.
[54] Chaudhry V, Corse AM, Cornblath DR et al. Multifocal motor neuropathy: electrodiagnostic features. *Muscle Nerve* 1994; 17: 198-205.
[55] Nobile-Orazio E. Multifocal motor neuropathy. *J. Neurol. Neurosurg. Psychiatry* 1996; 60: 599-603.
[56] Leger JM, Younes-Chennoufi AB, Chassande B et al. Human immunoglobulin treatment of multifocal motor neuropathy and polyneuropathy associated with monoclonal gammopathy. *J. Neurol. Neurosurg. Psychiatry* 1994; 57 Suppl: 46-49.
[57] Brown MJ, Asbury AK. Diabetic neuropathy. *Ann. Neurol.* 1984; 15: 2-12.

[58] Vinik AI, Holland MT, Le Beau JM et al. Diabetic neuropathies. *Diabetes Care* 1992; 15: 1926-1975.
[59] Simmons Z, Feldman EL. Update on diabetic neuropathy. *Curr. Opin. Neurol.* 2002; 15: 595-603.
[60] Dyck PJ, Carter RE, Litchy WJ. Modeling nerve conduction criteria for diagnosis of diabetic polyneuropathy. *Muscle Nerve* 2011; 44: 340-345.
[61] Andersen H, Stalberg E, Falck B. F-wave latency, the most sensitive nerve conduction parameter in patients with diabetes mellitus. *Muscle Nerve* 1997; 20: 1296-1302.
[62] Pastore C, Izura V, Geijo-Barrientos E, Dominguez JR. A comparison of electrophysiological tests for the early diagnosis of diabetic neuropathy. *Muscle Nerve* 1999; 22: 1667-1673.
[63] Karsidag S, Morali S, Sargin M et al. The electrophysiological findings of subclinical neuropathy in patients with recently diagnosed type 1 diabetes mellitus. *Diabetes Res. Clin. Pract.* 2005; 67: 211-219.
[64] Gibbons CH, Freeman R, Veves A. Diabetic neuropathy: a cross-sectional study of the relationships among tests of neurophysiology. *Diabetes Care* 2010; 33: 2629-2634.
[65] Soliven B, Maselli R, Jaspan J et al. Sympathetic skin response in diabetic neuropathy. *Muscle Nerve* 1987; 10: 711-716.
[66] Krarup C, Crone C. Neurophysiological studies in malignant disease with particular reference to involvement of peripheral nerves. *J. Neurol.* 2002; 249: 651-661.
[67] Argyriou AA, Chroni E, Koutras A et al. Vitamin E for prophylaxis against chemotherapy-induced neuropathy: a randomized controlled trial. *Neurology* 2005; 64: 26-31.
[68] Argyriou AA, Koutras A, Polychronopoulos P et al. The impact of paclitaxel or cisplatin-based chemotherapy on sympathetic skin response: a prospective study. *Eur. J. Neurol.* 2005; 12: 858-861.
[69] Argyriou AA, Polychronopoulos P, Iconomou G et al. Paclitaxel plus carboplatin-induced peripheral neuropathy. A prospective clinical and electrophysiological study in patients suffering from solid malignancies. *J. Neurol.* 2005; 252: 1459-1464.
[70] Graus F, Delattre JY, Antoine JC et al. Recommended diagnostic criteria for paraneoplastic neurological syndromes. *J. Neurol. Neurosurg. Psychiatry* 2004; 75: 1135-1140.
[71] Olney RK. AAEM minimonograph #38: neuropathies in connective tissue disease. *Muscle Nerve* 1992; 15: 531-542.
[72] de Groot K, Schmidt DK, Arlt AC et al. Standardized neurologic evaluations of 128 patients with Wegener granulomatosis. *Arch. Neurol.* 2001; 58: 1215-1221.
[73] Mori K, Iijima M, Koike H et al. The wide spectrum of clinical manifestations in Sjogren's syndrome-associated neuropathy. *Brain* 2005; 128: 2518-2534.
[74] Reilly MM. Classification of the hereditary motor and sensory neuropathies. *Curr. Opin. Neurol.* 2000; 13: 561-564.
[75] Parman Y. Hereditary neuropathies. *Curr. Opin. Neurol.* 2007; 20: 542-547.
[76] Reilly MM. Sorting out the inherited neuropathies. *Pract. Neurol.* 2007; 7: 93-105.
[77] Krajewski KM, Lewis RA, Fuerst DR et al. Neurological dysfunction and axonal degeneration in Charcot-Marie-Tooth disease type 1A. *Brain* 2000; 123 (Pt 7): 1516-1527.

[78] Nicholson GA. Penetrance of the hereditary motor and sensory neuropathy Ia mutation: assessment by nerve conduction studies. *Neurology* 1991; 41: 547-552.
[79] Kane NM, Oware A. Nerve conduction and electromyography studies. *J. Neurol.* 2012.
[80] Lenssen PP, Gabreels-Festen AA, Valentijn LJ et al. Hereditary neuropathy with liability to pressure palsies. Phenotypic differences between patients with the common deletion and a PMP22 frame shift mutation. *Brain* 1998; 121 (Pt 8): 1451-1458.
[81] Verhagen WI, Gabreels-Festen AA, van Wensen PJ et al. Hereditary neuropathy with liability to pressure palsies: a clinical, electroneurophysiological and morphological study. *J. Neurol. Sci.* 1993; 116: 176-184.

In: Contemporary Issues in Peripheral Neuropathy
Editor: Daniel L. Menkes
ISBN: 978-1-62948-681-9

Chapter II

Role of Genetic Testing in Peripheral Neuropathy

Charles H. Whitaker[1,2]
[1]Director, Muscular Dystrophy Association Clinic for Children
Neuromuscular Center at the Hospital for Special Care
New Britain, CT, US
[2]Assistant Professor of Neurology
University of Connecticut Health Center
Farmington, CT, US

Abstract

Physicians who assess patients presenting with signs or symptoms of a peripheral neuropathy must consider the possibility that it is genetic in origin. Most of these patients present with a longstanding, progressive clinical course. The importance of taking a comprehensive history that includes a comprehensive pedigree cannot be overemphasized. Nonetheless, the absence of a family history does not exclude the possibility of an inherited neuropathy as spontaneous mutations occur. This chapter reviews the clinical approach to patients suspected of having an inherited neuropathy. Classical Mendelian genetics are reviewed along with atypical patterns of inheritance such as mitochondrial disorders and triplet repeat diseases that manifest the phenomenon of anticipation. This chapter also addresses the means by which DNA codes for RNA molecules that are translated into their end products. This chapter concludes with an approach to the patient with a suspected inherited neuropathy such that results in the judicious use of confirmatory testing.

Introduction

Gregor Mendel, an Augustinian monk and scientist, is generally credited with performing the first controlled genetic experiments while at St Thomas's Abbey in Brno. [1] Between

1856 and 1863, Mendel performed experiments of plant hybridization, wherein he cultivated and tested 29,000 pea plants. Seven observable traits were used to demonstrate the outcomes of cross hybridization. From the collected data, he was able to conclude that traits could be expressed as either dominant or recessive. He reported that one in four pea plants had purebred dominant alleles, two out of four were hybrids and one out of four was purebred recessive. These observations lead to the formulation of the fundamental rules of genetics, the Law of Segregation and the Law of Independent Assortment, which later became known as Mendel's Laws of Inheritance. [2] Mendel's work suggested that heredity was not acquired, and that the inheritance patterns of many traits could be explained through simple rules and ratios.

Mendel's data were published in 1865-1866 at which time his work was viewed primarily as a contribution to the study of plant hybridization. It was not until 35 years later with its rediscovery that this seminal paper became the foundation of classical genetics. The concept of the gene could be inferred from Mendel's cross fertilization experiments. Nonetheless it was the work of Thomas Hunt Morgan and others on drosophila (fruit flies), which have a short generation time and a relatively simple genome that allowed further application of these principles to the animal kingdom and helped to support the chromosome theory of inheritance. [3] Through the application of linkage analysis, it could be demonstrated that genes were linearly arranged on chromosomes. The actual molecule that carries genetic information was not evident until experimentation demonstrated that transformation of bacteria requires DNA rather than protein. In 1953, the correct structure of DNA was determined by Watson and Crick. [4] Further work regarding replication, transcription and translation of the DNA molecule would follow.

The hereditary neuropathies represent a large proportion of referrals to neuromuscular centers. Thus, a comprehensive understanding of basic genetic principles is necessary for the diagnosis of these and other hereditary conditions. A family pedigree analysis is necessary in order to determine the precise inheritance pattern. Although basic, this is absolutely required before more specific genetic testing as it allows for a more focused search by eliminating unlikely conditions. Even with negative genetic testing, the knowledge gained from pedigree analysis is paramount for risk assessment and genetic counseling. This chapter reviews patterns of inheritance and basic molecular genetics as it applies to the evaluation of patients with hereditary neuropathy. The hereditary neuropathies are discussed in greater detail in another chapter.

Modes of Inheritance

Mendelian disorders are caused by a mutation in a single gene that results in a clear effect on the phenotype. They are inherited in the simple patterns similar to those described by Mendel. Mendelian disorders are *autosomal* if encoded by a gene on one of the 22 non-sex chromosomes, and *X-linked* if encoded by a gene on the X chromosome. The nomenclature used when describing these conditions is interchangeable and may be confusing. It is important to be familiar with this terminology as it is essential when interpreting the results of genetic testing. A genetic *locus* is a specific position on a chromosome. Alternate forms of a gene at a particular locus are referred to as *alleles*. If both alleles are the same they are *homozygous* at the locus and if both alleles are different they are *heterozygous*. An individual may be either homozygous or heterozygous. However, if one has two different mutant alleles at a locus he or she is referred to as a *compound heterozygote*.

Dominant conditions are those which are expressed in the heterozygous state. Dominant disorders occur with one mutated allele associated with a disease and one normal or wild-type allele. *Recessive* conditions are only expressed in either the homozygous or compound heterozygous state. Thus, recessive conditions require a disease associated mutation on both alleles. X-linked conditions result from mutant genes on the X chromosome such that they are fully expressed in males given that they have one X chromosome such that they are designated *hemizygous*. Most X-linked conditions are recessive such that carrier females rarely manifest any signs of the disease. X-linked dominant conditions are less common. Such conditions affect both genders although males are more severely affected. X-linked disorders do not demonstrate male to male transmission as a father only transmits a Y chromosome to his sons. Chromosomal abnormalities or genomic disorders caused by duplications or deletions of genetic material that span more than one gene may also manifest a dominant inheritance pattern.

Gene mutations cause disease by altering the function of the encoded protein product. In dominant disorders, wherein only one allele is affected, this change results in a toxic gain of function or "haploinsufficiency." In contrast, recessive conditions are typically due to a loss of function. An exception to Mendel's laws of inheritance is observed in the inheritance pattern of the mitochondrial disorders that result from mutations in the mitochondrial genome. This follows a maternal pattern of inheritance given that mitochondria are strictly maternally inherited. The mitochondrial genome encodes for only a fraction of the proteins necessary for oxidative phosphorylation. Therefore, many diseases that affect mitochondrial function are due to mutations in the nuclear DNA and will follow an autosomal pattern of inheritance. [5]

Autosomal Dominant Inheritance

These disorders are caused by a single gene mutation located on one allele. Individuals heterozygous for the mutation develop disease. Pedigree analysis reveals that autosomal dominant inheritance is *vertical* and therefore should not skip generations. However, there are instances when this may seem to be the case. Both males and females are affected and have an equal probability of transmitting the trait. There may be differences that are influenced by the sex of the individual. Normal alleles and mutant alleles are distributed equally in the formation of the gametes. Therefore, the inheritance of a mutant allele is fifty percent with each offspring produced. According to the independence principle, the probability of two or more independent events is the product of their separate probabilities. For example, the probability of having three affected siblings is $\frac{1}{2} \times \frac{1}{2} \times \frac{1}{2} = \frac{1}{8}$ or 12.5%.

There are exceptions to the rule regarding the vertical inheritance pattern of autosomal dominant conditions. Sporadic mutations may occur despite neither parent being affected. For some disorders, the *spontaneous mutation* rates may be quite high. This is more common in conditions that affect life expectancy or reproductive fitness. Autosomal dominant disorders typically manifest either complete or incomplete *penetrance*. With complete penetrance, all persons that carry the mutation manifest signs of the disease. In conditions with *incomplete penetrance*, a mutation carrier may not manifest any signs of this disorder. Nonetheless, the mutant gene will pass with the same frequency and may be expressed in subsequent generations. In some dominant disorders, there is delayed onset such that the carrier of the mutation could still reproduce, transmit the disorder, and expire from an unrelated cause. Additionally, many dominant conditions are *variably expressed.* While this may be confused with incomplete penetrance, all individuals that carry the mutant gene will manifest some evidence of being affected to a variable degree. Affected individuals within a family who carry the same mutant allele may vary from mild or few symptoms to a more severe expression of the genetic defect. In some cases, the expression is mild or unrecognized by the individual. Charcot-Marie-Tooth disease type 1A (CMT1A) is one of the most common genetic disorders seen in neuromuscular practice. These cases show an autosomal dominant pattern of inheritance which is variably expressed within the family. It is not unusual that a patient presenting with the typical signs and symptoms of CMT1A has a mildly affected parent with the same demyelinating changes noted on nerve conduction studies. In this example there is complete penetrance of the genetic mutation with demyelination noted on nerve conduction studies and variable expression within the family ranging from mild to severe. [6]

There are several conditions encountered in a neuromuscular practice that result from unstable *trinucleotide repeat expansions*. Although not commonly associated with an isolated polyneuropathy, there are conditions with associated polyneuropathy resulting from either translated or non-translated trinucleotide repeat expansions that result in abnormal gene expression. The adult onset autosomal dominant spinocerebellar ataxias may have an associated polyneuropathy. Many of these conditions produce proteins with long expansions of the amino acid glutamine. This alters the protein sequence creating a toxic change that ultimately leads to neurodegeneration. [7] In some of these conditions, the phenomenon of *anticipation*, where each successive generation is more affected than the proceeding, may occur. This is the direct result of an increasing the number of repeats in successive generations and may be dependent on the gender of the contributing parent, a sex-specific expansion. For example, severe congenital myotonic dystrophy type one is always inherited from the mother. [8] In contrast, juvenile onset Huntington disease is almost invariably paternally inherited. [9]

Autosomal Recessive Inheritance

Autosomal recessive disorders present in individuals homozygous for the mutant gene or compound heterozygotes for two different mutant alleles at the same locus. Persons heterozygous for the mutation, that is those with one normal or wild type allele, are carriers and do not have signs or symptoms of the condition. The characteristic pedigree pattern is *horizontal* with affected individuals limited to a single sibship rather than multiple generations. Autosomal recessive conditions are due to loss of function mutations. Both parents are clinically unaffected and must be heterozygous carriers for the mutant allele. Male and female offspring are affected with equal probability with ¼ homozygous affected, $^2/_4$ or ½ heterozygous carriers, and ¼ homozygous for the normal or "wild type" allele.

The frequency of heterozygotes within a given population determines the probability that two heterozygote carriers will mate. This is increased within isolated populations where there is a high incidence of the mutation or within certain groups where consanguineous mating is more common. Given that the average American family is relatively small (2-3 children), an autosomal recessive condition may only be seen in one child, which may give the appearance of a sporadic mutation. Therefore, it is important not to disregard a possible genetic etiology of a condition in such cases. All the offspring of a homozygous affected individual will be obligate carriers presuming that the mate is homozygous for the normal alleles. If the mate happened to be a heterozygous carrier of a mutation at the same allele, then the pairing will result in a 50 percent risk of having an affected child. If two homozygous affected individuals produce offspring, then all of them will be affected. This uncommon situation arises when the children are the products of parental consanguinity or if the mutant allele is common.

X-linked Inheritance

These disorders result from mutations in genes located on the X chromosome; the majority of which are X-linked recessive. X-linked recessive conditions affect males from multiple generations of a family, but never demonstrate male-to-male transmission. Female carriers either show no signs of the condition or minimal signs if the process of random X inactivation results in a disproportionate inactivation of the normal allele. [10] X-linked dominant disorders manifest in both heterozygous females and hemizygous males although males are more severely affected.

With mating of a heterozygous carrier female to normal male, there is a fifty percent risk of having an affected son and a fifty percent risk of having a carrier daughter. An affected male paired with an unaffected female will result in all daughters being obligate carriers whereas all sons will be unaffected. When there is a high frequency of the abnormal X allele in a population, the probability of an affected male and a carrier female coupling is increased. In this instance, their daughters will have an equal chance of being carriers or homozygous affected while their sons will have the same odds of being affected or receiving the normal allele from the mother. This would appear to break the hallmark rule of no male to male inheritance of an X-linked condition even though the X inheritance from the mother is independent of the father being affected.

Rarely, an X-linked recessive disorder will be observed in a female. This may occur when two abnormal X-chromosomes are transmitted or in females with Turner syndrome (45XO) who are *hemizygous* for the X-chromosome. [11] As previously stated, partial expression of the mutant allele, the *manifest carrier* state may result from skewed X inactivation of more X chromosomes that possess the normal allele which produces a disproportionate number of cells with the mutant allele.

A number of X-linked conditions result from a spontaneous mutation. For instance, one third of all new cases of Duchenne muscular dystrophy are the result of a spontaneous mutation. [12] X-linked CMT (CMTX) is the prototypical X-linked dominant disorder wherein all individuals who possess the mutant allele are affected. Males are more affected than their sisters as they lack a protective normal allele. A pedigree analysis is needed to confirm X-linked inheritance by the absence of male-to-male transmission of the abnormal gene. [13]

Mitochondrial Inheritance

Mitochondrial inheritance represents the exception to Mendel's rules. All cells, with the exception of mature erythrocytes, contain between 2-100 mitochondria. Each mitochondrion contains between five and ten circular chromosomes. Mitochondria are subcellular organelles responsible for oxidative metabolism and energy production, which is accomplished through oxidative phosphorylation. Tissues differ in their dependence on oxidative phosphorylation. Those with the highest dependence include the heart, skeletal muscle, and the central nervous system. Therefore, mitochondrial disorders will disproportionately affect these organs resulting in encephalopathies, myopathies, or encephalomyopathies. The 16.5-kb mitochondrial chromosome encodes for protein translation machinery, two ribosomal RNAs and 22 transfer RNAs, as well as the 13 proteins involved in oxidative phosphorylation. [14] Because of its cytoplasmic location, the inheritance of mitochondria is exclusively maternal as mature sperm have little cytoplasm and few mitochondria. Therefore, only women can transmit mitochondrial disorders and all of their offspring will inherit the disorder. Mitochondria replicate separately from the nucleus and segregate into daughter cells independently. Therefore, the number of mitochondria with mutated DNA may vary between cells and tissues. The relative proportion of normal to abnormal mitochondria, known as *heteroplasmy*, determines disease severity and phenotypic variability within a family. [15]

Flow of Genetic Information

Genetic information is stored within the DNA molecules situated in the chromosomes that are located in the cell nucleus and mitochondria. Each individual chromosome contains one long supercoiled DNA molecule. All cells, with the exception of mature erythrocytes, contain the information of the entire person's genome. By definition, genes are the portion of the DNA molecule that encodes for a functional gene product. The majority of these are proteins. However, it should be recalled that functional RNA molecules such as ribosomal RNA (rRNA), transfer RNA (tRNA) and small nuclear RNA (snRNA) molecules are also encoded by genes. Only 1-2 percent of the entire human genome codes for proteins while the remaining non-coding regions are responsible for gene regulation. The nucleic acids, both DNA and RNA, are polymers of individual *nucleotides* composed of a deoxyribose (DNA) or ribose (RNA) sugar, a phosphate, and either a purine (adenine or guanine) or pyrimidine (thymine, cytosine or uracil) base. The backbone is formed by linking the individual nucleotides from 5' to 3' through covalent bonds between the sugar phosphate molecules. The sequence is interpreted in a 5' to 3' order, 5' being *upstream* and 3' being *downstream*. Base pairings are specific. In DNA, adenine (A) is paired with thymine (T) and guanine (G) is paired with cytosine (C). In RNA, in which cytosine (C) is substituted by uracil (U), guanine (G) is paired with uracil (U). The sequence of one strand determines the sequence of the other as they are *complementary*. It is the order of the bases, specifically a three base sequence known as a *codon* that encodes for the twenty amino acids used to create proteins. There are also three base sequences known as "stop codons" that signal when the translation process is complete.

The flow of genetic information originates in the nucleus and is completed with the formation of the protein at the ribosome in the endoplasmic reticulum. DNA serves as a template for transcription into messenger RNA (mRNA). This is the primary transcript or the pre-mRNA which must be modified prior to its transport to the ribosome for protein translation. This is a three step process divided into *splicing*, *capping*, and *polyadenylation*. The pre-mRNA is spliced at specific sites removing *introns* (non-coding portions of the DNA molecule) and connecting the neighboring *exons* (coding portions of the DNA molecule) together. The addition of the 5' 7-methylguanisine cap and the 3'poly-A tail prevents degradation by enzymes and facilitates transport of the *mature transcript* from the nucleus to the cytoplasm. The mature transcript is composed of a 5' untranslated region (5'UTR), an open reading frame (ORF) and a 3' untranslated region (3'UTR). The triplet coding sequence is interpreted at the ribosome by transfer RNA molecules. There is a translational start site, which is important to establish the proper *reading frame*. Each of the 20 amino acids is carried by a specific tRNA. The tRNA has a triplet *anticodon* which is the complement of the codon on the mRNA molecule. This aligns the amino acid in the proper sequence at the ribosome where a peptide bond is formed. The process is repeated until the termination codon appears stopping the process. As there are 64 possible codons but only 20 amino acids, some amino acids are encoded by more than one codon. Therefore, the triplet genetic code is *degenerate*, as the third base in the codon may be substituted without a corresponding amino acid change. In addition, there are three *stop codons* which terminate protein translation. [16]

Types of Mutations

A mutation is any permanent heritable change in the sequence of genomic DNA. The types of mutations vary from a single base pair substitution to large deletions or duplications within genes. Large chromosomal mutations may also result in altered gene expression. This occurs during the first meiotic division of gametogenesis during a process known as *crossing over*. In meiosis I, homologous chromosomes align in pairs; a process designated as synapsis. Genetic material is exchanged by reciprocal breaking and rejoining of chromosome segments. The advantage of this process is that it increases the genetic diversity of the gametes and is site specific. The disadvantage is that a misalignment may result in the addition or deletions of entire genes. [17]

Mutations that affect single genes are most commonly located in the coding region of genes, at the intron-exon boundaries, or in regulatory sequences. These changes may result from changes of single base pair known as a point mutation. Insertions or deletions of one or multiple base pairs may also result in an altered protein product by substituting or removing an amino acid or by changing the reading frame, which alters the entire protein downstream from the mutation site. Larger duplications or deletions of entire genes alter the quantity of the protein produced.

Single base pair substitution or point mutations, wherein one base pair is replaced by another, may not necessarily result in a protein alteration. A mutation may be *silent* if it does not result in an amino acid change. If there is an amino acid substitution, then it is designated as a *missense* mutation. A change that inserts a termination or stop codon is known as a *non-sense* mutation. A *stop codon* mutation may occur wherein the stop codon is replaced by an amino acid codon allowing for continued protein translation. *Frameshift* mutations occur as a result of a deletion or insertion of bases that are not multiples of three. These result in an abnormal protein. Frameshift mutations often result in premature termination and are typically more severe in comparison to a deletion or duplication, neither of which affects the reading frame. [5]

Transformation of the protein product may lead to abnormal function and thereby cause disease. With non-sense, stop codon read through, and frameshift mutations, the predicted protein product would be either be truncated or distorted beyond recognition, such that it would be non-functional. A simple amino acid substitution may have a profound effect on protein function if it occurs in a critical site that is essential for normal function. This is in contrast to an amino acid substitution that represents a benign change or polymorphism. Therefore, point mutations must be interpreted based on known disease causing mutations or suspected disease causing mutations versus benign polymorphisms based on previously documented cases.

Microdeletions or chromosome duplications alter the quantity of protein produced. CMT1A is the result of a duplication of the gene *PMP22* that occurs during crossing over. This illustrates how an uneven exchange of chromosome material can result in a duplication of a single gene.

During meiosis I, there is misalignment of repetitive units flanking the *PMP22* gene altering the site for normal crossing over to occur. This results in an unbalanced exchange of genetic material with two copies of PMP 22 located on one chromosome 17 while the other chromosome 17 contains no copies of PMP22. The net result is a duplication and reciprocal deletion of *PMP22*. The duplication of *PMP22* is responsible for the uniform demyelination noted in CMT1A. In contrast, a deletion of this gene results in the segmental demyelination at common entrapment sites and pressure points seen in hereditary neuropathy with predisposition to pressure palsies (HNPP). [18] The *PMP22* gene encodes a critical protein for compact myelin formation. It is the alteration of the amount of protein produced that leads to the changes in myelin observed in these disorders; a gene dosage effect. [19] Both conditions are autosomal dominant, although CMT1A is much more common. The overwhelming majority of CMT1A patients will have an affected first degree relative whereas only 10 percent of cases result from *de novo* mutations.

Trinucleotide repeat disorders are conditions that result from large expansions of normally repeated elements. These expanses may be found in exons, introns, or untranslated regions of the gene. When found in exons, the expansion of amino acids that results alters the function of the protein in a negative way that is designated as a toxic gain of function. There are other conditions that have non-translated repeat elements found in either introns or untranslated regions of the gene. In these instances, the elongated mRNA is the toxic element as it interferes with normal mRNA splicing mechanisms, which may impact the expression of more than one gene. [20]

There are those mutations that may affect gene regulation by altering regulatory regions of DNA required for normal expression or in some cases suppression of a gene. These conditions are *epigenetic* as the effect is a result of gene regulation that occurs from either activating or silencing a gene. [21]

Molecular Diagnostic Techniques

With the advent of automated sequencing, clinical molecular diagnostic testing has become more available to assist in the diagnosis of a number of different genetic disorders. A basic understanding of the techniques used and the data that is generated aids the clinician in interpreting the results of testing. The common methods used by these laboratories will be reviewed in this section.

The Southern blot is a method used to detect large duplications or deletions in the DNA molecule. A modified version of this technique is used in the diagnosis of the duplication and conversely the deletion seen in CMT1A and HNPP. The Southern blot involves the use of restriction enzymes derived from bacteria. There are a number of restriction enzymes, each of which recognize a specific sequence of nucleotides and produce a double-stranded cut in the DNA. These sites are typically palindromic with the sequence on one strand reading the same in the reverse direction on the complementary strand. These sequences vary between 4 and 8 nucleotides in length.

A restriction digest, adding specific restriction enzymes to a reaction mixture of DNA, is required before the separation of DNA fragments by gel electrophoresis. As restriction sites are specific, the digestion results in variable but predictable lengths of DNA fragments. Gel electrophoresis is a technique used for the separation of DNA, RNA or protein using an electric current applied to a gel matrix. DNA which is rich in phosphate residues carries a negative charge and therefore travels toward the anode. The smaller fragments of DNA will travel farther over time in the gel than will the large fragments.

In order to analyze the DNA, it must first be transferred to a solid substrate such as a nylon membrane. This is accomplished with simple diffusion by placing the membrane over the gel and covering it with absorbent blotting papers. This draws the DNA out of the gel. The buffering solution passes through the membrane and the DNA becomes fixed to the membrane. The membrane-bound DNA can now be analyzed using a specific labeled DNA probe that is complementary to the area of interest. This requires the application of heat in order to break the hydrogen bonds connecting the two strands of DNA. [22] The labeled DNA probe will adhere to the area of interest revealing a discrete band at this site. Any gene rearrangement larger than 50-100 base pairs that either creates or destroys a restriction site will be detected by this technique. This includes a deletion, an insertion, or any point mutation.

Polymerase chain reaction (PCR) is a method used to amply a single or a few copies of DNA in order to create multiple copies of a particular sequence in a short time period. The method relies on thermal cycling, which consists of repeated episodes of heating and cooling that allow for repeated replication of a specific DNA segment. This is performed by using oligonucleotide primers, both sense and antisense, which are complementary to the target region. In addition, this method requires a thermostable DNA polymerase, a mixture of the reaction for DNA melting and enzymatic replication of the DNA. The DNA generated is used as a template for replication. The process is repeated for many cycles such that the DNA template is amplified exponentially. The reaction mixture requires several components. The first is a DNA template, which contains the region of the DNA fragment to be amplified. The second is two specific oligonucleotide primers, which determine the beginning and end of the region to be amplified. Other requirements include a thermostable polymerase, deoxynucleotide triphosphates (e.g., ATP, TTP, GTP, CTP), buffer solution, magnesium ions, potassium ions, and a thermal cycler.

Amplification of a specific DNA segment requires two specific oligonucleotide DNA (cDNA) primers complementary to the 5' and 3' ends of the segment to be copied. The cDNA that binds to the 5' end is sense and cDNA that binds to 3' or downstream end is antisense. After the reaction mixture is prepared, the vial is placed in the thermal cycler. The initial step involves denaturing the DNA by heating to the mixture to 95°C. This breaks the hydrogen bonds connecting the two strands. The mixture is then allowed to cool to a temperature that the sense and antisense primers can anneal to their complement. This temperature may vary but it is usually between 50 and 65°C. Then, the temperature is raised to 72°C, which is the optimal temperature of the thermostable DNA polymerase. Elongation of both strands of the DNA molecule occurs from the primer binding sites. The process is repeated for several cycles thus amplifying the segment of DNA between and including the two cDNA primer binding sites. [23]

The amplified segment may be further analyzed by direct DNA sequencing. The classical or Sanger method uses four reaction mixtures, each one containing a specific dideoxyneucleotide (ddATP, ddGTP, ddCTP or ddTTP). The incorporation of a dideoxynucleotide into the DNA molecule terminates the reaction. The reaction is designed as follows: DNA is denatured and divided into four separate reaction vial containing a primer, four deoxynucleotides (dATP, dGTP, dCTP and dTTP), DNA polymerase, and only one of the four dideoxynucleotides (ddATP, ddGTP, ddCTP and ddTTP). A radiolabeled dNTP (deoxyribonucleotide triphosphate) is added to each reaction mixture. After the reaction is complete, each reaction mixture is separated by gel electrophoresis in parallel columns. After separation, the gel is placed adjacent to an x-ray film wherein each mark indicates incorporation of the specific ddNTP (dideoxyribonucleotide triphosphate) into the corresponding column. [24, 25]

Automated sequencing uses the same technique but it does not require a radiolabeled nucleotide. Instead, it uses four different fluorescent dyes that correspond to the different ddNTPs. This is referred to as dye terminator sequencing. The advantage of this technique is that the complete sequencing set can be performed in a single reaction vial rather than the four needed with the labeled-primer approach. As each of the ddNTP chain terminators are labeled with a separate fluorescent dye that fluoresce at a different wavelengths, the labeled molecule can be separated through one column. Subsequently, the DNA sequence is interpreted using a computer that detects the differences in wavelength fluorescence at each termination site. [26]

Evaluation of Patients with a Suspected Hereditary Neuropathy

The diagnosis of hereditary neuropathy is suspected in patients with any of the following; a family history of neuropathy, high arches, hammertoes, or an abnormal gait. All evaluations should begin with a pedigree analysis in order to determine the pattern of inheritance as autosomal dominant, recessive or X-linked. The index of suspicion for a diagnosis of a genetically determined neuropathy, when there is no family history, include the following;

presentation in early childhood, slow progression, foot deformities, and weakness out of proportion to the sensory loss. Nerve conduction studies are then performed in order to separate the inherited neuropathy into demyelinating, intermediate, and axonal subtypes as will be discussed in a subsequent chapter. [27] Nonetheless, it should be stated that a uniform pattern of profound nerve conduction velocity slowing supports the diagnosis of an inherited dysmyelinating or "demyelinating" phenotype. The term "dysmyelinating" is preferred as the myelin has been abnormal since its inception. As molecular genetics of the hereditary neuropathies were being defined in the 1990s, it was clear that both CMT1 and CMT2, while often clinically similar, were genetically heterogeneous. An increasing number of genetic subtypes have been described, which have clarified the role of various proteins involved in the physiology of peripheral nerve conduction in health and in disease. [28] Given this heterogeneity, it is important to know the relative frequency of each mutation or subtype. This allows for judicious use of genetic testing.

CMT is among the most common heritable neurologic disorders with approximately 1 in 2500 persons being affected. CMT is found worldwide in people of all races and ethnic groups. CMT subtypes may be inherited in an autosomal dominant, autosomal recessive or an X-linked pattern. The most common CMT subtypes are as follows: CMT1A 55%, CMT1X 15.2%, HNPP 9.1%, CMT1B 8.5% and CMT2A2 4.0%. All other subtypes account for less than 1% apiece. [29] When the clinical and neurophysiologic phenotype and the family history suggest CMT, the patient should undergo molecular genetic testing. It is important to establish a precise diagnosis given the overlap between clinical syndromes and the significant variability between family members. [30] The importance of genotyping is that it facilitates informed genetic and prognostic counseling while advancing the scientific understanding of the different phenotypes of CMT.

Genetic Testing for Hereditary Neuropathy

One-third of all CMT mutations arise *de novo* and appear as a chronic sporadic neuropathy. [31] Molecular diagnostic testing in these cases provides a specific diagnosis and information regarding treatment and prognosis. It also allows for genetic counseling for family members who may be at risk of inheriting the gene. Advances in molecular diagnostic testing have made the definitive diagnosis of this expanding list of genetic neuropathies possible [16]. Given the lack of specific therapies, the value of determining the specific genetic mutation responsible in each case may not justify the expense of molecular diagnostic testing. As this is a genetically heterogeneous group of disorders with more than 40 different genes or loci identified, knowledge of the relative frequencies of the various subtypes is crucial prior to embarking upon extensive genetic testing.

A rational approach to the diagnosis of a suspected genetic disorder requires that an extensive family history and a pedigree analysis be obtained for anyone who is suspected to have a hereditary neuropathy. Determining the mode of inheritance will help to direct the next step in the diagnostic evaluation. The second step is to classify the presumptive inherited neuropathy based on the median motor nerve forearm motor conduction velocity into one of the following subtypes; dysmyelinating, intermediate, or axonal. A dysmyelinating (inherited demyelinating) subtype is diagnosed when the median motor nerve conduction velocity

[MNCV] in the forearm is less than 38 m/s. An intermediate form is diagnosed when the median MNCV forearm conduction velocity is 38-45 m/s. An axonal form is diagnosed when the median sensory nerve action potential [SNAP] is absent, the median motor nerve conduction study to the APB manifests a reduced compound muscle action potential [CMAP] but the MNCV in the forearm exceeds 45 m/s. Thus, a nerve conduction velocity of less than 38 m/s and in a uniform in pattern is consistent with dysmyelinating CMT (CMT1). Testing in this instance should commence with the most common genetic mutation, the *PMP22* gene duplication, which results in CMT type 1A. A negative result may be followed by sequencing the MPZ gene as this is responsible for the next most common demyelinating CMT, type 1B. When pedigree analysis is consistent with an X-linked pattern of inheritance, testing for CMTX should be performed first. With axonal CMT (CMT2), sequencing of the MFN2 gene associated with CMT type 2A2 should be considered. This targeted approach is preferable and is more cost effective than ordering the full genetic panels offered by some laboratories.

Genotyping facilitates discussions regarding prognosis, genetic counseling of family members, and will allow for inclusion in clinical trials as they become available. In cases of suspected hereditary neuropathy in the absence of a family history, testing may confirm the diagnosis. In addition to confirming a genetic etiology of the condition, these results provide an opportunity for genetic screening of other family members who may be at risk. In apparent sporadic cases, genetic testing will unequivocally establish the correct diagnosis.

Conclusion

A working knowledge of genetics is necessary to evaluate patients with a suspected hereditary neuropathy. The first step is to obtain a comprehensive family history to generate a pedigree. This should allow for characterization of the condition as autosomal, X-linked, dominant, or recessive such that focused genetic testing can be employed. Nonetheless, the results of molecular diagnostic testing may be misleading as not every identified mutation results in disease. Therefore, basic knowledge of gene expression and mutation is needed to allow for critical interpretation of genetic testing.

CMT is a common genetic disorder which shows marked genetic heterogeneity and phenotypic variability such that this diagnosis may be challenging. Correct classification relies on phenotypic recognition along with the support of ancillary studies such as electrodiagnostic studies and molecular diagnostic testing. Nerve conduction studies differentiate between the dysmyelinating (inherited demyelinating), intermediate, and axonal subtypes. This determination, along with family history, focuses genetic testing. Given the vast genetic heterogeneity of the hereditary neuropathies, it is important to devise a strategy of testing based on mutation frequency rather than relying upon a battery of hereditary neuropathy panels. In demyelinating CMT (CMT1) it is preferable to test for the *PMP* duplication observed in type 1A as it is causative in approximately 80% of cases. If negative, the next most frequent mutation is that of the *MPZ* gene observed in type 1B. If the pedigree is consistent with X-linked inheritance, genetic testing for CMTX is indicated. With axonal CMT (CMT2), testing for the *MFN2* gene mutation associated with CMT type 2A2 should be performed.

As there are no specific therapies directed at the individual subtypes of CMT, genotyping may seem academic. Genetic testing advances knowledge and the recognition of the subtypes that a single gene mutation confers upon a group of patients. Additionally, advances in basic science will likely lead to clinical trials, which will require genotyping in order to participate. A specific diagnosis empowers the affected individual as it provides further understanding of the condition and the disease prognosis, knowledge of supportive therapies, genetic counseling and testing of at risk family members.

References

[1] Mendel G, Corcos AF, Monaghan FV, Weber MC. Gregor Mendel's Experiments on Plant Hybrids: A Guided Study. New Brunswick, NJ: Rutgers University Press, 1993.

[2] Mendel G. Versuche über Pflanzenhybriden Verhandlungen des naturforschenden Vereines in Brünn, Bd. IV für das Jahr, 1865 Abhandlungen: 3–47. For the English translation, see: Druery CT, Bateson W. Experiments in plant hybridization. *Journal* of the Royal Horticultural Society. 1901; 26: 1–32. Accessed on 5/30/13 at http://www.esp.org/foundations/genetics/classical/gm-65.pdf.

[3] Morgan TH, Sturtevant AH, Muller HJ, Bridges CB. The Mechanism of Mendelian Heredity. New York: Henry Holt, 1915.

[4] Watson JD, Crick FHC. A structure for deoxyribose nucleic acid. *Nature* 1953; 171:737-738.

[5] Gelehrter TD, Collins FS, Ginsburg D. Principles of Medical Genetics, Philadelphia: Lippincott Williams & Wilkins, 1998.

[6] Lupski JR, Garcia CA, Parry GJ, Patel PI. Charcot-Marie-Tooth polyneuropathy syndrome: clinical, electrophysiological, and genetic aspects. In: Appel, S. *Current Neurology*. Chicago: Mosby-Yearbook (pub.) 1991. p. 1-25.

[7] van de Warrenburg BPC, Notermans NC, Schelhaas HJ, van Alfen N, Sinke RJ, Knoers NVAM, Zwarts MJ, Kremer BPH. Peripheral nerve involvement in spinocerebellar ataxias. Arch. Neurol. 2004; 61:257-261.

[8] Fu YH, Pizzuti A, Fenwick RG, King J, Rajnarayan S, Dunne PW, Dubel J, Nasser GA, Ashizawa T, de Jong P, Wieringa B, Korneluk R, Perryman MB, Epstein HF, Caskey CT. An unstable triplet repeat in a gene related to myotonic muscular dystrophy. Science 1992; 255: 1256-1258.

[9] Ridley RM, Frith CD, Crow TJ, Conneally PM. Anticipation in Huntington's disease is inherited through the male line but may originate in the female. J. Med. Genct. 1988; 25: 589-595.

[10] Yoshioka, M., Yorifuji, T., Mituyoshi, I. Skewed X inactivation in manifesting carriers of Duchenne muscular dystrophy. Clin. Genet. 1998; 53: 102-107.

[11] Kelsey G, Monagle P, Barnes C. Delayed diagnosis of congenital factor IX deficiency (Christmas disease) in a girl with Turner's syndrome. *Clin. Lab. Haematol.* 2006; 28:355-6.

[12] Caskey CT, Nussbaum RL, Cohan LC, Pollack L. Sporadic occurrence of Duchenne muscular dystrophy: evidence for new mutation. Clin. Genet. 1980; 18:329-341.

[13] Bergoffen J, Trofatter J, Pericak-Vance MA, Haines JL, Chance PF, Fischbeck KH. Linkage localization of X-linked Charcot-Marie-Tooth disease. Am. J. Hum. Genet. 1993; 52:312-318.

[14] Smeitink J, van den Heuvel L, DiMauro S. The genetics and pathology of oxidative phosphorylation. *Nat. Rev. Genet.* 2001; 2:342-352.

[15] Holt IJ, Harding AE, Petty RKH, Morgan-Hughes JA. A new mitochondrial disease associated with mitochondrial DNA heteroplasmy. Am. J. Hum. Genet. 1990; 46: 428-433.

[16] Berg JM, Tymoczko JL, Stryer L, Clarke ND. I. 5. DNA, RNA, and the Flow of Genetic Information: Amino Acids Are Encoded by Groups of Three Bases Starting from a Fixed Point. Biochemistry (5th ed.). New York: W. H. Freeman and Company, 2002.

[17] Griffiths WM., Miller JH, Suzuki DT. et al., eds. Nature of crossing-over: An Introduction to Genetic Analysis (7th ed.). New York: W. H. Freeman and Company, 2000.

[18] Lupski JR, Montes de Oca-Luna R, Slaugenhaupt S, Pentao L, Guzzetta V, Trask BJ, Saucedo-Cardenas O, Barker DF, Killian JM, Garcia CA, Chakravarti A, Patel PI. DNA duplication associated with Charcot-Marie-Tooth disease type 1A. Cell 1991; 66: 219-232.

[19] Lupski JR, Wise CA, Kuwano A, Pentao L, Parke JT, Glaze DG, Ledbetter DH, Greenberg F, Patel PI. Gene dosage is a mechanism for Charcot-Marie-Tooth disease type 1A. Nature Genet. 1992; 1:29-33.

[20] Botta A, Rinaldi F, Catalli C, Vergani L, Bonifazi E, Romeo V, Loro E, Viola A, Angelini C, Novelli G. The CTG repeat expansion size correlates with the splicing defects observed in muscles from myotonic dystrophy type 1 patients. J. Med. Genet. 2008; 45: 639-646.

[21] Castaldo I, Pinelli M, Monticelli A, Acquaviva F, Giacchetti M, Filla A, Sacchetti S, Keller S, Avvedimento VE, Chiariotti L, Cocozza S. DNA methylation in intron 1 of the frataxin gene is related to GAA repeat length and age of onset in Friedreich ataxia patients. J. Med. Genet. 2008; 45: 808-812.

[22] Southern EM. Detection of specific sequences among DNA fragments separated by gel electrophoresis. Journal of Molecular Biology 1975; 98(3):503–517.

[23] Saiki RK, Gelfand DH, Stoffel S, Scharf SJ, Higuchi R, Horn GT, Mullis KB, Erlich HA. Primer-directed enzymatic amplification of DNA with a thermostable DNA polymerase. *Science* 1988; 239(4839):487-491.

[24] Sanger F, Coulson AR. A rapid method for determining sequences in DNA by primed synthesis with DNA polymerase. J. Mol. Biol. 1975; 94:441–8.

[25] Sanger F, Nicklen S, Coulson AR. DNA sequencing with chain-terminating inhibitors. Proc. Natl. Acad. Sci. U.S.A. 1977; 74:5463–7.

[26] Bentley DR, Balasubramanian S, Swerdlow HP, Smith GP, Milton J, Brown CG, Hall KP, Evers DJ. et al. Accurate whole human genome sequencing using reversible terminator chemistry. Nature 2008; 456: 53–59.

[27] Dyck PJ, Lambert EH. Lower motor and primary sensory neuron diseases with peroneal muscular atrophy. I. Neurologic, genetic, and electrophysiologic findings in hereditary polyneuropathies. *Arch. Neurol.* 1968; 18:603-18.

[28] Online Mendelian Inheritance in Man, OMIM®. McKusick-Nathans Institute of Genetic Medicine, Johns Hopkins University (Baltimore, MD), 2013. World Wide Web URL: http://omim.org/Ann Neurol.

[29] Saporta ASD, Sottile SL, Miller LJ, Feely SME, Siskind CE, Shy ME. Charcot-Marie-Tooth disease subtypes and genetic testing strategies. Ann. Neurol. 2011; 69: 22-33.

[30] Patzko A, Shy ME. Charcot-Marie-Tooth disease and related genetic neuropathies. *Continuum*. 2012; 18:39-59.

[31] Boerkoel CF, Takashima H, Garcia CA, Olney RK, Johnson J, Berry K, Russo P, Kennedy S, Teebi AS, Scavina M, Williams LL, Mancias P, Butler IJ, Krajewski K, Shy M, Lupski JR. Charcot-Marie-Tooth disease and related neuropathies: mutation distribution and genotype-phenotype correlation. 2002; 51:190-201.

In: Contemporary Issues in Peripheral Neuropathy
Editor: Daniel L. Menkes
ISBN: 978-1-62948-681-9

Chapter III

Hereditary Peripheral Neuropathies

***Meriem Tazir*[1,2,*]*, Mounia Bellatache*[1,2]**
***and Sonia Nouioua*[1,2]**
[1]Service de Neurologie, CHU Mustapha Bacha, Algiers, Algeria
[2]Laboratoire de Neurosciences, Université d'Alger, Algiers, Algeria

Abstract

This chapter will summarize the recent developments regarding inherited neuropathies with a focus on "pure" hereditary neuropathies in which a peripheral neuropathy is the salient clinical feature. Thus, this chapter will not address any neurodegenerative disorders associated with peripheral neuropathy such as leukodystrophies, familial amyloidosis and cerebellar ataxia. Hereditary peripheral neuropathies (HPN) are classified by the fiber types that are affected clinically such that they are subdivided into the hereditary motor and sensory neuropathies (HMSN), the hereditary motor neuropathies (HMN) and the hereditary sensory and autonomic neuropathies (HSAN). The most frequent entity is HMSN, which is also known as Charcot-Marie-Tooth (CMT) disease. As the medical literature uses these terms interchangeably, the authors will use them in this same context throughout this chapter. HMSN is a heterogeneous group of disorders that are classified on the basis of their clinical, neurophysiological, genetic and pathological features. Charcot-Marie-Tooth disease is characterized by a chronic sensorimotor polyneuropathy. Patients usually present with distal muscle weakness and atrophy that is often associated with a similar clinical picture of a mild to moderate sensory loss, depressed tendon reflexes and skeletal deformities. These skeletal deformities usually consist of high-arched feet and "hammertoes," although some patients also manifest scoliosis. It should be understood that many disorders present with a similar phenotype such that its presentation should not be considered to be pathognomonic of an HMSN. Moreover, HMSN phenotypic variability is common in that some patients develop severe disability in infancy

* Address: Service de Neurologie et Laboratoire de Neurosciences, CHU Mustapha Bacha, 1 place de la Concorde, Algiers 16000, Algeria. Mob: 00 213 771 625 470, Tel/fax: 00 213 21 235 640, E-mail address: meriem.tazir@sante.dz.

(Dejerine-Sottas Disease or congenital hypomyelination) whereas others manifest few or no symptoms of this disorder. The term CMT is currently used for the classification of HMSN. On the basis of electrophysiological data, the major subtypes of CMT may be divided into demyelinating (CMT1), axonal (CMT2) and intermediate CMT (CMTI) forms. The genetic mutations that result in HPNs may be autosomal dominant (most common), autosomal recessive or X-linked. Over the past two decades, remarkable progress has been made with respect to the genetic etiologies of these disorders. More than forty genetic abnormalities are associated with CMT whereas approximately twenty such mutations have been associated with HMN and HSAN. A clinical, electrophysiological, and pathological description of the most frequent forms of HPNs along with a phenotype/genotype correlation will assist the clinician in narrowing the differential diagnosis such that focused genetic testing may be performed. While no specific therapies are currently available, the patient's quality of life may be maximized through a multidisciplinary team composed of neurologists, physiatrists, and orthopedic surgeons. Genetic counseling is recommended such that the clinician can provide individuals and their families with comprehensive information regarding these genetic disorders such that may make informed medical and personal decisions.

Introduction

Hereditary peripheral neuropathies (HPN) are the most common inherited disorder that affects the peripheral nervous system. They constitute a complex, clinically and genetically heterogeneous group of disorders. These may be subdivided into those in which the neuropathy is most prominent or sole clinical manifestation (HPN) and those wherein the neuropathy presents as part of a multisystemic disease process as is observed with the leukodystrophies, familial amyloidosis and cerebellar ataxia. This chapter will focus solely on the HPN. Hereditary peripheral neuropathies (HPN) include the hereditary motor and sensory neuropathies (HMSN), the hereditary motor neuropathies (HMN) that are also known as the distal spinal muscular atrophies [SMAs] and the hereditary sensory and autonomic neuropathies (HSAN). Despite this heterogeneity, HPN are a group of disorders that share characteristic clinical phenotypes that manifest as a peripheral neuropathy with a chronic progressive course. The most frequent entity, HMSN, also known by the eponym "Charcot-Marie-Tooth (CMT)," is a heterogeneous group of disorders which can be classified on the basis of their clinical, neurophysiological, genetic and pathological features. The wide variation in the age of onset and severity of these disorders is highly correlated with the severity of the underlying genetic abnormality. Despite this genetic diversity, it is possible to make a clinical distinction between HMSN with its manifest motor and sensory findings from HSAN with predominant sensory and autonomic features and from HMN in which only motor fibers are involved. Recent advances in molecular genetics as well as molecular and cell biology have revolutionized our understanding of HPN. More than forty genetic abnormalities are associated with CMT whereas there are approximately twenty genetic abnormalities that are associated with HMN and HSAN. Moreover, it has become apparent that certain subtypes of HMSN, HSAN and HMN are difficult to differentiate clinically. This is because different genetic mutations may produce the same clinical phenotype. Therefore, the authors recommend that these disorders be approached in a systematic manner rather than labeling all disorders as "Charcot-Marie-Tooth" disease.

1. Hereditary Motor and Sensory Neuropathies [Charcot-Marie-Tooth disease]

The hereditary motor and sensory neuropathies [HMSN], which are also known by the eponym Charcot-Marie-Tooth disease, are the most common degenerative disorders of the peripheral nervous system. Nonetheless, the frequency of the different subtypes varies within different populations. Cases of an inherited peripheral neuropathy manifesting with distal weakness and wasting in the limbs were reported in 1886 as "peroneal muscular atrophy" nearly simultaneously by the British physician Tooth and the French physicians Charcot and Marie such that this syndrome bore their names. Clinically, Charcot-Marie-Tooth [CMT] diseases or syndromes included progressive distal motor and sensory loss associated with foot deformities such as high arched feet (pes cavus) and hammertoes. Two major subtypes, demyelinating (CMT-I) and axonal (CMT-II) were subsequently distinguished by electrophysiological and nerve biopsy studies [1, 2, 3]. Patients were diagnosed with HMSN type I (demyelinating subtype), when a median nerve motor nerve conduction velocity (MCVs) <38 m/s was identified [1, 2]. Nerve biopsies of patients with HMSN I revealed histological findings of demyelination and remyelination known as "onion bulb" formations. In contrast, HMSN type II (axonal subtype), was defined as a median MCVs >38 m/s. Nerve biopsy specimens revealed axonal degeneration without onion bulb formation. Severely affected children with delayed walking and electrophysiological evidence of profound myelinopathy (median MCV< 15m/s) were classified as HMSN type III, which had been previously designated "Dejerine-Sottas syndrome (DSS) or congenital hypomyelination neuropathy (CHN)"; although CHN had been considered as a separate entity by some authors. Some authors prefer the term "dysmyelinating neuropathy" as opposed to the term "inherited demyelinating neuropathy" as patients with CMTI have a genetically determined, uniform myelin sheath pathology such that features of acquired demyelination (e.g. conduction block) are hardly ever observed. Despite all the recent genetic advances, electrodiagnostic studies should be the first diagnostic test used in order to classify the subtype of HMSN as primarily myelinopathic, intermediate or axonopathic such that directed genetic testing can be pursued. HMSN I and II are usually inherited as an autosomal dominant trait, but autosomal recessive and X-linked inheritance has also been reported [4, 5, 6]. In Western Europe, the United States and Japan, the dominant forms are the most frequent [7]. In other countries, such as those in the Mediterranean basin that have a high prevalence of consanguineous marriages, autosomal recessive inheritance may account for more than 50% of all forms [8].

Genetic testing of HMSN began in 1991 with the identification of the 1.4-Mb duplication of chromosome17 containing the peripheral myelin protein 22 (PMP22) gene as the cause of the most frequent form of CMT1 [9, 10]. Since that time, there have been additional advances in understanding the molecular basis for many forms, of HMSN such that approximately 40 genes have been identified.

Classical CMT Phenotype

As previously stated, HMSN is clinically and genetically heterogeneous with a variable age of onset, clinical progression, and electrodiagnostic findings. Most cases of HMSN are slowly progressive disorders that usually present in the first or second decades, although earlier or later initial presentations may occur depending on the underlying genetic abnormality. The more common phenotype includes steppage gait, pes cavus, distal sensory loss, and distal lower amyotrophy giving an aspect of "stork legs" or an inverted champagne bottle (Figure 1). A similar pattern of atrophy and sensory loss in the hands occurring may occur at a later point in the condition known as "main en griffe" or "claw hand." The typical neurologic examination reveals decreased or absent deep tendon reflexes in a distal symmetric pattern (e.g. Achilles reflex is lost first). Gait and balance are usually impaired because of proprioceptive loss and skeletal deformities that result in pes cavus and hammertoes (Figure 2).

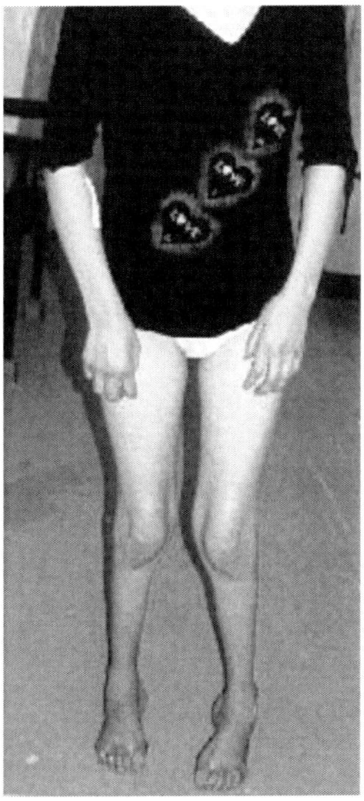

Figure 1. Common CMT phenotype in a young adult with distal limb wasting and foot deformities.

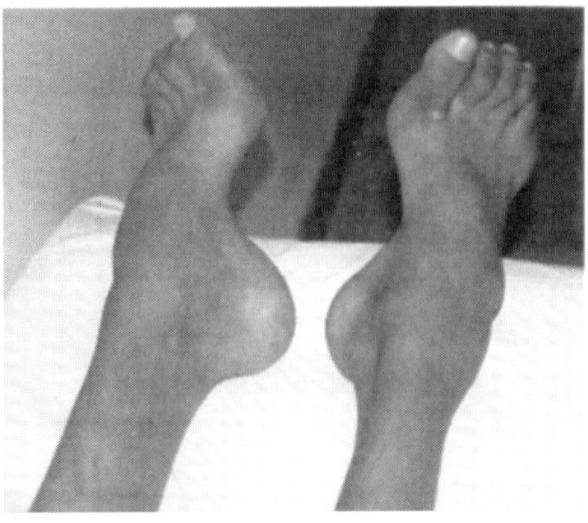

Figure 2. Pes cavus in a CMT patient.

The electrophysiological examination is the first important step in separating myelinopathies from neuronopathies or axonopathies. Nerve conduction studies (NCS) allow for a preliminary subtype classification into demyelinating, axonal or intermediate forms. In most cases, motor nerve conduction velocities (MNCV) and compound muscle action potential amplitudes (CMAP) in the upper extremities are required since the lower extremity nerves often demonstrate absent responses. When the median MNCV is <38m/s HMSN I or CMT-I is diagnosed whereas if the median MNCV is > 45m /s with the finding of a decreased CMAP and an absent median sensory nerve action potential (SNAP), HMSN-II or CMT-II is diagnosed. Intermediate HMSN or CMTI is diagnosed if the median MNCV falls in the range of 38-45 m/s). Although not necessary for diagnosis, needle electromyography (EMG) often demonstrates electrophysiological changes of both acute and chronic denervation.

Subtype classification is also based on the pattern of inheritance in addition to the motor NCVs. The myelin dysfunction variants of CMT, CMT1 and CMT2, are autosomal dominant (AD) disorders, whereas CMTX is an X-linked disorder. In contrast, autosomal recessive HMSN variants (AR CMT) are classified as CMT4 if they have demyelinating features and ARCMT2 if they have axonal findings.

Diagnosis of CMT and Classification

The diagnosis of CMT is relatively straightforward when there is a family history of progressive peroneal atrophy. When both a parent and a child are affected then an AD form of CMT is highly likely especially when the affected persons are father and son. Otherwise, it could be either due to AD or X-linked inheritance. Autosomal recessive CMT should be suspected when two or more siblings are affected and have phenotypically normal consanguineous parents.

The diagnosis of CMT is more challenging when there is no family history. In such cases, an inherited neuropathy should be suspected when the onset is in infancy or childhood, the signs and symptoms are slowly progressive over many years and if pes cavus is present bilaterally. Electrodiagnostic studies are also useful given that most inherited myelin dysfunction neuropathies present with uniformly slow MNCV as opposed to acquired chronic demyelinating neuropathies which may manifest asymmetric slowing, temporal dispersion or conduction block [11]. While most sporadic cases represent de novo AD mutations, others may be also X-linked or AR, especially when the parents are related. Nerve biopsy is no longer recommended for AD CMT1 and X-linked CMT, but it may be considered as a means of characterizing the underlying pathology in less common forms of CMT, (e.g. CMT2 and AR CMT), for the purposes of focused molecular testing [12, 13]. Nerve biopsy findings in such instances may be sufficiently characteristic such that the underlying genetic abnormality can be inferred such as those associated with mutations in *MPZ, GJB1, GDAP1, MTMR2, SH3TC2, PRX, FGD4*, and *LMNA* [12, 13].

CMT may be further subdivided on the basis of the underlying genetic abnormality as listed in Table 1. At the present time, more than 40 different genetic abnormalities have been shown to result in a CMT phenotype. Furthermore, this genetic classification has some limitations as there is some genetic overlap of CMT with the distal hereditary motor neuropathies (dHMNs), also known as “spinal CMT”, the hereditary sensory and autonomic neuropathies (HSANs) and the hereditary sensory neuropathies (HSNs). For all these reasons, the authors recommend that the classification system should be based on the clinically affected nerve fibers types instead of the non-descriptive eponym CMT.

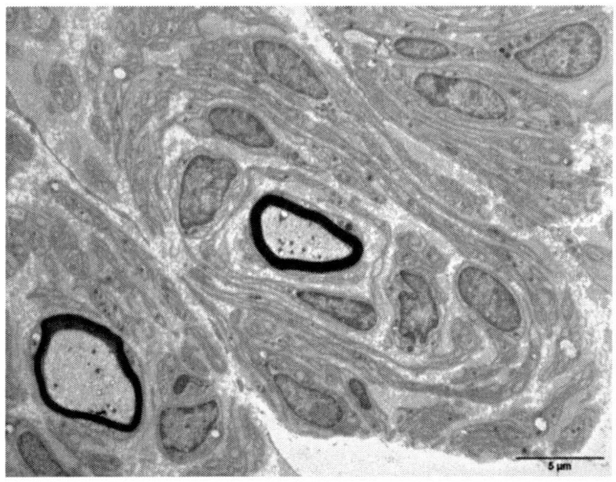

Figure 3. Electron micrograph. Transverse section. *PMP22* duplication (CMT1A). Around two myelinated fibers, there is an intense proliferation of Schwann cells, (i.e. onion bulbs). The myelinated fiber on the left appears to be hypomyelinated.

Genetic testing should not be considered obligatory. The physician should inform the patient or the parents that there are no known treatments for these inherited disorders. The patient should be also informed that the outcome of this test would be used primarily for family planning purposes.

The Different Subtypes of CMT

Autosomal Dominant CMT

CMT1

AD CMT1 is the most common form of HMSN that is not associated with consanguineous marriage. Most patients with AD CMT1 have the classic CMT phenotype. Nerve biopsy reveals extensive segmental demyelination combined with concentric proliferation of Schwann cells (hypertrophic neuropathy) resulting in the formation of "onion bulbs" (Figure 3).

CMT1A

In European populations, CMT1A accounts for about 70% of all CMT1 cases [14, 15]. CMT1A results from 1.4-Mb duplication on 17p11.2 containing the gene encoding a 22 kD peripheral myelin protein (PMP22). This duplication results from an unequal translocation of homologous chromosomes such that affected individuals have three copies of this chromosome. It is noteworthy that a deletion of the identical 1.5 Mb region containing PMP22, in which an affected individual has only one copy of 17p11.2, results in a related condition known as hereditary neuropathy with liability to pressure palsies (HNPP).

Patients with CMT1A have a characteristic length-dependent sensorimotor dysmyelinating neuropathy, a term used to indicate that the myelin sheath is uniformly affected along the entire nerve. Therefore, temporal dispersion, conduction block, and asymmetric MNCVs should not be observed as might be noted in an acquired demyelinating polyneuropathy. Although affected persons walk at the same age as unaffected persons, they develop progressive symptoms in the first two decades. Enlarged nerves may be palpable, especially the ulnar nerve at the elbow. When associated with postural tremor and ataxia, it is designated the Roussy-Levy syndrome.

Given the chronic course of this condition, very few patients become non-ambulatory. Nerve biopsy demonstrates a significant reduction of myelinated axons that become less numerous later in the course of the disease. The "onion bulbs" depicted in figure three are composed of several layers of basal lamina, connective tissue and Schwann cells around thinly myelinated axons.

Given its autosomal dominant inheritance pattern, approximately 90% of patients will have a family history. The other 10% are considered to be sporadic mutations.

Other mutations in the *PMP22* gene may result in other phenotypes including the more severe CMT1 resembling Dejerine-Sottas Syndrome associated with hearing loss, currently classified as CMT1E [16].

Hereditary Neuropathy with Liability to Pressure Palsies (HNPP)

HNPP is caused by a deletion in *PMP22* gene, the same region that is duplicated in CMT1A. A small percentage of people with HNPP have this phenotype due to a frameshift, splice site, or point mutation of the *PMP22* gene. This condition is relatively frequent as it is the third most common type of inherited dysmyelinating neuropathy. HNPP affects 9.1% of persons classified as having an inherited myelinopathy or dysmyelinating neuropathy [15].

The clinical pattern is usually that of multiple compression mononeuropathies. Patients with HNPP present with focal symptoms of weakness or sensory loss following compression of individual nerves. Most of these symptoms are transient, lasting from hours to days. Peripheral nerves which are susceptible to pressure along their path are most likely to be involved (e.g. ulnar nerve across the elbow and fibular nerve at the fibular head). While patients may only note that one nerve territory is symptomatic, electrodiagnostic studies may demonstrate multiple compression neuropathies with associated conduction slowing. Nerve conduction velocities are particularly asymmetric in HNPP [17]. Nerve biopsies from HNPP patients demonstrate segmental demyelination, remyelination, and the loss of large diameter axons together with "sausage shaped swellings" at the site of compression known as "tomaculi" on teased fibers, which is the hallmark of this condition. As such, some authors have referred to this condition as "tomaculous neuropathy."

CMT1B

CMT1B is the second most common cause of AD CMT1. It results from mutations in the myelin protein zero (*MPZ*) gene located at chromosome 1q22. CMT1B represents approximately about 8 to10% of AD CMT1. Myelin protein zero is an important constituent of the myelin sheath.

Mutations in *MPZ* associated with CMT1B are characterized by a classical CMT phenotype with progressive slowing of nerve conduction velocities due to hypertrophy of

Schwann cells [12]. Other mutations in *MPZ* may also result in more severe phenotypes such as, Dejerine-Sottas syndrome, congenital hypomyelinating neuropathy with early onset disease and delayed age of walking, as well as axonal CMT [18, 19]. Patients with later-onset CMT1B and a normal age of walking tend to have an intermediate or axonal CMT as classified by nerve conduction studies [15]. Nerve pathology show mainly two types of lesions depending on the mutation site. Some mutations lead to the formation of onion bulbs and uncompacted myelin (Figure 4). Other mutations result in the other pathological finding of focal folding and myelin thickening in additional to onion bulb formation and axonal loss [12].

CMT1C

The rare CMT1C results from mutations in lipopolysaccharide-induced tumor necrosis factor (*LITAF*), also referred to as *SIMPLE*, at chromosome 16p13.3-p12 [20]. The *LITAF* gene encodes a transcription factor, which is a regulator of TNF-alpha gene expression [21]. LITAF may play a role in protein degradation pathways [20].

CMT1C patients frequently resemble those with CMT1A with symptom onset between the first and the third decade, MNCV between 16 and 25 m/s and a progressive dysmyelinating sensorimotor polyneuropathy [15, 22].

CMT1D

CMT1D, another rare cause of AD CMT1, is caused by mutations in the early growth response gene-2 (*EGR2*) gene at chromosome 10q21 [23]. While some patients may present with a classical CMT phenotype resembling CMT1A, most present with a severe phenotype in infancy. Such patients may have a congenital hypomyelination or a DSS with hypotonia, delayed motor milestones and MNCV<15m/s. Mutations in EGR2 may also result in an AR hypomyelination neuropathy designated CMT4E [23] (see description later in this chapter).

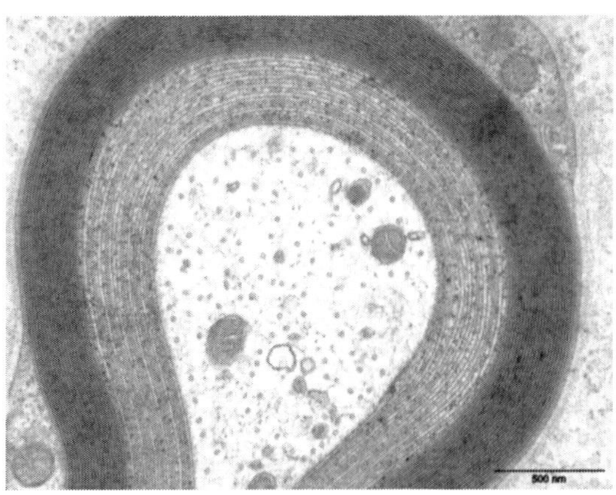

Figure 4. Electron micrograph. Transverse section. *P0* mutation (CMT1B). Abnormal myelin compaction induced by a P0 mutation. The inner myelin lamellae of this myelin sheath are regularly and abnormally widened whereas the external lamellae are normally compacted.

A CMT1 form associated with macular degeneration and hyperelastic skin, allelic to distal HMN, linked to Fibulin-5 (*FBLN5*) mutations has recently been reported [24].

CMT2

Autosomal dominant axonal CMT (CMT2/HMSN type 2) is relatively frequent as it may represent a third of AD CMT cases [15]. Most CMT2 patients have a classical CMT phenotype but they have a wider range of age of onset than CMT1A patients. Moreover, in some subtypes of CMT2, atypical signs such as brisk reflexes, a Babinski sign or optic atrophy may be observed. In CMT2, NCV in the upper limbs are greater than 38m/s, the CMAP amplitudes are reduced or absent in severe cases and the median SNAP is often absent. Consistent with the electrophysiological features, sural nerve biopsy findings demonstrate axonal loss often with a cluster of regeneration (axonal sprouting), without pathological evidence of primary demyelination.

To date, causative gene mutations have been identified in 25% to 35% of CMT2 patients [15]. Mutations in 16 genes/loci have been identified as the etiology of CMT2 although some mutations may also cause a dysmyelinating form of CMT. Currently CMT2 are classified from CMT2A to CMT2P (Table 1). With the notable exception of the CMT2A subtype, which is relatively frequent, all the other CMT2 subtypes identified to date have a low prevalence.

CMT2A

CMT2A is caused by mutations in *MFN2* the gene encoding Mitofusin 2, which is a mitochondrial protein located on chromosome 1p36.2 [25]. Most disease-causing mutations are in the GTPase domain, coiled-coil domains, or in other conserved regions of the protein.

This is the most frequent type of CMT2 and accounts for about 21% of axonal CMT [26]. *MFN2* mutations are present in 3.4 to 4% of all genetically defined CMT patients in Norwegian [27] and North American [15] populations.

Most of CMT2A patients are severely affected such that they are non-ambulatory before age 20 [26]. A minority of patients may present with a later onset and more moderate CMT phenotype [28, 29]. *MFN2* linked families with autosomal recessive inheritance have also been described [29, 30]. CMT2A can be associated with pyramidal signs, bilateral optic atrophy and/or periventricular and subcortical hyperintense lesions on brain MRI [25, 26, 28]. In a recent study of 6 MFN2 patients, nerve pathology was characterized by a marked decrease in the density of myelinated fibers, primarily the large diameter fibers. Although neurophysiologic findings were more suggestive of axonal degeneration, some onion bulbs were present.

Axonal mitochondria were smaller than normal, round, and abnormally aggregated. These changes may result from abnormal mitochondrial fusion and fission [31].

Previously, a Japanese family with AD CMT2 due to a Q98L mutation in *KIF1B* was reported. This gene encodes the kinesin family member 1B (KIF1B) which is a protein that transports mitochondria and synaptic vesicle precursors in neuronal cells [32]. However, this locus has not been validated in other CMT2A families.

Table 1. Classification of HMSN or Charcot-Marie-Tooth (CMT) diseases

Type	Gene	Age of onset	Specific phenotypes	Nerve biopsy features
Autosomal dominant CMT1				
CMT1A	*PMP22* Dup17p11	All ages	Classic form/DSS/CHN Hypertrophy of nerves	Segmental demyelination / remyelination. OB formations and axonal loss.
HNPP	*PMP22* Deletion	2 to 64 years	Recurrent entrapment neuropathies. Multifocal neuropathies	Focal thickening (tomaculae) and folding of myelin sheath
CMT1B	*MPZ*	1st -2nd decade	Clinically more severe than CMT1A. DSS/CHN/CMT2 Abnormal gait. Occasional nerve hypertrophy Rarely deafness	Uncompacted myelin. Occasional myelin outfolding.
CMT1C	*LITAF*	Childhood		Segmental demyelination / remyelination. OB formations
CMT1D	*EGR2*	1st -2nd decade	Classic form/DSS/CHN Possible cranial nerve involvement	Severe loss of myelinated and unmyelinated fibers, OB formations
CMT1E	*PMP22*	Childhood	Associated with deafness	Demyelination; tomaculae
CMT1F	*NEFL*	1-13 years	CMT1 with early onset, severe disease/CMT2	Reduced MF density, loss of large diameter myelinated fibers, clusters of axonal regeneration.
Autosomal dominant CMT2				
CMT2A	*MFN2*	6 months to 50 years	Prominent distal weakness, late proximal weakness. Optic atrophy, CNS involvement.	Axonal atrophy, decrease of large myelinated fiber density, small OB. Abnormal mitochondria.
CMT2B	*RAB7*	Second decade	Severe sensory loss. Foot ulcers, arthropathy and amputations.	Axon degeneration: large and small sensory fibers and unmyelinated axons. Axonal regeneration
CMT2C	*TRPV4*	Birth to 60 years	Younger more severe. Vocal cord, diaphragm, respiratory involvement.	Axonal degeneration.
CMT2D	*GARS*	16 to 30 years	Distal upper limb predominance	-
CMT2E	*NEFL*	1st -5th decade	CMT2 phenotype Hearing loss Hyperkeratosis	Giant fibers: neurofilament accumulation. Axonal atrophy

Type	*Gene*	Age of onset	Specific phenotypes	Nerve biopsy features
CMT2F	*HSPB1*	Adult	CMT2 phenotype/distal HMN	
X linked CMT dominant				
CMT X1	*GJB1*	1st-2nd decade	Males more affected than carrier females. Occasional deafness	Axonal degeneration and regeneration with some segmental demyelination. Occasional cluster formations. Few OB.
CMT X5	*PRPS1*	Childhood	Mild-moderate neuropathy. Deafness. Late optic atrophy.	Axonal neuropathy. Mild demyelinating changes.
Dominant intermediate CMT				
DI-CMTB (CMT2M)	*DNM2*	1st-2nd decade	Classic CMT/with neutropenia and early onset cataract.	Loss of large MF, rare segmental demyelination/remyelination. OB formations. Axonal degeneration.
DI-CMTC	*YARS*	7-59 years	Classic CMT.	Axonal regeneration (clusters), decreased nerve fiber density and thickness.
DI-CMTD	*MPZ*	30-50 years	Sensory loss and weakness Range in clinical severity. Deafness/Pupil disorders	Axonal loss and regeneration, segmental. Unmyelinated fiber loss demyelination/remyelination.
Autosomal recessive CMT1/CMT4				
CMT4A	*GDAP1*	< 2 years	Severe, progressive. Vocal cord and diaphragm paralysis in some cases.	Demyelinated fibers, segmental demyelination, OB formation. Axonal loss
CMT4B1	*MTMR2*	3 years	Severe CMT1. Facial/bulbar weakness. Scoliosis.	Myelin outfolding. Loss of MF.
CMT4B2	*MTMR13* *SBF2*	4-13 years	Severe CMT1. Glaucoma. Kyphoscoliosis.	Similar to CMT4B1.
CMT4C	*SH3TC2*	Early onset 1st-2nd decade	Severe to moderate CMT1 Scoliosis. Deafness.	Increase of basal membranes around several demyelinated and unmyelinated axons with supernumerary extensions
CMT4D	*NDRG1*	<10 years	Severe CMT1/ deafness/tongue atrophy.	OB formations, myelin decompaction. Severe axonal loss of MF. Axonal inclusions. Regenerating clusters

Table 1. (Continued)

Type	Gene	Age of onset	Specific phenotypes	Nerve biopsy features
CMT4E	*EGR2*	Birth	Congenital hypotonia, respiratory failure. Arthrogryposis.	Severe loss of myelinated and unmyelinated fibers, OB formations
CMT4F	*PRX*	Birth to first decade	CMT1/ prominent sensory involvement.	Severe loss of myelinated fibers. Congenital hypomyelination.
CMT4G HMSN-Russe	*HK1*	8-16 years	Severe to moderate CMT1	Hypomyelination, regenerating clusters.
CMT4H	*FDG4*	< 2 years	Delayed milestones. Scoliosis, severe course.	Hypomyelination. Small OB.
CMT4J	*FIG4*	Congenital, Childhood or Adult	Severe disorder. Similarities to motor neuron disease.	Profound axonal loss, thinly myelinated fibers. Small OB
Autosomal recessive CMT2/AR CMT2				
CMT2B1	*LMNA*	Second decade	Severe course. Distal and Proximal weakness	Severe decrease of MF density.
CMT2B2	*MED25*	28 to 42 years	Classic CMT2 (Costa-Rican family)	-
CMT2H	*GDAP1*	1st decade	Pyramidal involvement. Vocal cord involvement.	Reduced MF density. Thin myelin. Rare axonal degeneration.
CMT2K Rarely AD	*GDAP1*	Severe early-onset form	Severe form. Vocal cord paralysis. Skeletal deformities. Milder dominant form.	Reduced MF density. Axonal degeneration. Pseudo OB formations.

AD, autosomal dominant; AR, autosomal recessive; CHN, congenital hypomyelinating neuropathy; DNM2,dynamin2; DSS, Dejerine Sottas Syndrome; Dup, duplication; EGR2, early growth response2; FGD4, actin filament-binding protein frabin; FIG4, FIG4homologSAC1 lipid phosphatase domain containing; GARS, glycyl-tRNA synthetase; GDAP1, ganglioside-induced differentiation-associated protein1; GJB1, gap-junction proteinβ-1; HK1, hexokinase1; HSPB1, heat shock27-kDa protein1; HSPB8, heat shock22-kDa protein8; LITAF, lipopolysaccharide-induced tumor necrosis factor; LMNA, lamin A/C; MF: myelinated fibers; MED25, mediator complex subunit25; MFN2, mitofusin2; MPZ, myelin protein zero; MTMR2, myotubularin-related protein2; MTMR13, myotubularin-related protein13; NDRG1, N-myc downstream-regulated gene1 protein; NEFL, neurofilament light chain polypeptide68kDa; OB: onion bulbs; PMP22, peripheral myelin protein22; PRPS1, phosphoribosyl pyrophosphate synthetase1; PRX, periaxin; RAB7, RAS-associated protein RAB7 ; SH3TC2, SH3 domain and tetratricopeptides repeats2 ; SPTLC1, serine palmitoyl transferase long-chain base subunit1; TRPV4, transient receptor potential cation channel subfamily V member4; YARS, tyrosyl-tRNA synthetase.

CMT2B

CMT2B results from mutations in the *RAB7* gene located on Chromosome 3q21.3 [33]. RAB 7 is a member of the RAB family of RAS associated GTP binding proteins, which are essential for the regulation of the major steps involved in intracellular trafficking [34]. This subtype of CMT is characterized by distal sensory loss that often leads to foot ulcerations followed by infections and subsequent amputations. Other features include mild scoliosis, absent ankle reflexes, decreased distal sensation, lateral-gaze nystagmus, and cerebellar degeneration on MRI. Nerve conduction studies demonstrate a chronic sensory neuropathy with axonal features whereas sural nerve biopsies display axonal degeneration with prominent regeneration [35]. Given the prominent feature of distal sensory loss and trophic complications in CMT2B patients, it is difficult to distinguish this condition from HSAN1 due to *SPTLC1* mutations. However, it should be recalled that many patients with HSAN1 associated with SPTLC1 have associated neuropathic pain [36].

CMT2C

CMT2C results from a mutation in the *TRPV4* gene on chromosome 12q24 [37, 38]. This form is distinguished by vocal cord and diaphragmatic paresis, often presenting with hoarseness or stridor in addition to the typical CMT phenotype [39]. Other prominent features include bilateral sensorineural hearing loss, bladder urgency and incontinence, as well as cold-induced exacerbations of hand muscle weakness. One family with a mild neuropathy had pronounced short stature [40]. Allelic disorders have been described such as scapuloperoneal spinal muscular atrophy, spondylometaphyseal dysplasia, metatropic dysplasia and brachyolmia [41, 42, 43]. Thus, patients with *TRPV4* mutations may be distinguished from other forms of axonal CMT in the presence of skeletal abnormalities such as short stature and scoliosis in association with variable degrees of vocal cord dysfunction.

CMT2D

CMT2D results from mutations in the Glycyl tRNA Synthetase (*GARS*) gene located on Chromosome 7p14.3. GARS is a member of the family of aminoacyl-tRNA synthetases responsible for charging tRNAs with their cognate amino acids; a critical step in protein translation [44]. Patients with CMT2D typically manifest more weakness and wasting in the hands than in the legs. CMT2D is allelic to hereditary motor neuropathy type V (HMN VA). Lack of sensory involvement differentiates HMN VA from CMT2D. Patients with this unusual CMT phenotype of severe hand weakness manifesting before leg weakness may also have mutations in the *BSCL2* gene causing HMN VB and Silver spastic paraplegia syndrome [45]

CMT2E

CMT2E results from mutations in the Neurofilament Light Chain *(NEFL)* gene located on chromosome 8p21 [46]. The clinical picture is highly variable and ranges from severe CMT phenotypes with either intermediate or severely slowed nerve conduction velocities to moderate CMT phenotypes. Nerve biopsy may reveal a primary axonopathy characterized by "giant axons" (focally distributed axonal swellings containing accumulation of disorganized neurofilaments) as observed in giant axonal neuropathy (GAN) due to mutations in the *Gigaxonin* gene [47]. Patients with the classical GAN phenotype have a severe axonal neuropathy and an early onset central nervous system involvement including cerebellar and pyramidal signs, associated with kinky hair. However, a milder GAN form with an ARCMT2-like presentation has also been reported [48, 49]. Mutations in *NEFL* may rarely manifest as an AD demyelinating CMT, which is designated CMT1F [50].

CMT2F

CMT2F results from mutations in the *HSPB1* gene, a member of the heat shock protein superfamily. HSPB1, which is also known as *HSP27,* is located on chromosome 7q11.23 [51]. Most reported mutations involve the α-crystallin conserved domain. Such mutations may results in either a CMT2 phenotype, or a distal HMN with retained reflexes, which is a pure motor phenotype. These observations support the hypothesis of a continuum between CMT2 and dHMN forms [52].

The remainder of the CMT2 subtypes are either very rare or result from established genetic abnormalities. These CMT2 subtypes include CMT2G (12q12-q13.3) [53] and CMT2I/J (*MPZ*) with late onset sensory motor neuropathy associated with deafness (CMT2I) and pupillary abnormalities (CMT2J) [54]. CMT2K (*GDAP1*) which is allelic to CMT4A and is described later in the chapter, refers to a milder form of axonal CMT with variable age of onset that is sometimes associated with vocal paralysis and pyramidal features [55]. CMT2L (*HSPB8*), which is allelic to HMN IIA, was reported in a single Chinese family [56]. CMT2M (*DNM2)* is allelic to both autosomal dominant centronuclear myopathy (ADCNM) [57, 58] and to DI-CMTB [59]. CMT2N (*AARS)* is the second tRNA synthetase gene implicated in CMT2 after *GARS* [60]. CMT2O is linked to Dynein cytoplasmic 1 heavy chain 1(*DYNC1H1*), which has a key role in retrograde axonal transport in neurons. CMT2P is linked to Leucine-rich repeats and sterile alpha motif-containing 1 (*LRSAM1*); an E3ubiquitin ligase. These are the most recently described axonal dominant loci in a large British family (leucine-rich repeats) and a Canadian family (LRSAM1) [61, 62].

X-linked CMT

At present, two X-linked CMT disorders have been described; CMTX1 and CMTX5 (Table 1). X-linked CMT should be suspected when no father to son transmission is noted on pedigrees and when males are more impaired than females. CMTX1, which maps to chromosome Xq13, represents the second most frequent form of CMT after CMT1A. CMTX1results from mutations in the gap junction protein beta 1 (*GJB1*) gene encoding connexin 32 (Cx32) located on the X chromosome [63, 18]. Connexin 32, expressed in myelinated peripheral nerve at the nodes of Ranvier and Schmidt-Lanterman incisures, form intracellular gap junctions that connect to the folds of Schwann cell cytoplasm that allows for the transfer of ions and molecules to the innermost myelin layers [64]. It was demonstrated that most *GJB1*mutations cause neuropathy by a loss of normal connexin 32 function [65]. In males, the age of onset occurs within the first two decades of life with a predilection for early childhood. CMTX1 is characterized by atrophy and weakness of peroneal muscles and intrinsic hand muscles, sensory abnormalities and pes cavus. Asymmetry of signs is often observed in males whereas females tend to have mild or asymptomatic variant that is likely on the basis of random X-inactivation. Median motor nerve conduction velocities are in the intermediate range (25–40 m/s) in both men and women. A small subset of these patients manifests central nervous system involvement such as mild deafness and /or abnormal brainstem-evoked potentials. Nerve biopsy studies demonstrate either a primary axonopathy [66] or a primary myelinopathy [67]. Nevertheless, both axonal and demyelinating features were present in all nerve biopsies to some extent [68].

In contrast to CMTX1, CMTX5 is a very rare axonal form of CMT. It has also been designated as the Rosenberg-Chutorian syndrome. CMTX5 results from a mutation in the gene encoding phosphoribosylpyrophosphate synthetase I (*PRPS1*). CMTX5 is associated with an early onset of hearing loss, lower leg weakness and atrophy beginning in childhood, with subsequent progressive visual loss secondary to optic atrophy that manifests around age 20 [69].

Dominant Intermediate CMT

Autosomal dominant intermediate CMT (DI-CMT) is characterized by a classic, mild to moderately severe CMT phenotype and median motor NCVs overlapping those observed in CMT1 and CMT2 with a range from 25 to 50 m/s [70]. The mean age at onset is 16 years with a range from age two to 59 years. Five clinical forms have been identified. DI-CMTA is linked to 10q24.1-q25.1 whose gene and protein product remain unknown [71]. DI-CMTB is caused by *DNM2* (Dynamin 2) mutations [59] and is allelic to CMT2M [57]. DI-CMTC results from Tyrosyl-tRNA synthetase *(YARS)* mutations [72] whereas DI-CMTD results from *MPZ* mutations [73]. Of note, the recently described intermediate CMT, subtype DI-CMTE, results from abnormalities of Inverted formin 2 (INF2) and is associated with focal segmental glomerulosclerosis and proteinuria.This new discovery may lead to additional insights into the pathophysiological mechanisms linking formin proteins to podocyte and Schwann-cell functions [74].

Autosomal Recessive CMT

Autosomal recessive Charcot- Marie Tooth (ARCMT) disorders were once considered to be extremely rare. However, more recent clinical and molecular investigations of CMT families with autosomal recessive inheritance from countries around the Mediterranean basin allowed for the identification of many gene mutations and their corresponding proteins. This led to a more comprehensive understanding of these hereditary conditions as well as their pathophysiology. Autosomal recessive CMT disorders include demyelinating (AR CMT1 or CMT4) and axonal forms (AR CMT2).

CMT4

The designation CMT4 is applied to autosomal recessive forms of dysmyelinating Charcot-Marie-Tooth disease. Autosomal recessive CMT cases are characterized by earlier onset, (usually before age 2 years), and more rapid clinical progression that results in more marked distal limb deformities such as pes equino-varus (Figure 5), claw-like hands (mains en griffe), and major spinal deformities. Several different subtypes of autosomal recessive demyelinating CMT have been identified (CMT4A to CMT4J), each with its own particular clinical, pathological, and ethnic characteristics. However, DSS or CHN phenotypes may be the clinical presentation of many of these subtypes (Table 1). Nerve biopsy studies demonstrate prominent demyelinating lesions responsible for marked secondary axonal loss along with subtype-specific myelin abnormalities [75].

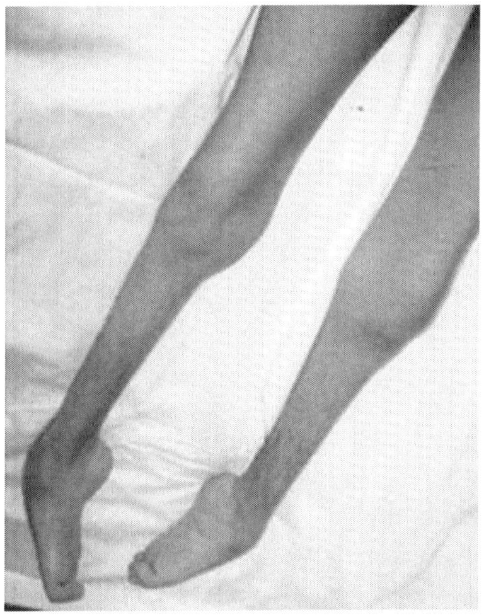

Figure 5. Pes equino-varus in a CMT4 adolescent patient.

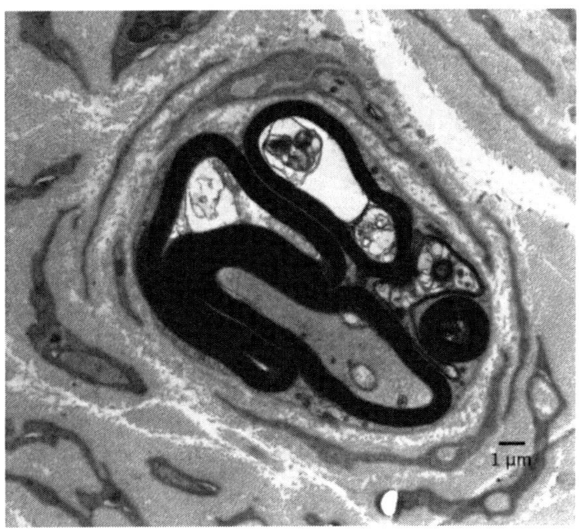

Figure 6. Electron microscopy. Transverse section. *MTMR2* mutation (CMT4B1 or AR-CMT1B1). Numerous outfoldings of the myelin sheath. There is a concentric proliferation of flattened Schwann cell cytoplasm around the myelinated Schwann cell.

CMT4A

CMT4A, the first AR locus described, is linked to *GDAP1* gene on 8q13-q21 and was reported in four Tunisian families [76, 77]. This subtype is characterized by an early onset, (before 2 years of age), severe neuropathy manifesting as a rapidly progressive distal weakness and atrophy of the limbs associated with marked foot deformities leading to an inability to walk in late childhood or adolescence. There may also be an associated paralysis of the vocal cords and the diaphragm. [78]. Mutations in Ganglioside-induced differentiation-associated protein 1 (*GDAP1)* have been reported to cause both demyelinating [77], and axonal CMT (CMT2H and CMT2K) [78, 79, 80, 81]. GDAP1has been hypothesized to be part of a putative signal transduction pathway in neuronal development. GDAP1 is expressed in both Schwann cells and neurons of human and rat peripheral nerve as well as in various regions of the central nervous system. GDAP1 is an integral membrane protein of the outer mitochondrial membrane and plays a role in mitochondrial dynamics by promoting fission events [82].

CMT4B1

CMT4B1 results from mutations in Myotubularin-related protein-2 (*MTMR2)* located on chromosome 11q22. It was first reported in a large Italian family with 10 affected members. CMT4B1 presents clinically as a severe early onset sensorimotor polyneuropathy and is characterized pathologically a demyelination in the presence of focally folded myelin [83]. We reported on three siblings with a homozygous insertion of adenine detected in *MTMR2* exon 4: c.331dupA (p.Arg111LysfsX24) [84]. They had a typical phenotype of an early and severe onset of a sensorimotor neuropathy with nerve biopsy features of typical focally folded myelin (Figure 6). Other unusual associated clinical features in this family included vocal cord paresis, prominent chest deformities and claw hands. The *MTMR2* gene encodes a protein that belongs to the myotubularin family characterized by the presence of a phosphatase domain. Loss of the phospholipid phosphatase MTMR2 results in CMT4B1 with myelin outfoldings in humans and mice [85]. It was demonstrated that MTMR2 has a predicted role in membrane trafficking, which is crucial for myelin membrane biogenesis and homeostasis [86].

CMT4B2

Mutations in *MTMR13* (or *SBF2:* SET binding factor 2) on chromosome11p15 result in CMT4B2, a demyelinating sensory neuropathy with myelin outfoldings. Like MTMR2, MTMR13 belongs to a family of ubiquitously expressed proteins sharing homology with protein tyrosine phosphatases (PTPs). Both proteins may regulate vesicular trafficking in Schwann cells such that their their loss could lead to uncontrolled folding of myelin observed in the CMT4B phenotype [87].

A consanguinous Turkish family with four affected adult individuals presented with a severe sensorimotor neuropathy phenotype. Disease onset occurred at age five such that they were only able to ambulate with the help of assistive devices given the severity of distal muscle wasting and foot deformities. Neurophysiologic examination revealed severely reduced median motor NCVs. Sural nerve biopsies revealed a severe loss of myelinated fibers and focally folded myelin protrusions. A homozygous in-frame deletion of exons 11 and 12 of the *SBF2* gene was identified in this family [88]. Two other consanguineous families from Tunisia and Morocco presented with a similar phenotype with a demyelinating sensorimotor polyneuropathy associated with early-onset glaucoma [89].

CMT4C

The gene mutated in CMT4C disease, SH3 domain and tetratricopeptide repeat domain 2 (*SH3TC2* or *KIAA1985)* is located on chromosome 5q32. This gene encodes a protein expressed in Schwann cells of peripheral nerves. It is associated with the plasma membrane and the perinuclear endocytic recycling compartment such that it may be associated with myelination and maintaining the integrity of the node of Ranvier [90].

The locus for CMT4C was identified in two large consanguineous Algerian families, by homozygosity mapping, to chromosome5q23-33. In addition to the demyelinating CMT phenotype, all patients had foot deformities and prominent scoliosis requiring surgery with a relatively slow progression of motor deficits [91, 92]. Subsequently, CMT4C European cases were identified and such that the neuropathological features could be established. They were characterized by an increase of basal membranes around several demyelinated and unmyelinated axons with relatively few classic onion bulbs. CMT4C cases also typically manifested long cytoplasmic extensions of the Schwann cells that were more prominent in unmyelinated fibers than in myelinated fibers [93]. A cohort of 17 CMT4C patients was subsequently reported, which emphasizes the relatively high frequency of this form [94]. Recurrent mutations were recognized in some additional populations; R1109X in Spanish Roma (formerly Gypsy) [95, 96, 97], R954X in European, and 01 in Algerian and many French Canadian families [98, 99, 100, 101].

CMT4D

A mutation in the N-myc downstream-regulated gene-1(*NDRG-1*) located on chromosome 8q24 results in CMT4D [102]. It is also designated as the Lom type of hereditary motor and sensory neuropathy (HMSNL) in that Lom is the Bulgarian city where it was first described. CMT4D demonstrates Schwann cell dysfunction and early onset of severe axonal loss; features that suggest impairment of axon-glial interaction as the main cause of this condition. Recent studies suggested that impaired Schwann cell trafficking failing to meet the considerable demands of nerve growth is the likely pathogenetic mechanism of NDRG1 deficiency [103].

CMT4D is characterized by a severe distal sensorimotor neuropathy with distal limb deformities and associated deafness; a pathognomonic feature that is usually present by the third decade. Onset typically occurs in the first decade and most patients become non-ambulatory in the fifth decade. Nerve biopsies demonstrate typical lesions of demyelination and remyelination associated with severe axonal loss [102].

The disease-causing founder mutation in the Roma (Gypsy) population is a premature termination signal at codon 148 (R148X) of NDRG1 [102].The disorder was diagnosed in several Rom populations across Europe. HMSNL is phenotypically similar to the Russe form of hereditary motor and sensory neuropathy (CMT4G/HMSN-R), which is also common in the Roma population and has been diagnosed in patients from Spain, Romania and France. The clinical phenotype of HMSN-R shares the general features of CMT4D (HMSN-Lom), except that the associated sensorial deafness occurs later in life and there is a slower rate of disease progression [104]. The gene has recently been identified as affecting the function of hexokinase1 (HK1) [105].

In addition to CMT4D (HMSNL) and CMT4G (HMSN-R), a third syndrome found in European Roma populations known as CCFDN is characterized by a syndrome of congenital cataracts, facial dysmorphism and a neuropathy. CCFDN is caused by a single-nucleotide substitution in intron 6 of the c-terminal domain of RNA polymerase in subunit A phosphatase of subunit 1 (*CTDP1*) gene [106]. Otherwise, CCFDN is genetically distinct from Marinesco-Sjogren syndrome although these two conditions share some overlapping features, including congenital cataracts, delayed psychomotor development, ataxia and mild cognitive impairment [107].

CMT4E

CMT4E is a rare neuropathy that results from a homozygous mutation of the *EGR2* gene located on chromosome 10q21, which causes a congenital hypomyelination neuropathy (CHN). CMT4E presents clinically with an early onset of hypotonia, areflexia, distal muscle weakness, and profoundly slow nerve conduction velocities (NCV) [108]. The early growth response 2 gene (*EGR2)* is part of a multigene family encoding Cys2His2 type zinc-finger proteins. EGR2 may play a role in the regulation of peripheral nervous system myelination proteins such as myelin protein zero, connexin 32 and periaxin [109]. Animal models studies established that Krox20 (Egr2) is not only required for the onset of myelination but that it is also crucial for maintaining the myelinated state [110]. In addition to CMT4E, defects in this gene are also associated with the previously described Charcot-Marie-Tooth disease type 1D (CMT1D), and with the Dejerine-Sottas syndrome (DSS). Thus, it became clear that mutations affecting Krox20/EGR2 result in a large spectrum of HMSN severity depending on the mutation site [111].

Originally, DSS (or HMSN type III) was defined as an early onset of an autosomal recessive severe dysmyelinating polyneuropathy whereas CHN was considered to be the result of congenital impairment in myelin formation. Nevertheless both DSS and CHN disorders may be inherited either as as an autosomal recessive or autosomal dominant trait [111]. Genetic heterogeneity of DSS and CHN is currently well established given that mutations in *PMP22, P0, EGR2* and *PRX* genes are known to cause these two syndromes [16, 18, 111, 112].

CMT4F

The CMT4F locus was mapped to 19q13.1-13.3 in a large consanguineous Lebanese family with a severe Dejerine–Sottas-like phenotype [112]. The periaxin gene (*PRX*) encodes two PDZ-domain proteins; S (small)- and L (long)-periaxin. Both periaxins are thought to be essential for the formation and maintenance of peripheral nerve myelin [113]. Most of the reported CMT4F patients had an early onset with a DSS phenotype associated with a neuropathy manifesting more sensory than motor impairment [114].

Nonetheless, there is some phenotypic variability in CMT4F in that the authors reported a CMT4F consanguineous family in which a novel homozygous mutation in the *PRX* gene, c.1090C>T (p.Arg364X), was identified [84]. The four patients of this CMT4F family had a relatively late onset and slow progression of their neuropathy that presented with a moderate sensory ataxia and mild distal motor dysfunction associated with prominent spine deformities. Nerve biopsies demonstrated severe loss of myelinated and unmyelinated fibers as well as rare myelin outfoldings. The remaining fibers were surrounded by onion bulb Schwann cell proliferations [84].

The clinical heterogeneity observed in this CMT4F family, as in other CMT4 patients, demonstrate a variable functional impairment that may be correlated with different mutations in a given gene that lead to a wide spectrum of illness [115].

CMT4H

Mutations in the *Frabin (FGD4)* gene on chromosome 12q12 are responsible for CMT4H [116, 117]. This was demonstrated in two families, one Lebanese and one Algerian, including 10 individuals who presented with a severe form with early-onset demyelinating CMT. The age at onset varied between 10 and 24 months. The affected individuals presented with moderate muscle weakness associated with amyotrophy in the distal portions of their extremities, mild symmetrical stocking-type hypesthesia and absent deep tendon reflexes. The majority of patients had associated skeletal deformities including severe scoliosis and pes equinus with toe retraction. Disease progression was slow in both families. Subsequently, other patients with *Frabin* mutations had a moderate to severe demyelinating sensorimotor polyneuropathy and numerous myelin outfoldings on sural nerve biopsy [115, 118]. Patients diagnosed with CMT4H had variable functional impairment, which suggested that Frabin plays a crucial role during myelin formation [119].

CMT4J

Mutations in the lipid phosphatase *FIG4* on chromosome 6 q21, causes CMT4J, a severe recessive subtype of CMT. Initially CMT4J phenotype was described as a severe early onset ARCMT [120]. Further studies demonstrated that this form was characterized by a highly variable age of onset (early childhood to the sixth decade) and severity [121]. Muscle weakness was typically distal and proximal as well as asymmetric. Two of these affected individuals demonstrated additional evidence of cranial nerve involvement manifesting as impaired right eye abduction in one and tongue function in the other. The majority of the unrelated patients with CMT4J were compound heterozygotes carrying one unique null allele of *FIG4* in combination with the shared ancestral missense allele FIG4-I41T [120, 121]. Furthermore, *FIG4* heterozygote mutations have been demonstrated to be associated with amyotrophic lateral sclerosis [122]. FIG4 is a phosphatase which removes the 5-phosphate from the low abundance signaling phosphoinositide PI (3, 5) P2 that is localized on the cytoplasmic surface of vesicles of the endosome/lysosome pathway. It is noteworthy that phosphoinositide signaling has previously been implicated in CMT disorder types 4B1, 4B2 and 4H. A generated double Mtmr2/Fig4-null mouse model demonstrated that Mtmr2 and Fig4 interact in neurons and Schwann cells in order to control phospholipid metabolism [123].

ARCMT2

To date, the autosomal recessive axonal CMT linked to specifically identified genes are either rare or restricted to geographical areas such as North-Africa (CMT2B1) and Costa-Rica (CMT2B2).

ARCMT2A (CMT2B1)

ARCMT2 A was mapped to the 1q21.2 region in a large multigeneration consanguineous Moroccan family with nine affected siblings. They presented with a severe distal motor and sensory axonal neuropathy with early proximal lower limb muscle involvement in many cases [124]. A unique R298C mutation in the *LMNA* gene encoding the lamin A/C in five patients from two Algerian AR-CMT2 families was identified [125]. Subsequently, the authors reported a group of 21 ARCMT2 patients from seven unrelated Algerian families with the same R298C mutation in the lamin A/C gene and a marked variability of the clinical phenotype [126]. Four patients in one ARCMT2A family manifested marked proximal muscular atrophy involving the scapular and pelvic girdle [127]. Nerve biopsy data in all six patients revealed that myelinated fibers were severely reduced in number without evidence of demyelination and remyelination or of active axonal regeneration [126].

The genetic abnormality is a unique homozygous missense mutation c.892C>T (p.Arg298Cys) in the *LMNA* gene. To date, this mutation has only been found in affected individuals originating from a restricted region of Northwest Africa (northwest of Algeria and east of Morocco), implicating a founder effect. The authors reported that the affected individuals share a common ancestral haplotype in a region of about 1.0 Mb (1 cM) such that the most recent common ancestor would have lived approximately 800-900 years ago (95% confidence interval: 550 to 1300 years) [128]. In this geographical context, this *LMNA* mutation is the most likely etiology of either a sporadic or a familial case of ARCMT2. Otherwise, *LMNA* mutations may be responsible for "axonal neuropathies plus" syndromes. One is an autosomal dominant axonal neuropathy associated with muscular dystrophy, cardiac disease, and leuconychia [129] whereas the other is a scapuloperoneal myopathy associated with an axonal neuropathy [130]. Furthermore, *LMNA* mutations may be responsible for about 10 different other diseases including dilated cardiomyopathy 1A, AD and AR Emery-Dreifuss muscular dystrophy 2 and 3, Hutchinson-Gilford progeria, familial partial lipodystrophy 2 , mandibuloacral dysplasia, congenital muscular dystrophy, limb-girdle muscular dystrophy type 1B, lethal restrictive dermopathy, and congestive cardiomyopathy associated with hypergonadotropic hypogonadism known as Malouf syndrome [131, 132].

ARCMT2B (CMT2B2)

A large consanguineous Costa Rican family with adult onset ARCMT2 has been reported [133, 134]. Affected members present with distal symmetrical weakness and atrophy along with sensory deficits in the four limbs. Motor nerve conduction velocities were normal or slightly reduced, which is consistent with an axonal degenerative process. A homozygous 1004C-T transitionin the *MED25* gene, resulting in an ala335-to-val (A335V) substitution was identified in the affected members of this family [135].

Two more forms of ARCMT2 were recently identified; one linked to *LRSAM1* coding for an E3 Ubiquitin ligase, allelic to CMT2P, that was identified in a large Canadian family [136] and ARCMT2 linked to *MFN2*, allelic to CMT2A presenting as an early onset CMT associated with optic atrophy [29, 30].

2. Hereditary Motor Neuronopathy (HMN)

Hereditary motor neuronopathics (HMN) are a heterogeneous group of disorders that include the proximal HMNs with spinal muscular atrophies SMA1 (Werdnig-Hoffman disease) and SMA2 (Kugelberg-Welander disease), as well as X-linked bulbo-spinal neuronopathy (Kennedy's disease). These are considered to be motor neuron disorders such that they will not be discussed in this chapter. This chapter will focus on the distal HMNs (dHMN), often referred to as "spinal forms of CMT." These are group of clinically and genetically heterogeneous diseases that occur from degeneration of spinal motor neurons, leading to distal muscle weakness and wasting.

Distal HMNs, which are much less common than HMSN, are characterized by a very slowly progressive length-dependant motor neuropathy. They usually present in the first two decades as a CMT-like clinical phenotype (Figure 7). Hereditary transmission is usually autosomal dominant although autosomal recessive [137] and X-linked [138] inheritance has been described. Sporadic cases also occur [137]. Affected persons often report a history of poor athletic performance with an insidious progression. As such, a history of a chronic progressive motor weakness would help to differentiate these disorders from sporadic motor neuron diseases. Clinical examination usually reveals distal amyotrophy associated with reduced or absent deep tendon reflexes in the absence of sensory deficits.

In dHMN, neurophysiology testing confirms normal NCV with reduced CMAPs and normal sensory nerve action potentials (SNAP). Needle electromyography (EMG) demonstrates abnormalities consistent with chronic denervation that is distally predominant [139]. Normal SNAPs exclude the diagnosis of CMT2. Needle electromyography may help differentiate dHMN from a distal hereditary myopathy such as Myoshi myopathy, which may mimic a CMT like disorder. In 1993, Harding et al. proposed a classification of distal HMN into seven types based on clinical presentation, age of onset and mode of inheritance [140]. Four of the subtypes have autosomal dominant inheritance patterns, (type I, II, V and VII), whereas three are autosomal recessive forms (type III, IV and VI). Type I (juvenile onset) and II (adult onset) present with distal leg weakness and wasting. Type V is characterized by onset in the arms whereas type VII manifests vocal cord paralysis in addition to distal weakness.

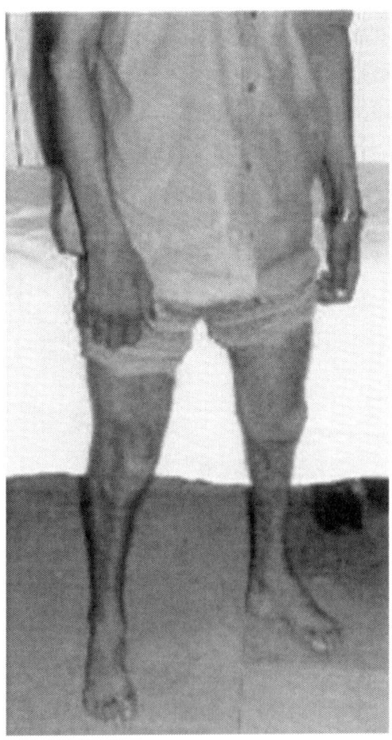

Figure 7. Distal HMN patient: distal four limbs wasting associated with moderate foot and hand deformities.

Table 2. Classification of distal hereditary motor neuropathies (dHMN)

Type	Inheritance	Gene/locus	Age of onset	Clinical features
dHMN I	AD	HSPB8 /12q24.3 HSPB1 /7q11-q21 TRPV4 / 12q24.1 Unknown / 7q34-q36 BSCL2 / 11q12-q14	1st decade	Juvenile onset with distal leg wasting and weakness. Slow progression.
dHMN IIA dHMN IIB dHMN IIC	AD	HSPB8 /12q24.3 HSPB1 /7q11-q21 HSPB3 / 5q11 BSCL2 / 11q12-q14	2nd decade	Progressive wasting and weakness in distal lower extremities without pyramidal involvement. Delayed proximal wasting. No orthopedic deformities.
dHMN III	AR	Unknown / 11q13	Infancy	Distal leg weakness without pyramidal involvement. Kyphoscoliosis, diaphragmatic paresis. More severe form with early onset and respiratory failure has been reported.
dHMN IV	AR	Unknown / 11q13	Adult	Slow progressive wasting and weakness in distal lower limbs.
dHMN VA	AD	GARS / 7p15	Adult	Upper-limb predominant distal motor neuropathy with mild sensory symptoms (allelic to CMT2D).
dHMN VB	AD	REEP1 / 2p11.2	Adult	Upper limb onset.
dHMN VC	AD	BSCL2 / 11q12-q14	Adult	Upper-limb onset, brisk reflexes. Silver syndrome. Hereditary spastic paraplegia.
dHMN VI	AR	IGHMBP2 / 11q13.2-13.4	Childhood	Upper-limb prominent distal weakness with diaphragmatic palsy. Severe course.
dHMN VIIA dHMN VIIB	AD	Unknown / 2q14 DCTN1 / 2q13 TRPV4 / 12q24.1	Adult	Upper limb wasting and vocal cord paralysis.
X-linked dHMN	X-linked	ATP7A / Xq13-q21	1st decade	Slow progressive wasting and weakness in distal lower limbs.
dHMN with pyramidal tract features	AD	SETX / 9q34 BSCL2 / 11q12-q14	1st-2nd decade	Lower-limb onset with wasting and pyramidal signs.
Congenital distal spinal muscular atrophy	AD	TRPV4 /12q24.1	Birth	Distal leg weakness and arthrogryposis.

AD, autosomal dominant; AR, autosomal recessive; BSCL2, Berardinelli-Seip congenital lipodystrophy type 2; DCTN1, P150 subunit of dynactin; DYNC1H1, cytoplasmic dynein heavy chain 1; GARS, glycyl-tRNA synthetase; HSPB1, heat-shock protein B1; HSPB3, heat-shock protein B3; HSPB8, heat-shock protein B8; IGHMBP2, immunoglobulin μ binding protein 2; SETX, senataxin; TRPV4, transient receptor vallanoid 4 gene.

Currently, the identification of related gene mutations in some of these subtypes allows for a more detailed classification with the main clinical subtype characteristics as noted in table 2. HMN type I (childhood onset) and HMN type II (adult onset) are typical distal motor neuropathies beginning in the lower limbs. There is genetic heterogeneity as both may result from mutations in either *HSPB1* or *HSPB8*. [141]. It is noteworthy that these two genes are also mutated in CMT2F *(HSPB1)* and CMT2L (*HSPB8*). HMN type II is further subdivided into IIA, IIB and IIC. HMN IIA is linked to Heat-shock 22-kD protein 8 *(HSPB8; HSP22)* [142], HMN IIB is linked to Heat-shock 27-kD protein 1 (*HSPB1; HSP 27*) [51] and HMN IIC is linked to Heat-shock 27-kd protein 3 (*HSPB3*) also termed heat-shock protein 27-like protein (*HSPL27*) [143]. Mutations of *HSPB8, HSPB1, BSCL2* and *TRPV4* are also implicated in dHMN-I (Table 2). There is a significant clinical and genetic overlap between dHMN-I and dHMN-II, such that they are distinguished only by their age at onset; dHMN-I in the first decade, dHMN-II in the second. HMN V with upper limb predominance is linked to three genes. The first is Glycyl tRNA Synthetase (*GARS*, HMN VA) [44]. The second is Bernardinelli-Seip congenital lipodystrophy 2 (*BSCL2),* encoding Seipin (HMN VB), which is allelic to Silver syndrome [144]. The third is Receptor expression–enhancing protein 1 gene (*REEP1*, HMN VC), which is allelic to SPG31 a subtype of hereditary spastic paraplegia [145]. HMN VII with vocal cord paralysis is subdivided into HMN VIIA linked to 2q14 (unknown gene) and HMN VIIB linked to Dynactin 1 [146]. *TRPV4* is a gene implicated in three distinct phenotypes: CMT2C, scapuloperoneal spinal muscular atrophy and congenital distal spinal muscular atrophy [41]. It is also mutated in this subtype of HMN associated with vocal cord palsy. Otherwise striking phenotypic variability between and within *TRPV4* linked families is observed [147].

In recessive HMN, only one gene has been identified; immunoglobulin μ-binding protein 2 (*IGHMBP2*, HMN VI) [148]. The sole gene identified in X-linked HMN is *ATP7A*, a copper transporter ATPase allelic to Menkes disease [149]. Otherwise, some rare subtypes of HMN linked to *BSCL2* and *SETX* are associated with upper motor neuron involvement, overlapping with juvenile familial forms of amyotrophic lateral sclerosis (ALS) such as ALS4 that is also linked to Senataxin (*SETX*) [150, 151]. Notably, homozygous and compound heterozygous mutations in *SETX* are associated with Ataxia with Oculomotor Apraxia type 2 (AOA2); a condition characterized by cerebellar atrophy, sensorimotor axonal neuropathy and oculomotor apraxia [152].

Notwithstanding these advances, approximately 80% of HMN cases have not been genetically characterized [153, 154].

In summary, the concept of dHMN is defined as a hereditary distal amyotrophy characterized electrophysiologically by a pure motor axonal involvement without associated sensory abnormalities. It has been postulated that this occurs from the death of lower motor neurons likely because their large axons have a greater metabolic demand. The known dHMN genes encode for proteins with diverse functions in motor nerve disease including protein misfolding (HSPB1, HSPB8, BSCL2), cellular protection against oxidative stress (HSPB1, HSPB8), RNA metabolism (IGHMBP2, SETX, GARS), axonal transport (HSPB1, DCTN1) and cation-channel dysfunction (ATP7A and TRPV4) [154, 155].

Despite the great number of identified dHMN modified genes, genotype/phenotype correlations are not easy to establish as inter and intra familial variability are very common. There is also significant overlap with genetic abnormalities that result in CMT2. Thus, clinicians have to be as accurate as possible when defining the phenotypic presentation.

3. Hereditary Sensory and Autonomic Neuropathies (HSAN)

Hereditary sensory and autonomic neuropathies (HSAN) are a clinically and genetically heterogeneous group of inherited peripheral neuropathies in which the peripheral sensory and autonomic fibers are primarily affected [156]. They are also referred to as hereditary sensory neuropathies (HSN) [157].

The major clinical feature is that of a distal, symmetric predominantly sensory axonal neuropathy characterized by loss of pain and temperature. In some patients pain and paresthesias may be present while others manifest insensitivity to pain; previously described as "indifference to pain." This degree of sensory loss predisposes these patients to recurrent painless limb injuries such that ulcerations may occur. This may be followed by complications such as infections or osteomyelitis that leads to spontaneous or surgical amputations of fingers and toes.

Autonomic dysfunction may be present in some patients manifesting as anhidrosis, fever, blood pressure fluctuations and gastro-intestinal disturbances. Electrophysiology confirms reduced or absent SNAP and reduced CMAP amplitude while the MNCVs remain normal or only moderately reduced [157]. Sural nerve biopsy reveals a markedly decreased number of sensory fibers with the unmyelinated fibers and the small diameter myelinated fibers affected to the greatest degree and the large diameter myelinated fibers to the least degree [156].

HSAN can be subdivided into two major groups according to the mode of inheritance, either autosomal dominant [AD] or autosomal recessive [AR], although some cases may occur through spontaneous mutations [156, 158, 159]. In general, HSAN patients with AD forms present with a later onset (second to fifth decade) of their symptoms that is characterized by a profound sensory neuropathy, mild autonomic signs and variable degrees of motor involvement. By contrast, patients with AR forms have an early or congenital onset of a severe sensory neuropathy with mutilating complications and marked autonomic involvement. In 1993, Dyck classified HSAN into five groups (HSAN I to V) based on the mode of inheritance and the subtype's clinical features [156]. This classification has been updated such that the genes underlying these disorders have been incorporated (see Table 3).

The most common subtype, HSAN type I, is a dominant form presenting with perforating ulcers of the feet, lancinating pain, mutilating acropathy, and neurotrophic arthropathy. The age of onset ranges from 15 to 50 years, although congenital or childhood onset of HSAN-I has been reported [158]. The most common presentation is usually with hyperkeratosis (e.g. a "corn") on a great toe followed by a painless ulcer with bony debris. Neurologic examination demonstrates absent lower extremity reflexes with a loss of pain, touch, heat and cold sensation over the feet with these sensory modalities preserved in the upper extremities. The cranial nerves are usually unaffected although deafness may occur in later stages. Nerve conduction studies demonstrate low amplitude or absent SNAPs in the affected limbs whereas motor studies are typically normal. Autopsy data have revealed marked loss of ganglion cells in the lumbosacral dorsal root ganglia [160]. In mild cases, "burning feet" may be the sole manifestation of a dominantly inherited sensory neuropathy. Such patients may manifest with symptoms of burning pain, restless legs, and lancinating pain, rather than with signs of a mutilating acropathy or severe distal sensory loss [161, 162].

Table 3. Classification of the hereditary sensory and autonomic neuropathies (HSAN)

Type	Inheritance	Gene/Locus	Age of onset	Clinical features
HSAN IA	AD	SPTLC1 9q22	2nd-5th decade	Predominant loss of pain, preservation of vibration sense, lancinating pain, frequent later motor involvement and ulcero-mutilating complications
HSAN IB	AD	3p22-p24	20 – 40 years	Sensory neuropathy. Cough and gastro-esophageal reflux.
HSAN IC	AD	SPTLC2 14q24	2nd-5th decade	Similar to SPTLC1.
HSAN ID	AD	ATL1 14q11	Early adult	Sensory neuropathy without motor involvement, mutilating acropathy. Reflexes may be brisk and spasticity has been described.
HSAN IE	AD	DNMT1 19p13	16-35 years	Sensory neuropathy, deafness with dementia developing in 4th decade.
HSAN IIA	AR	HSN2/WNK1 12p13	Infancy to first two decades	Mutilating acropathy, often unrecognized fractures, marked sensory loss affecting all modalities. Autonomic dysfunction less marked.
HSAN IIB	AR	FAM134B 5p15	Childhood	Childhood onset impaired sensation, ulcers and arthropathy. Autonomic dysfunction with hyperhidrosis, urinary incontinence and slow pupillary light reflex.
HSAN IIC	AR	ATSV(KIF1A) 2q37	1-2nd decade	Sensory neuropathy, severe ulcero-mutilating complications, mild motor involvement.
HSAN III	AR	IKBKAP 9q31	Birth	Riley-Day syndrome. Failure to produce tears, absent corneal reflexes, postural hypotension, relative indifference to pain, absence of fungiform papillae on tongue, normal intelligence. (Ashkenazi Jewish patients).
HSAN IV	AR	NTRK1 1q21	Infancy	Congenital insensitivity to pain with anhydrosis. High fevers during hot weather. Lack of pain sensation. Inability to distinguish hot and cold, self mutilation. Mild mental retardation.
HSAN V	AR	NGFB 1p13	Early childhood to adult	Rare disorder. Painless injuries of the extremities, lack of pain and thermal sensitivity in the limbs but preservation of response to tactile and mechanical stimuli, distal anhidrosis. Normal intelligence.
HSAN VI	AR	Dystonin 6p12	Congenital	Absent tears. Sensory neuropathy.
HSAN with spastic paraplegia	AR	CCT5	Infancy to adult	Mutilating sensory neuropathy with spastic paraplegia.

AD autosomal dominant, AR autosomal recessive, SPTLC1 serine palmitoyltransferase, long chain base subunit-1, SPTLC2 serine palmitoyl-transferase, long chain base subunit-2, ATL1 atlastin1, DNMT1 DNA methyltransferase1, HSN2/WNK1 nerve specific isoform of WNK lysine deficient protein kinase1, FAM134B family with sequence similarity 134, member B, KIF1A kinesin family member1 A, IKBKAP inhibitor of kappa light polypeptide gene enhancer in B- cells, kinase complex-associated protein, NTRK1 neurotrophic tyrosine kinase receptor type1, NGFB nerve growth factor beta polypeptide.

In contrast to HSAN-I, HSAN-II (AR inheritance), manifests in infancy or early childhood with distal sensory loss as well as impaired pain, temperature and touch sensation.

Other characteristics of HSAN-II include Charcot arthropathy, severe ulcerations, auto-amputations, trophic changes of skin and nails, diminished taste sensation, and loss of tendon reflexes.

Sural nerve biopsy studies from HSAN-II patients display loss of large and small myelinated fibers to a greater extent than unmyelinated fibers [163].

To date, 12 genes have been identified to be the cause of these disorders. Table 3 displays the HSAN known subtypes with their main clinical characteristics. HSAN type IA is caused by mutations in the serine palmitoyltransferase subunit-1 (*SPTLC1*) gene on chromosome 9q22, which encodes the rate limiting enzyme in ceramide synthesis [164, 165]. HSAN I is genetically heterogeneous as four additional genetic loci were identified. HSAN IC, which is similar to HSANIA, results from mutations in *SPTLC2* [166]. As mentioned earlier in this chapter, patients with CMT2B caused by mutations in *RAB7* demonstrate considerable phenotypic overlap with those who have mutations in *SPTLC1* and *SPTLC2*. In addition to the symptoms previously described, patients with these mutations may present with distal lancinating pain. HSAN IB is a rare subtype associated with cough and gastroesophageal reflux that has been linked to 3p24 [167]. HSAN ID is due to mutations in *ATL1* which encodes the large dynamin-related GTPase atlastin-1, allelic to an early onset hereditary spastic paraplegia [168]. HSAN IE is associated with dementia and hearing loss and results from mutations in *DNMT1* encoding DNA methyltransferase 1 [169]. Autosomal recessive inheritance of HSAN type II is genetically heterogeneous as well, with congenital to early childhood onset. Mutations on three genes have been identified: *WNK1* [170], *FAM134B* [171] and *ATSV* (*KIF1A*) [172]. HSAN III is also known as familial dysautonomia or Riley Day syndrome, (*IKBKAP*) [173]. Other HSAN subtypes that are of autosomal recessive inheritance include HSAN IV or congenital insensitivity to pain with anhidrosis (*NTRK1*) [174], HSAN V (*NGF-b*) [175], and HSAN VI (*Dystonin*) [176]. Finally, an AR form of HSAN associated with spastic paraplegia, is a complex phenotype characterized by an early-onset sensory neuropathy accompanied by acral mutilations resulting from a homozygous missense mutation in *CCT5*; the gene encoding T-complex protein 1 subunit ε (TCP-1 ε) [177].

Despite of the numerous mutated genes implicated in HSAN, the overall mutation rate is relatively low, less than 20%, which suggests that other genes must be involved in the pathogenesis of HSAN [158, 159]. Currently, the precise molecular mechanism underlying these diseases is unknown, but emerging evidence suggests that axonal transport, control of neuronal membrane excitability and neuronal development are some of the likely candidates [178].

Further identification of causative genes and functional studies may provide further insight into the pathophysiology of these disorders. This may help to determine the common pathways that underlie HSANs that might lead to effective therapies that will improve these patients' quality of life.

Management

There are no known treatments for any of these disorders that will reverse the disease course much less slow its progression [179, 180]. Nonetheless, it is well-recognized that symptomatic treatment is necessary for management of these disorders.

[5] Bergoffen J, Scherer SS, Wang S. et al. Connexin mutations in X-linked Charcot-Marie-Tooth disease. *Science* 1993; 262: 2039–2042.
[6] Birouk N, LeGuern E, Maisonobe T. et al. X-linked Charcot-Marie-Tooth disease with connexin 32 mutations: clinical and electrophysiologic study. *Neurology* 1998; 50: 1074-1082.
[7] Siskind CE, Shy ME. Genetics of neuropathies. *Semin. Neurol.* 2011; 31: 494-505.
[8] Dubourg O, Azzedine H, Verny C et al. Autosomal-recessive forms of demyelinating Charcot-Marie-Tooth disease. *Neuromolecular Med.* 2006; 8: 75-86.
[9] Lupski JR, de Oca-Luna RM, Slaugenhaupt S. et al. DNA duplication associated with Charcot-Marie-Tooth disease type 1A. *Cell* 1991; 66: 219– 232.
[10] Raeymaekers P, Timmerman V, Nelis E. et al. Duplication in chromosome 17p11.2 in Charcot-Marie-Tooth neuropathy type 1a (CMT 1a). *Neuromuscul. Disord.* 1991; 1: 93–97.
[11] Lewis RA, Sumner AJ. The electrodiagnostic distinctions between chronic familial and acquired demyelinative neuropathies. *Neurology* 1982; 32: 592.
[12] Vallat JM. Dominantly inherited peripheral neuropathies. *J. Neuropathol. Exp. Neurol.* 2003; 62: 699-714.
[13] Vallat JM, Grid D, Magdelaine C. et al. Autosomal recessive forms of Charcot-Marie-Tooth disease. *Bull. Acad. Nat. Med.* 2005 Jan; 189: 55-68.
[14] Nelis E, Van Broeckhoven C, De Jonghe P. et al. Estimation of the mutation frequencies in Charcot-Marie-Tooth disease type 1 and hereditary neuropathy with liability to pressure palsies: a European collaborative study. *Eur. J. Hum. Genet.* 1996; 4: 25–33.
[15] Saporta AS, Sottile SL, Miller LJ et al. Charcot-Marie-Tooth disease subtypes and genetic testing strategies. *Ann. Neurol.* 2011; 69: 22-33.
[16] Kovach MJ, Lin J P, Boyadjiev S. et al. A unique point mutation in the PMP22 gene is associated with Charcot-Marie-Tooth disease and deafness. *Am. J. Hum. Genet.* 1999; 64: 1580-1593.
[17] Andersson PB, Yuen E, Parko K, So YT. Electrodiagnostic features of hereditary neuropathy with liability to pressure palsies. *Neurology* 2000; 54: 40–44.
[18] Boerkoel C F, Takashima H, Garcia C. A. et al. Charcot-Marie-Tooth disease and related neuropathies: mutation distribution and genotype-phenotype correlation. *Ann. Neurol.* 2002; 51: 190-201.
[19] Shy ME, Jani A, Krajewski K. et al. Phenotypic clustering in MPZ mutations. *Brain* 2004; 127: 371-384.
[20] Street VA, Bennett CL, Goldy JD et al. Mutation of a putative protein degradation gene LITAF/SIMPLE in Charcot-Marie-Tooth disease 1C. *Neurology* 2003; 60: 22 - 26.
[21] Takashiba S, Van Dyke TE, Shapira L, Amar S. Lipopolysaccharide-inducible and salicylate-sensitive nuclear factor(s) on human tumor necrosis factor alpha promoter. *Infect. Immun.* 1995; 63: 1529-34.
[22] Latour P, Gonnaud PM, Ollagnon E. et al. SIMPLE mutation analysis in dominant demyelinating Charcot-Marie-Tooth disease: three novel mutations. *J. Peripher. Nerv. Syst.* 2006; 11: 148–55.
[23] Warner LE, Mancias P, Butler IJ et al. Mutations in the early growth response 2 (EGR2) gene are associated with hereditary myelinopathies. *Nat. Genet.* 1998; 18: 382-4.

[24] Auer-Grumbach M, Weger M, Fink-Puches R. et al. Fibulin-5 mutations link inherited neuropathies; age-related macular degeneration and hyperelastic skin. *Brain* 2011; 134: 1839-52.

[25] Zuchner S, Mersiyanova IV, Muglia M. et al. Mutations in the mitochondrial GTPase mitofusin 2 cause Charcot-Marie-Tooth neuropathy type 2A. *Nat. Genet.* 2004; 36: 449–451.

[26] Feely SM, Laura M, Siskind CE et al. MFN2 mutations cause severe phenotypes in most patients with CMT2A. *Neurology* 2011; 76: 1690–96.

[27] Braathen GJ, Sand JC, Lobato A, Høyer H, Russell MB. MFN2 point mutations occur in 3.4% of Charcot-Marie-Tooth families. An investigation of 232 Norwegian CMT families. *BMC Med. Genet.* 2010; 11: 48.

[28] Chung KW, Kim SB, Park KD et al. Early onset severe and late-onset mild Charcot-Marie-Tooth disease with mitofusin 2 (MFN2) mutations. *Brain* 2006; 129: 2103-18.

[29] Calvo J, Funalot B, Ouvrier R. A. et al. Genotype-phenotype correlations in Charcot-Marie-Tooth disease type 2 caused by mitofusin 2 mutations. *Arch. Neurol.* 2009; 66: 1511-1516.

[30] Polke JM, Laurá M, Pareyson D. et al. Recessive axonal Charcot-Marie-Tooth disease due to compound heterozygous mitofusin 2 mutations. *Neurology* 2011; 77: 168-73.

[31] Vallat JM, Ouvrier RA, Pollard JD et al. Histopathological findings in hereditary motor and sensory neuropathy of axonal type with onset in early childhood associated with mitofusin 2 mutations. *J. Neuropathol. Exp. Neurol.* 2008; 67: 1097-102.

[32] Zhao C, Takita J, Tanaka Y. et al. Charcot-Marie-Tooth disease type 2A caused by mutation in a microtubule motor KIF1Bbeta. *Cell* 2001; 105: 587-97.

[33] Kwon J M, Elliott JL, Yee W-C, Ivanovich J, Scavarda N. Charcot-Marie-Tooth type II locus to chromosome 3q. *Am. J. Hum. Genet.* 1999; 57: 853-858.

[34] Verhoeven K, De Jonghe P, Coen K. et al. Mutations in the small GTP-ase late endosomal protein RAB7 cause Charcot-Marie-Tooth type 2B neuropathy. *Am. J. Hum. Genet.* 2003; 72: 722–727.

[35] Houlden H, King RH, Muddle JR et al. A novel RAB7 mutation associated with ulcero-mutilating neuropathy. *Ann. Neurol.* 2004; 56: 586-90.

[36] Houlden H, King R, Blake J. et al. Clinical pathological and genetic characterization of hereditary sensory and autonomic neuropathy type 1 (HSAN I). *Brain* 2006; 129: 411–425.

[37] Klein CJ, Cunningham JM, Atkinson EJ et al. The gene for HMSN2C maps to 12q23-24: a region of neuromuscular disorders. *Neurology* 2003; 60: 1151–56.

[38] Landoure G, Zdebik AA, Martinez TL et al. Mutations in TRPV4 cause Charcot-Marie-Tooth disease type 2C. *Nat. Genet.* 2010; 42: 170-174.

[39] Dyck PJ, Litchy WJ, Minnerath S. et al. Hereditary motor and sensory neuropathy with diaphragm and vocal cord paresis. *Ann. Neurol.* 1994; 35: 608-615.

[40] Chen DH, SulY, Weiss M. et al. CMT2C with vocal cord paresis associated with short stature and mutations in the TRPV4 gene. *Neurology* 2010; 75: 1968–75.

[41] Auer-Grumbach M, Olschewski A, Papic L. et al. Alterations in the ankyrin domain of TRPV4 cause congenital distal SMA, scapuloperoneal SMA and HMSN2C. *Nature Genet.* 2010; 42: 160-164.

[42] Deng HX, Klein CJ, Yan J. et al. Scapuloperoneal spinal muscular atrophy and CMT2C are allelic disorders caused by alterations in TRPV4. *Nature Genet.* 2010; 42: 165-169.

[43] Unger S, Lausch E, Stanzial F. et al. Fetal akinesia in metatropic dysplasia: the combined phenotype of chondrodysplasia and neuropathy. *Am. J. Med. Genet.* 2011; 155: 2860-2864.

[44] Antonellis A, Ellsworth RE, Sambuughin N et al. Glycyl tRNA synthetase mutations in Charcot-Marie-Tooth disease type 2D and distal spinal muscular atrophy type V. *Am. J. Hum. Genet.* 2003; 72: 1293–99.

[45] Windpassinger C, Auer-Grumbach M, Irobi J. et al. Heterozygous missense mutations in BSCL2 are associated with distal hereditary motor neuropathy and Silver syndrome. *Nature Genet.* 2004; 36: 271-276.

[46] Mersiyanova IV, Perepelov AV, Polyakov AV et al. A new variant of Charcot-Marie-Tooth disease type 2 is probably the result of a mutation in the neurofilament-light gene. *Am. J. Hum. Genet.* 2000; 67: 37–46.

[47] Bomont P, Cavalier L, Blondeau F. et al. The gene encoding gigaxonin; a new member of the cytoskeletal BTB/kelch repeat family; is mutated in giant axonal neuropathy. *Nature Genet.* 2000; 26: 370-374.

[48] Zemmouri R, Azzedine H, Assami S. et al. Charcot-Marie-Tooth 2-like presentation of an Algerian family with giant axonal neuropathy. *Neuromuscul. Disord.* 2000; 10: 592-8.

[49] Tazir M, Nouioua S, Magy L. et al. Phenotypic variability in giant axonal neuropathy. *Neuromuscul. Disord.* 2009; 19: 270-4.

[50] Jordanova A, De Jonghe P, Boerkoel CF et al. Mutations in the neurofilament light chain gene (NEFL) cause early onset severe Charcot-Marie-Tooth disease. *Brain* 2003; 126: 590-7.

[51] Evgrafov OV, Mersiyanova I, Irobi J. et al. Mutant small heat-shock protein 27 causes axonal Charcot-Marie-Tooth disease and distal hereditary motor neuropathy. *Nat. Genet.* 2004; 36: 602–606.

[52] Solla P, Vannelli A, Bolino A. et al. Heat shock protein 27 R127W mutation: evidence of a continuum between axonal Charcot-Marie-Tooth and distal hereditary motor neuropathy. *J. Neurol. Neurosurg. Psychiatry* 2010; 81: 958–62.

[53] Nelis E, Berciano J, Verpoorten N. et al. Autosomal dominant axonal Charcot-Marie-Tooth disease type 2 (CMT2G) maps to chromosome 12q12-q13.3. *J. Med. Genet.* 2004; 41: 193–7.

[54] Shy ME, Jani A, Krajewski K. et al. Phenotypic clustering in MPZ mutations. *Brain* 2004; 127: 371–84.

[55] Crimella C, Tonelli A, Airoldi G. et al. The GST domain of GDAP1 is a frequent target of mutations in the dominant form of axonal Charcot Marie Tooth type 2 K. *J. Med. Genet.* 2010; 47: 712–6.

[56] Tang BS, Zhao GH, Luo W. et al. Small heat-shock protein 22 mutated in autosomal dominant Charcot-Marie-Tooth disease type 2L. *Hum. Genet.* 2005; 116: 222–4.

[57] Fabrizi GM, Ferrarini M, Cavallaro T. et al. Two novel mutations in dynamin-2 cause axonal Charcot-Marie-Tooth disease. *Neurology* 2007; 69: 291–5.

[58] Bitoun M, Maugenre S, Jeannet PY et al. Mutations in dynamin 2 cause dominant centronuclear myopathy. *Nat. Genet.* 2005; 37: 1207-9.

[59] Zuchner S, Noureddine M, Kennerson M. et al. Mutations in the pleckstrin homology domain of dynamin 2 cause dominant intermediate Charcot-Marie-Tooth disease. *Nature Genet.* 2005; 37: 289-294.

[60] Latour P, Thauvin-Robinet C, Baudelet-Mery C. et al. A major determinant for binding and aminoacylation of tRNA (Ala) in cytoplasmic Alanyl-tRNA synthetase is mutated in dominant axonal Charcot-Marie-Tooth disease. *Am. J. Hum. Genet.* 2010; 86: 77–82.

[61] Weedon MN, Hastings R, Caswell R. et al. Exome sequencing identifies a DYNC1H1 mutation in a large pedigree with dominant axonal Charcot-Marie-Tooth disease. *Am. J. Hum. Genet.* 2011; 89: 308-12.

[62] Weterman MA, Sorrentino V, Kasher PR et al. A frameshift mutation in LRSAM1 is responsible for a dominant hereditary polyneuropathy. *Hum. Molec. Genet.* 2012; 21: 358-370.

[63] Bergoffen J, Scherer SS, Wang S et al. Connexin mutations in X-linked Charcot-Marie-Tooth disease. *Science* 1993; 262: 2039-42.

[64] Bone LJ, Deschenes SM, Balice-Gordon RJ Fischbeck KH, Scherer SS. Connexin32 and X-linked Charcot-Marie-Tooth disease. *Neurobiol. Dis.* 1997; 4: 221–230.

[65] Shy ME, Siskind C, Swan ER et al.CMT1X phenotypes represent loss of GJB1 gene function *Neurology* 2007; 68: 849-55.

[66] Birouk N, LeGuern E, Maisonobe T et al. X-linked Charcot-Marie-Tooth disease with connexin 32 mutations: clinical and electrophysiologic study. *Neurology* 1998; 50: 1074-82.

[67] Tabaraud F, Lagrange E, Sindou P. et al. Demyelinating X-linked Charcot-Marie-Tooth disease: unusual electrophysiological findings. *Muscle Nerve* 1999; 22: 1442-7.

[68] Hattori N, Yamamoto M, Yoshihara T. et al. Study Group for Hereditary Neuropathy in Japan. Demyelinating and axonal features of Charcot-Marie-Tooth disease with mutations of myelin-related proteins (PMP22, MPZ and Cx32): a clinicopathological study of 205 Japanese patients. *Brain* 2003; 126: 134-51.

[69] Kim HJ, Sohn KM, Shy ME et al. Mutations in PRPS1, which encodes the phosphoribosyl pyrophosphate synthetase enzyme critical for nucleotide biosynthesis, cause hereditary peripheral neuropathy with hearing loss and optic neuropathy (cmtx5). *Am. J. Hum. Genet.* 2007; 81: 552-8.

[70] Nicholson G, Myers S. Intermediate forms of Charcot-Marie-Tooth neuropathy: a review. *Neuromolecular Med.* 2006; 8: 123–30.

[71] Verhoeven K, Villanova M, Rossi A. et al. Localization of the gene for the intermediate form of Charcot-Marie-Tooth to chromosome 10q24.1-q25.1. *Am. J. Hum. Genet.* 2001; 69: 889-894.

[72] Jordanova A, Irobi J, Thomas FP et al. Disrupted function and axonal distribution of mutant tyrosyl-tRNA synthetase in dominant intermediate Charcot-Marie-Tooth neuropathy. *Nature Genet.* 2006; 38: 197-202.

[73] Mastaglia FL, Nowak KJ, Stell R. et al. Novel mutation in the myelin protein zero gene in a family with intermediate hereditary motor and sensory neuropathy. *J. Neurol. Neurosurg. Psychiat.* 1999; 67: 174-179.

[74] Boyer O, Nevo F, Plaisier E. et al. INF2 mutations in Charcot-Marie-Tooth disease with glomerulopathy. *N. Engl. J. Med.* 2011; 365: 2377-88.

[75] Vallat JM, Tazir M, Magdelaine C, Sturtz F, Grid D. Autosomal-recessive Charcot-Marie-Tooth diseases. *J. Neuropathol. Exp. Neurol.* 2005; 64: 363-70.

[76] Ben Othmane K, Hentati F, Lennon F. et al. Linkage of a locus (CMT4A) for autosomal recessive Charcot-Marie-Tooth disease to chromosome 8q. *Hum. Mol. Genet.* 1993; 2: 1625-8.

[77] Baxter RV, Ben Othmane K, Rochelle JM et al. Ganglioside-induced differentiation-associated protein-1 is mutant in Charcot-Marie-Tooth disease type 4A/8q21. *Nature Genet.* 2002; 30: 21-22.

[78] Cuesta A, Pedrola L, Sevilla T. et al. The gene encoding ganglioside-induced differentiation-associated protein 1 is mutated in axonal Charcot-Marie-Tooth type 4A disease. *Nature Genet.* 2002; 30: 22-24.

[79] Birouk N, Azzedine H, Dubourg O. et al. Phenotypical features of a Moroccan family with autosomal recessive Charcot-Marie-Tooth disease associated with the S194X mutation in the GDAP1 gene. *Arch. Neurol.* 2003; 60: 598-604.

[80] Claramunt R, Pedrola L, Sevilla T et al. Genetics of Charcot-Marie-Tooth disease type 4A: mutations, inheritance, phenotypic variability, and founder effect. *J. Med. Genet.* 2005; 42: 358-365.

[81] Crimella C, Tonelli A, Airoldi G. et al. The GST domain of GDAP1 is a frequent target of mutations in the dominant form of axonal Charcot Marie Tooth type 2K. *J. Med. Genet.* 2010; 47: 712-716.

[82] Pedrola L, Espert A, Valdés-Sánchez T. et al.Cell expression of GDAP1 in the nervous system and pathogenesis of Charcot-Marie-Tooth type 4A disease. *J. Cell Mol. Med.* 2008; 12: 679-89.

[83] Bolino A, Muglia M, Conforti FL et al. Charcot-Marie-Tooth type 4B is caused by mutations in the gene encoding myotubularin-related protein-2. *Nat. Genet.* 2000; 25: 17-9.

[84] Nouioua S, Hamadouche T, Funalot B. et al. Novel mutations in the PRX and the MTMR2 genes are responsible for unusual Charcot-Marie-Tooth disease phenotypes. *Neuromuscul. Disord.* 2011; 21: 543-50.

[85] Previtali SC, Quattrini A, Bolino A. Charcot-Marie-Tooth type 4B demyelinating neuropathy: deciphering the role of MTMR phosphatases. *Expert Rev. Mol. Med.* 2007; 9: 1-16.

[86] Bolis A, Coviello S, Visigalli I. et al. Dlg1, Sec8, and Mtmr2 regulate membrane homeostasis in Schwann cell myelination. *J. Neurosci.* 2009; 29: 8858-70.

[87] Bolis A, Zordan P, Coviello S, Bolino A. Myotubularin-related (MTMR) phospholipid phosphatase proteins in the peripheral nervous system. *Mol. Neurobiol.* 2007; 35: 308-16.

[88] Senderek J, Bergmann C, Weber S. et al. Mutation of the SBF2 gene, encoding a novel member of the myotubularin family, in Charcot-Marie-Tooth neuropathy type 4B2/11p15. *Hum. Mol. Genet.* 2003; 12: 349-56.

[89] Azzedine H, Bolino A, Taïeb T. et al. Mutations in MTMR13; a new pseudophosphatase homologue of MTMR2 and Sbf1; in two families with an autosomal recessive demyelinating form of Charcot-Marie-Tooth disease associated with early-onset glaucoma. *Am. J. Hum. Genet.* 2003; 72: 1141-53.

[90] Arnaud E, Zenker J, de Preux Charles AS et al. SH3TC2/KIAA1985 protein is required for proper myelination and the integrity of the node of Ranvier in the peripheral nervous system. *Proc. Natl. Acad. Sci. U. S. A.* 2009; 106: 17528-33.

[91] Kessali M, Zemmouri R, Guilbot A. et al. A clinical; electrophysiologic; neuropathologic; and genetic study of two large Algerian families with an autosomal recessive demyelinating form of Charcot-Marie-Tooth disease. *Neurology* 1997; 48: 867-73.

[92] LeGuern E, Guilbot A, Kessali M. et al. Homozygosity mapping of an autosomal recessive form of demyelinating Charcot-Marie-Tooth disease to chromosome 5q23-q33. *Hum. Mol. Genet.* 1996; 5: 1685-8.
[93] Gabreëls-Festen A, van Beersum S, Eshuis L. et al. Study on the gene and phenotypic characterisation of autosomal recessive demyelinating motor and sensory neuropathy (Charcot-Marie-Tooth disease) with a gene locus on chromosome 5q23-q33. *J. Neurol. Neurosurg. Psychiatry* 1999; 66: 569-74.
[94] Senderek J, Bergmann C, Stendel C et al. Mutations in a gene encoding a novel SH3/TPR domain protein cause autosomal recessive Charcot-Marie-Tooth type 4C neuropathy. *Am. J. Hum. Genet.* 2003; 73: 1106-19.
[95] Gooding R, Colomer J, King R. et al. A novel Gypsy founder mutation; p. Arg1109X in the CMT4C gene; causes variable peripheral neuropathy phenotypes. *J. Med. Genet.* 2005; 42: e69.
[96] Colomer J, Gooding R, Angelicheva D. et al. Clinical spectrum of CMT4C disease in patients homozygous for the p. Arg1109X mutation in SH3TC2. *Neuromuscul. Disord.* 2006; 16: 449-53.
[97] Claramunt R, Sevilla T, Lupo V. et al. The p.R1109X mutation in SH3TC2 gene is predominant in Spanish Gypsies with Charcot-Marie-Tooth disease type 4. *Clin. Genet.* 2007; 71: 343-9.
[98] Azzedine H, Ravisé N, Verny C. et al. Spine deformities in Charcot-Marie-Tooth 4C caused by SH3TC2 gene mutations. *Neurology* 2006; 67: 602-6.
[99] Gosselin I, Thiffault I, Tétreault M. et al. Founder SH3TC2 mutations are responsible for a CMT4C French-Canadians cluster. *Neuromuscul. Disord.* 2008; 18: 483-92.
[100] Houlden H, Laura M, Ginsberg L. et al. The phenotype of Charcot-Marie-Tooth disease type 4C due to SH3TC2 mutations and possible predisposition to an inflammatory neuropathy. *Neuromuscul. Disord.* 2009; 19: 264-9.
[101] Laššuthová P, Mazanec R, Vondráček P. et al. High frequency of SH3TC2 mutations in Czech HMSN I patients. *Clin. Genet.* 2011: 1399-0004.
[102] Kalaydjieva L, Gresham D, Gooding R. et al. N-myc downstream-regulated gene 1 is mutated in hereditary motor and sensory neuropathy-Lom. *Am. J. Hum. Genet.* 2000; 67: 47-58.
[103] King RH, Chandler D, Lopaticki S. et al. Ndrg1in development and maintenance of the myelin sheath. *Neurobiol. Dis.* 2011; 42: 368-80.
[104] Navarro C, Teijeira S. Neuromuscular disorders in the Gypsy ethnic group. A short review. *Acta Myol.* 2003; 22: 11-4.
[105] Hantke J, Chandler D, King R. et al. A mutation in an alternative untranslated exon of hexokinase 1 associated with hereditary motor and sensory neuropathy Russe (HMSNR). *Eur. J. Hum. Genet.* 2009; 17: 1606-14.
[106] Varon R, Gooding R, Steglich C. et al. Partial deficiency of the C-terminal-domain phosphatase of RNA polymerase II is associated with congenital cataracts facial dysmorphism neuropathy syndrome. *Nat. Genet.* 2003; 35: 185-9.
[107] Merlini L, Gooding R, Lochmuller H. et al. Genetic identity of Marinesco-Sjogren/myoglobinuria and CCFDN syndromes. *Neurology* 2002; 58: 231-236.
[108] Warner L. E, Mancias P, Butler I. J. et al. Mutations in the early growth response 2 (EGR2) gene are associated with hereditary myelinopathies. *Nature Genet.* 1998; 18: 382-384.

[109] Warner LE, Svaren J, Milbrandt J, Lupski JR. Functional consequences of mutations in the early growth response 2 gene (EGR2) correlate with severity of human myelinopathies. *Hum. Mol. Genet.* 1999; 8: 1245-51.

[110] Decker L, Desmarquet-Trin-Dinh C, Taillebourg E. et al. Peripheral myelin maintenance is a dynamic process requiring constant Krox20 expression. *J. Neurosci.* 2006; 26: 9771-9.

[111] Boerkoel CF, Takashima H, Bacino CA, Daentl D, Lupski JR. EGR2 mutation R359W causes a spectrum of Dejerine-Sottas neuropathy. *Neurogenetics* 2001; 3: 153-7.

[112] Delague V, Bareil C, Tuffery S. et al. Mapping of a new locus for 381autosomal recessive demyelinating Charcot-Marie-Tooth disease to 382 19q13. 1-13. 3 in a large consanguineous Lebanese family: exclusion of 383 MAG as a candidate gene. *Am. J. Hum. Genet.* 2000; 67: 236–43.

[113] Boerkoel CF, Takashima H, Stankiewicz P. et al. Periaxin mutations cause recessive Dejerine-Sottas neuropathy. *Am. J. Hum. Genet.* 2001; 68: 325-33.

[114] Takashima H, Boerkoel CF, De Jonghe P. et al. Periaxin mutations cause a broad spectrum of demyelinating neuropathies. *Ann. Neurol.* 2002; 51: 709-15.

[115] Fabrizi G. M, Taioli F, Cavallaro T. et al. Further evidence that mutations in FGD4/frabin cause Charcot-Marie-Tooth disease type 4H. *Neurology* 2009; 72: 1160-1164.

[116] De Sandre-Giovannoli A, Delague V, Hamadouche T. et al. Homozygosity mapping of autosomal recessive demyelinating Charcot-Marie-Tooth neuropathy (CMT4H) to a novel locus on chromosome 12p11. 21-q13. 11. *J. Med. Genet.* 2005; 42: 260-5.

[117] Delague V, Jacquier A, Hamadouche T et al. Mutations in FGD4 encoding the Rho GDP/GTP exchange factor FRABIN cause autosomal recessive Charcot-Marie-Tooth type 4H. *Am. J. Hum. Genet.* 2007; 81: 1-16.

[118] Houlden H, Hammans S, Katifi H, Reilly MM. A novel frabin (FGD4) nonsense mutation p.R275X associated with phenotypic variability in CMT4H. *Neurology* 2009; 72: 617-620.

[119] Stendel C, Roos A, Deconinck T. et al. Peripheral nerve demyelination caused by a mutant Rho GTPase guanine nucleotide exchange factor; frabin/FGD4. *Am. J. Hum. Genet.* 2007; 81: 158-64.

[120] Chow CY, ZhangY, Dowling JJ et al. Mutation of FIG4 causes neurodegeneration in the pale tremor mouse and patients with CMT4J. *Nature* 2007; 448: 68-72.

[121] Nicholson G, Lenk GM, Reddel SW et al. Distinctive genetic and clinical features of CMT4J: a severe neuropathy caused by mutations in the PI (3;5) P phosphatase FIG4. *Brain* 2011; 134: 1959-71.

[122] Chow CY, Landers JE, Bergren SK et al. Deleterious variants of FIG4; a phosphoinositide phosphatase; in patients with ALS. *Am. J. Hum. Genet.* 2009; 84: 85-8.

[123] Vaccari I, Dina G, Tronchère H. et al. Genetic interaction between MTMR2 and FIG4 phospholipid phosphatases involved in Charcot-Marie-Tooth neuropathies. *PLoS Genet.* 2011; 7: e1002319.

[124] Bouhouche A, Benomar A, Birouk N. et al. A locus for an axonal form of autosomal recessive Charcot-Marie-Tooth disease maps to chromosome 1q21. 2-q21. 3. *Am. J. Hum. Genet.* 1999; 65: 722-7.

[125] De Sandre-Giovannoli A, Chaouch M, Kozlov S et al. Homozygous defects in LMNA; encoding lamin A/C nuclear-envelope proteins; cause autosomal recessive axonal neuropathy in human (Charcot-Marie-Tooth disorder type 2) and mouse. *Am. J. Hum. Genet.* 2002; 70: 726-36.

[126] Tazir M, Azzedine H, Assami S et al. Phenotypic variability in autosomal recessive axonal Charcot-Marie-Tooth disease due to the R298C mutation in lamin A/C. *Brain* 2004; 127: 154-63.

[127] Bouhouche A, Birouk N, Azzedine H et al. Autosomal recessive axonal Charcot-Marie-Tooth disease (ARCMT2): phenotype-genotype correlations in 13 Moroccan families. *Brain* 2007; 130: 1062-75.

[128] Hamadouche T, Poitelon Y, Genin E et al. Founder effect and estimation of the age of the c. 892C > T (p.Arg298Cys) mutation in LMNA associated to Charcot-Marie-Tooth subtype CMT2B1 in families from North Western Africa. *Ann. Hum. Genet.*, 2008; 72: 590-7.

[129] Goizet C, Yaou RB, Demay L. et al. A new mutation of the lamin A/C gene leading to autosomal dominant axonal neuropathy; muscular dystrophy; cardiac disease; and leuconychia. *J. Med. Genet.* 2004; 41: e29.

[130] Benedetti S, Bertini E, Iannaccone S. et al. Dominant LMNA mutations can cause combined muscular dystrophy and peripheral neuropathy. *J. Neurol. Neurosurg. Psychiatry* 2005; 76: 1019-21.

[131] Benedetti S, Merlini L. Laminopathies: from the heart of the cell to the clinics. *Curr. Opin. Neurol.* 2004; 17: 553-60.

[132] Bertrand AT, Chikhaoui K, Ben Yaou R, Bonne G. Laminopathies: one gene, several diseases]. *Biol. Aujourdhui* 2011; 205: 147-62.

[133] Leal A, Morera B, Del Valle G. et al. A second locus for an axonal form of autosomal recessive Charcot-Marie-Tooth disease maps to chromosome 19q13. 3. *Am. J. Hum. Genet.* 2001; 68: 269-274.

[134] Berghoff C, Berghoff M, Leal A. et al. Clinical and electrophysiological characteristics of autosomal recessive axonal Charcot-Marie-Tooth disease (ARCMT2B) that maps to chromosome 19q13. 3. *Neuromusc. Disord.* 2004; 14: 301-306.

[135] Leal A, Huehne K, Bauer F. et al. Identification of the variant Ala335Val of MED25 as responsible for CMT2B2: molecular data; functional studies of the SH3 recognition motif and correlation between wild-type MED25 and PMP22 RNA levels in CMT1A animal models. *Neurogenetics* 2009; 10: 275-287.

[136] Guernsey DL, Jiang, H, Bedard K. et al. Mutation in the gene encoding ubiquitin ligase LRSAM1 in patients with Charcot-Marie-Tooth disease. *PLoS Genet.* 2010; 6: e1001081.

[137] Harding A, Thomas PK. Hereditary distal spinal muscular atrophy. A report on 34 cases and a review of the literature. *J. Neurol. Sci.* 1980; 45: 337-48.

[138] Takata RI, Speck Martins CE, Passosbueno MR et al. A new locus for recessive distal spinal muscular atrophy at Xq13.1-q21. *J. Med. Genet.* 2004; 41: 224-9.

[139] De Jongue P, Timmerman V, Van Broeckoven C. 2nd Workshop of the European CMT Consortium: 53rd ENMC International Workshop on Classification and Diagnostic Guidelines for Charcot-Marie-Tooth Type 2 (CMT2-HMSN II) and Distal Hereditary Motor Neuropathy (distal HMN-Spinal CMT) 26-28 September 1997, Naarden, The Netherlands. *Neuromuscul. Disord.* 1998; 8: 426-31.

[140] Harding AE, Dyck PJ, Thomas PK, Griffin JW. Inherited neuronal atrophy and degeneration predominantly of lower motor neurons eds. Peripheral Neuropathy. Philadelphia: W. B. Saunders Company 1993; 1051e64.
[141] Irobi J, Dierick I, Jordanova A. et al. Unraveling the genetics of distal hereditary motor neuronopathies. *Neuromolecular Med.* 2006; 8: 131-46.
[142] Irobi J, Van Impe K, Seeman P. et al.Hot-spot residue in small heat-shock protein 22 causes distal motor neuropathy. *Nat. Genet.* 2004; 36: 597-601.
[143] Kolb SJ, Snyder PJ, Poi EJ. et al. Mutant small heat shock protein B3 causes motor neuropathy: utility of a candidate gene approach. *Neurology* 2010; 74: 502-506.
[144] Windpassinger C, Auer-Grumbach M, Irobi J. et al. Heterozygous missense mutations in BSCL2 are associated with distal hereditary motor neuropathy and Silver syndrome. *Nat. Genet.* 2004; 36: 271-6.
[145] Beetz C, Pieber TR, Hertel N. et al. Exome sequencing identifies a REEP1 mutation involved in distal hereditary motor neuropathy type V. *Am. J. Hum. Genet.* 2012; 91: 139-145.
[146] Puls I, Jonnakuty C, LaMonte BH et al. Mutant dynactin in motor neuron disease. *Nat. Genet.* 2003; 33: 455-6.
[147] Zimoń M, Baets J, Auer-Grumbach M. et al. Dominant mutations in the cation channelgene transient receptor potential vanilloid 4 cause an unusual spectrum of neuropathies. *Brain* 2010; 133: 1798-809.
[148] Grohmann K, Schuelke M, Diers A. et al. Mutations in the gene encoding immunoglobulin mu-binding protein 2 cause spinal muscular atrophy with respiratory distress type 1. *Nat. Genet.* 2001; 29: 75-7.
[149] Kennerson ML, Nicholson GA, Kaler SG et al. Missense mutations in the copper transporter gene ATP7A cause X-linked distal hereditary motor neuropathy. *Am. J. Hum. Genet.* 2010; 86: 343-52.
[150] Auer-Grumbach M, Löscher WN, Wagner K et al. Phenotypic and genotypic heterogeneity in hereditary motor neuronopathy type V: a clinical, electrophysiological and genetic study. *Brain* 2000; 123: 1612-23
[151] De Jonghe P, Auer-Grumbach M, Irobi J. et al. Autosomal dominant juvenile amyotrophic lateral sclerosis and distal hereditary motor neuronopathy with pyramidal tract signs: synonyms for the same disorder. *Brain* 2002; 125: 1320-5.
[152] Moreira MC, Klur S, Watanabe M. et al. Senataxin, the ortholog of a yeast RNA helicase, is mutant in ataxia-ocular apraxia 2. *Nat. Genet.* 2004; 36: 225-7.
[153] Dierick I, Baets J, Irobi J. et al. Relative contribution of mutations in genes for autosomal dominant distal hereditary motor neuropathies: a genotype-phenotype correlation study. *Brain* 2008; 131: 1217-27.
[154] Rossor AM, Kalmar B, Greensmith L, Reilly MM. The distal hereditary motor neuropathies. *J. Neurol. Neurosurg. Psychiatry* 2012; 83: 6-14.
[155] Devic P, Petiot P. Distal hereditary motor neuropathy. *Rev. Neurol.* 2011; 167: 781-90.
[156] Dyck PJ. Neuronal atrophy and degeneration predominantly affecting peripheral sensory and autonomic neurons. In: Dyck PJ, Thomas PK, Griffin JW, Low PA, Poduslo JF (eds) Peripheral neuropathy. W.B Saunders, Philadelphia 1993; 1065–1093.
[157] Houlden H, Blake J, Reilly MM. Hereditary sensory neuropathies. *Curr. Opin. Neurol.* 2004; 17: 569–577.

[158] Rotthier A, Baets J, De Vriendt E. et al. Genes for hereditary sensory and autonomic neuropathies: a genotype-phenotype correlation. *Brain* 2009; 132: 2699-711
[159] Davidson GL, Murphy SM, Polke JM et al. Frequency of mutations in the genes associated with hereditary sensory and autonomic neuropathy in a UK cohort. *J. Neurol.* 2012; 259:1673-85.
[160] Denny-Brown D. Hereditary sensory radicular neuropathy. *J. Neurol. Neurosurg. Psychiat.* 1951; 14: 237-252.
[161] Dyck PJ, Low PA, Stevens J. C. Burning feet' as the only manifestation of dominantly inherited sensory neuropathy. *Mayo Clin.* 1983; 58: 426-429.
[162] Stögbauer F, Young P, Kuhlenbäumer G. et al. Autosomal dominant burning feet syndrome. *J. Neurol. Neurosurg. Psychiatry* 1999; 67: 78-81.
[163] Axelrod FB, Gold-von SG. Hereditary sensory and autonomic neuropathies: types, II, III, and IV. *Orphanet. J. Rare Dis.* 2007; 2: 39.
[164] Bejaoui K, Wu C, Scheffler MD et al. SPTLC1 is mutated in hereditary sensory neuropathy type 1. *Nat. Genet.* 2001; 27: 261-2
[165] Dawkins JL, Hulme DJ, Brahmbhatt SB, Auer-Grumbach M, Nicholson GA. Mutations in SPTLC1 encoding serine palmitoyltransferase; long chain base subunit-1; cause hereditary sensory neuropathy type I. *Nat. Genet.* 2001; 27: 309-12
[166] Rotthier A, Auer-Grumbach M, Janssens K. et al. Mutations in the SPTLC2 subunit of serine palmitoyltransferase cause hereditary sensory and autonomic neuropathy type I. *Am. J. Hum. Genet.* 2010; 87: 513-522.
[167] Kok C, Kennerson M. L, Spring PJ et al. A locus for hereditary sensory neuropathy with cough and gastroesophageal reflux on chromosome 3p22-p24. *Am. J. Hum. Genet.* 2003; 73: 632-637.
[168] Guelly C, Zhu PP, Leonardis L. et al. Targeted high-throughput sequencing identifies mutations in atlastin-1 as a cause of hereditary sensory neuropathy type I. *Am. J. Hum. Genet.* 2011; 88: 99-105.
[169] Klein CJ, Botuyan MV, Wu Y. et al. Mutations in DNMT1 cause hereditary sensory neuropathy with dementia and hearing loss. *Nature Genet.* 2011; 43: 595-600.
[170] Shekarabi M, Girard N, Riviere JB et al. Mutations in the nervous system-specific HSN2 exon of WNK1 cause hereditary sensory neuropathy type II. *J. Clin. Invest.* 2008; 118: 2496-2505.
[171] Kurth I, Pamminger T, Hennings JC et al. Mutations in FAM134B, encoding a newly identified Golgi protein, cause severe sensory and autonomic neuropathy. *Nature Genet.* 2009; 41: 1179-1181.
[172] Riviere JB, Ramalingam S, Lavastre V. et al. KIF1A, an axonal transporter of synaptic vesicles, is mutated in hereditary sensory and autonomic neuropathy type 2. *Am. J. Hum. Genet.* 2011; 89: 219-230.
[173] Slaugenhaupt SA, Blumenfeld A, Gill SP et al. Tissue-specific expression of a splicing mutation in the IKBKAP gene causes familial dysautonomia. *Am. J. Hum. Genet.* 2001; 68: 598-605.
[174] Indo Y, Tsuruta M, Hayashida Y. et al. Mutations in the TRKA/NGF receptor gene in patients with congenital insensitivity to pain with anhidrosis. *Nature Genet.* 1996; 13: 485-488.
[175] Einarsdottir E, Carlsson A, Minde J. et al. A mutation in the nerve growth factor beta gene (NGFB) causes loss of pain perception. *Hum. Molec. Genet.* 2004; 13: 799-805.

[176] Edvardson S, Cinnamon Y, Jalas C. et al. Hereditary sensory autonomic neuropathy caused by a mutation in dystonin. *Ann. Neurol.* 2012; 71: 569-572.
[177] Bouhouche A, Benomar A, Bouslam N, ChkiliT, Yahyaoui M. Mutation in the epsilon subunit of the cytosolic chaperonin-containing t-complex peptide-1 (Cct5) gene causes autosomal recessive mutilating sensory neuropathy with spastic paraplegia. *J. Med. Genet.* 2006; 43: 441–443.
[178] Rotthier A, Baets J, Timmerman V, Janssens K. Mechanisms of disease in hereditary sensory and autonomic neuropathies. *Nat. Rev. Neurol.* 2012; 8: 73-85.
[179] Pareyson D, Reilly MM, Schenone A. et al. Ascorbic acid in Charcot-Marie-Tooth disease type 1A (CMT-TRIAAL and CMT-TRAUK): a double-blind randomised trial. *Lancet Neurol.* 2011; 10: 320-8.
[180] Garofalo K, Penno A, Schmidt BP et al. Oral L-serine supplementation reduces production of neurotoxic deoxysphingolipids in mice and humans with hereditary sensory autonomic neuropathy type 1. *J. Clin. Invest.* 2011; 121: 4735-45.
[181] Burns J, Ouvrier R, Estilow T. et al. Validation of the Charcot-Marie-Tooth disease pediatric scale as an outcome measure of disability. *Ann. Neurol.* 2012; 71: 642-52.
[182] Padua L, Aprile I, Cavallaro T. et al. Variables influencing quality of life and disability in Charcot Marie Tooth (CMT) patients: Italian multicentre study. *Neurol. Sci.* 2006; 27: 417-23.
[183] Padua L, Cavallaro T, Pareyson D. et al. Charcot-Marie-Tooth and pain: correlations with neurophysiological, clinical, and disability findings. *Neurol. Sci.* 2008; 29: 193-4.
[184] Ramirez JD, Barnes PR, Mills KR, Bennett DL. Intermediate Charcot-Marie-Tooth disease due to a novel Trp101Stop myelin protein zero mutation associated with debilitating neuropathic pain. *Pain* 2012; 153: 1763-8.
[185] Couzin-Frankel J. Chasing a disease to the vanishing point. *Science* 2010; 328: 298–300.

Reviewed by Jean-Michel Vallat, Centre de référence «Neuropathies Périphériques Rares», Service et Laboratoire de Neurologie, CHU de Limoges, Limoges, France.

In: Contemporary Issues in Peripheral Neuropathy
Editor: Daniel L. Menkes
ISBN: 978-1-62948-681-9

Chapter IV

Guillain–Barré Syndrome

***Akiyuki Hiraga*[1,2,*]*, Masahiro Mori*[1]**
***and Satoshi Kuwabara*[1]**
[1]Department of Neurology, Graduate School of Medicine,
Chiba University, Chiba, Japan
[2]Department of Neurology,
Chiba Rosai Hospital, Chiba, Japan

Abstract

Guillain–Barré syndrome (GBS) is the most frequent peripheral neuropathic cause of acute flaccid paralysis. GBS is currently classified into two major forms on the basis of the following pathological and electrophysiological criteria; acute inflammatory demyelinating polyneuropathy (AIDP), and acute motor axonal neuropathy (AMAN). AIDP is the most commonly encountered variant except in East Asia, (China and Japan), where the AMAN variant predominates. AMAN is characterized by electrophysiological and pathological changes that may reflect axonal degeneration of the motor nerves, functional conduction failure or other pathophysiology. An important cause of AMAN is the molecular mimicry between human gangliosides and bacterial lipo-oligosaccharides, possibly associated with anti-ganglioside antibodies. In particular, IgG antibodies to the gangliosides GM1, GM1b, GD1a and GalNAc-GD1a may be induced by infectious agents such as *Campylobacter jejuni* or *Haemophilus influenza.* In contrast, target molecules have not yet been identified for AIDP. Although AMAN and AIDP appear similar in their clinical features, there are important differences. AMAN presents clinically as a predominantly motor syndrome, with infrequent and mild involvement of the autonomic nervous system. When sensory fibers are also affected, this axonal subtype is designated acute motor and sensory axonal neuropathy (AMSAN). Patients with AMAN may manifest hyperreflexia during the recovery phase. AMAN progresses rapidly in its early stage and has an earlier nadir than AIDP. AMAN has two distinct

* Address correspondence to: Akiyuki Hiraga, MD, Department of Neurology, Chiba Rosai Hospital, 2-16 Tatsumidai-Higashi, Ichihara-shi, Chiba 290-0003, Japan. Telephone number: +81-436-74-1111, Fax number: +81-436-74-1151. e-mail: hiragaa@yahoo.co.jp.

patterns of clinical recovery; rapid and prolonged. This contrasts with the relatively uniform recovery observed in AIDP. Irrespective of the variant, electrophysiological evidence of axonal degeneration is thought to be an indicator of poor prognosis. However, even the most severely disabled patients with AMAN may walk independently within a few years, indicating that a diagnosis of AMAN in and of itself does not always imply a poor recovery. The efficacy of plasma exchange and intravenous immunoglobulin (IVIg) has been established in large international randomized trials. Nonetheless, IVIg is preferred because of its greater availability, comparative ease of administration and relatively lower complication rates. In contrast, corticosteroid treatments are ineffective. This review provides an update on the clinical features, pathogenesis and treatment of GBS.

Introduction

Guillain–Barré syndrome (GBS) is the leading cause of acute flaccid paralysis in developed countries that results from peripheral nerve system dysfunction. GBS was first described in 1916 by the French neurologists Guillain, Barré and Strohl. They reported two soldiers who developed acute paralysis with areflexia that was accompanied by the characteristic cerebrospinal fluid (CSF) findings that differentiated from poliomyelitis; an increased protein concentration with a normal cell count designated albuminocytological dissociation [1]. Although cases with similar clinical features has been previously reported by Landry in 1859 [2], the combination of these clinical features and pathological characteristics became known as the GBS.

Since its original description, GBS had been regarded as a demyelinating neuropathy on the basis of pathological and electrophysiological observations. In 1986, Feasby et al. identified a severe axonal type of GBS associated with poor recovery. These patients demonstrated severe Wallerian-like degeneration in the peripheral nerves at autopsy [3]. In the 1990s, a purely motor form of GBS, designated acute motor axonal neuropathy (AMAN), was recognized in northern China. AMAN was originally observed to occur in summer epidemics that affected primarily children and young adults [4-6]. Thereafter, it was reported in other countries as well [7-17]. GBS is currently divided into two major categories on the basis of the following pathological and electrophysiological criteria; acute inflammatory demyelinating polyneuropathy (AIDP, the classical demyelinating form) and AMAN (the predominantly motor form with axonal features on nerve conduction studies). Plasma exchange (PEX) and intravenous immunoglobulin (IVIg) are equally effective treatments [18]. This review summarizes the clinical features, pathogenesis and treatment of GBS.

Epidemiology

GBS has been reported worldwide. A systematic review showed that the annual incidence varies between 0.38/100, 000/year in Finland and 2.53/100, 000/year in Curaçao, with most studies reporting incidences between 1.1/100, 000 and 1.8/100, 000/year [19]. The lifetime likelihood of any individual acquiring GBS is 1:1000 [20, 21]. A recent systematic review reported a median incidence of 1.1/100, 000/year. The incidence of GBS increases by 20%

for every 10-year increase in age. The risk is higher for males than females, with a relative risk of 1.78 for males [22]. There is no clear seasonal association in Western countries, although this may be because the most frequent antecedent events, respiratory and enteric infections, occur at different times of the year. [23]. Summer epidemics of AMAN associated with *Campylobacter jejuni* infection have been shown to occur among children and young adults in northern China [4-6].

The incidence of AMAN varies according to location. AMAN accounted for only 7% of patients with GBS reported in a group of patients in the United Kingdom [24]. Only 3% of GBS patients were identified as AMAN in a multicenter study in 11 Western countries [25]. In contrast, AMAN constituted 65% of patients with GBS in a study in northern China [6], 56% in Bangladesh [17], and 39% in Japan [26]. Thus, AMAN is more frequently encountered in Asia than other regions of the world. The relative proportion of cases of AMAN of all GBS cases in other countries have been reported from various countries in their reported case series as follows: 31% in Pakistan [15], 29% in Argentina (pediatric ages) [11], 14.7% in Brazil [27], 10.6% in India [16] and 4% in Taiwan [9].

Antecedent Events

Two-thirds of patients with GBS report an antecedent infection such as an upper respiratory infection or gastroenteritis. Previous infection rates with *C. jejuni* (32%), cytomegalovirus (13%), Epstein–Barr virus (10%) and *Mycoplasma pneumoniae* (5%) were shown to be higher in patients who subsequently developed GBS than in controls as noted in a Dutch study [28]. In another report of 383 patients with GBS enrolled in 11 European countries, North America and Australia, patients reported these percentages of antecedent infections; *C. jejuni* (23%), cytomegalovirus (8%) and Epstein–Barr virus (2%) [29]. Similarly, 86 patients with GBS in Japan had a previous infection from *C. jejuni* (23%), cytomegalovirus (10%), *M. pneumoniae* (6%) and Epstein–Barr virus (3%) [12]. These studies indicate that *C. jejuni* is the most frequent cause of an antecedent infection in persons who subsequently develop GBS worldwide. Many other pathogens have been identified as potential triggers for GBS in anecdotal reports or in small samples. However, these studies lack statistical validation [30].

In 1976, concerns regarding vaccine-induced GBS were raised in the United States of America. A vaccine developed for swine influenza was associated with a slightly increased risk of GBS within the first 6–8 weeks after receiving the vaccine [31]. However, subsequent epidemiological studies have shown that influenza does not appear to increase the risk for developing GBS. Even studies that report an association note that this occurs in less than 1 case per million vaccine recipients [32]. Despite individual case reports suggesting an association, conventional vaccines have not generally been associated with a significant risk of GBS [33, 34].

GBS has also been reported following surgery and trauma [35-37]. A recent retrospective analysis showed that the relative risk of developing GBS during the 6-week period after surgery is 13.1 times higher than the normal incidence, which results in a relative risk of 4.1 cases per 100, 000 surgeries [37]. Notwithstanding, the mechanisms by surgery and trauma result in GBS have yet to be determined.

Pathophysiology

GBS is thought to be a post-infectious autoimmune disorder although AMAN and AIDP are presumed to have different immunopathogeneses. Previous studies have shown that AMAN may be associated with anti-ganglioside antibodies; specifically IgG antibodies to the gangliosides GM1, GM1b, GD1a and GalNAc-GD1a [12, 17, 38-46]. *C. jejuni* infection is the most common antecedent infection in patients who subsequently develop AMAN. As such, this bacterium may share epitopes homologous with gangliosides expressed on human peripheral motor axons (i.e. molecular mimicry) [26, 30, 33, 35 and 47]. In contrast to AMAN, target molecules in AIDP have not yet been identified.

AIDP

Pathological studies in AIDP reveal patchy multifocal mononuclear cell infiltrates throughout the peripheral nervous system, with the distribution of inflammation often corresponding to the pattern of clinical deficit. Activated macrophages invade the intact myelin sheaths resulting in myelin damage and demyelination [48]. These pathological changes in AIDP are similar to those seen in animal models of experimental autoimmune neuritis (EAN). The immunological mechanisms underlying the macrophage-mediated invasion of nerves remain elusive, although two potentially complementary mechanisms have been proposed [49]. According to the first hypothesis, activated helper T cells react against specific antigens on the surface of Schwann cells or the myelin sheath, thereby directing activated macrophages to this region. An alternative hypothesis focuses on humoral immunity in AIDP, especially in the early stages of the disease. It has been proposed that antibodies bind to epitopes on the outer surface of Schwann cells inciting complement activation and subsequent myelin destruction before macrophage invasion.

AMAN

Autopsy studies of patients with AMAN have revealed axonal degeneration of motor fibers without demyelination or lymphocytic inflammation [5]. Immunochemistry has demonstrated the presence of IgG and the complement activation product C3d bound to the axolemma of motor fibers [50]. These changes indicate that there may be an immune response directed primarily against the motor axonal membrane.

C. Jejuni Is Strongly Associated with AMAN

A serial electrodiagnostic study on *C. jejuni*-positive GBS reported that antecedent infection with *C. jejuni* is strongly associated with AMAN electrodiagnosis, in which *C. jejuni*-positive GBS initially mimics demyelination but does not ultimately result in the classic electrodiagnostic findings in AIDP [51]. Electrodiagnostic studies dmeonstrate that AMAN has electrophysiological features of axonal degeneration as well as reversible conduction block [12, 39 and 46]. Lipo-oligosaccharide (LOS) is one of the most important cell-surface structures expressed by *C. jejuni*, whereas GM1 and GD1a are major gangliosides in the peripheral nervous system [47]. Molecular mimicry, the sharing of homologous epitopes, between GM1 and GD1a gangliosides and LOS of *C. jejuni* strains isolated from AMAN subsequent to *C. jejuni* enteritis has been demonstrated [47, 52]. This molecular mimicry is the proposed pathogenic mechanism of AMAN, wherein antibodies to gangliosides attack motor nerves.

Animal Model of AMAN

An AMAN rabbit model was established by sensitization of Japanese white rabbits with a bovine brain ganglioside mixture that included GM1 [53]. This model had elevated anti-GM1 IgG antibodies as well as pathological findings of Wallerian-like degeneration in the peripheral nerves in the absence of lymphocytic infiltration or demyelination. IgG was deposited on the axons of ventral roots, internodal axolemmas and nodes of Ranvier. Cauda equina and spinal nerve root specimens from paralyzed rabbits demonstrated macrophage infiltration in the periaxonal space [54]. In contrast, the surrounding myelin sheaths remained mostly intact. These pathological findings correspond well with those observed in human AMAN. The immunization of animals with *C. jejuni* LOS also produces an AMAN-like neuropathy [52]. A study of an animal model of AMAN revealed important microstructural changes at and near the nodes of Ranvier (i.e. disruption of nodal sodium channel clusters and detachment of paranodal terminal myelin loops, mimicking paranodal demyelination) [55].

These findings are consistent with electrophysiological features of human AMAN, including rapidly reversible nerve conduction block and axonal degeneration [12, 39 and 46]. At the nodes or paranodes, deposition of anti-ganglioside antibodies causes initial reversible conduction block followed by axonal degeneration. In contrast, reversible antibody-mediated conduction block occurring before development of significant axonal degeneration appears to explain rapid symptomatic improvement.

C. Jejuni Sialyltransferase and AMAN

Genetic polymorphisms of *C. jejuni* determine the expression of gangliosides on the bacterial wall. *C. jejuni* sialyltransferase (cst-II), which functions in the biosynthesis of ganglioside-like LOSs, determines transferase activity. Strains with cst-II (Thr51) frequently express GM1 and GD1a epitopes, whereas patients with GBS infected by cst-II (Thr51) strains are frequently positive for anti-GM1 or anti-GD1a IgG antibodies [47, 56].

On the basis of these observations, *C. jejuni*-associated anti-GM1or GD1a-related GBS cases are thought to be true cases of a post-infectious, molecular mimicry-associated autoimmune disorder [47].

Table 1. Criteria for Guillain–Barré syndrome

1. Features required for diagnosis
   - A. Progressive motor weakness of more than one limb. The degree ranges from minimal weakness to total paralysis of the all four limbs, trunk and cranial nerves
   - B. Areflexia or distal areflexia with definite hyporeflexia of the biceps and knee jerk will suffice if other features are consistent
2. Features strongly supportive of diagnosis
   - A. Clinical features
     1. Symptoms and signs of motor weakness develop rapidly but cease to progress by 4 weeks into the illness
     2. Relative symmetry symptoms
     3. Mild sensory symptoms or signs
     4. Cranial nerve involvement
     5. Recovery usually begins 2 or 4 weeks after progression stops
     6. Autonomic dysfunction
     7. Absence of fever at the onset of neuritic symptoms
   - B. Cerebrospinal fluid (CSF) features strongly supportive of the diagnosis
     1. After the first week of symptoms, CSF protein is elevated or has been shown to rise in serial lumbar punctures
     2. Counts of 10 or fewer mononuclear leukocytes/mm^3 in CSF
   - C. Electrodiagnosis features strongly supportive of the diagnosis*
3. Features casting doubt on the diagnosis
   1. Marked, persistent asymmetry of weakness
   2. Persistent bladder or bowel dysfunction
   3. Bladder or bowel dysfunction at onset
   4. More than 50 mononuclear leukocytes/mm^3 in CSF
   5. Presence of polymorphonuclear leukocytes in CSF
   6. Sharp sensory level
4. Features that rule out a diagnosis
   1. A current history of hexacarbone abuse
   2. Abnormal porphyrin metabolism indicates acute intermittent porphyria
   3. A history or finding of recent diphtheric infection.
   4. Features clinically consistent with lead neuropathy
   5. The occurrence of a purely sensory syndrome
   6. A definite diagnosis of a condition such as poliomyelitis, botulism, hysteria, or toxic neuropathy

This table summarizes the original GBS criteria from Asbury and Cornblath [57] as well as original criteria 'Features that rule out the diagnosis', this (adapted table) shows differential diagnoses. *Electrodiagnostic features from the original criteria only described demyelinating pattern such as conduction velocity slowing or prolonged distal latencies or F-wave latency. Electrodiagnosis features are divided into 'axonal' or 'demyelinating' subtypes; so, the original description of electrodiagnosis features from Asbury and Cornblath are omitted from this table.

Diagnosis

Clinical diagnostic criteria of GBS proposed by Asbury and Cornblath in 1990 [57] are summarized in Table 1. Areflexia or decreased deep tendon reflexes (DTR) is a critical feature required for diagnosis. Nonetheless, the initial clinical features of GBS may be protean such that patients with the initial onset of hand weakness, asymmetric weakness or preserved tendon reflexes may be difficult to diagnose. For instance, some patients with AMAN have preserved DTRs, as described in the clinical features section. In addition, GBS with severe bowel dysfunction as well as asymmetric cases have also been reported. While patients with typical GBS presentations are usually correctly diagnosed, several other disorders can cause acute onset flaccid paralysis such that they must be considered. Table 2 summarizes the differential diagnoses of GBS.

Table 2. Differential diagnosis of acute onset flaccid paralysis (differential diagnosis of Guillain–Barré syndrome)

Peripheral neuropathy	
	Vasculitic neuropathy
	Diphtheric neuropathy
	Acute intermittent porphyria
	Critical illness neuropathy
	Lymphomatous neuropathy
	Heavy metal or drug intoxication
	Post-rabies vaccine neuropathy
	Diabetic–uremic neuropathy with acute peritoneal dialysis
	Beriberi neuropathy
	POEMS syndrome
	Chronic inflammatory demyelinating polyneuropathy
Disorders of the neuromuscular junction	
	Myasthenia gravis
	Lambert-Eaton myasthenic syndrome
	Botulism
	Biological or industrial toxin poisoning
Disorders of muscle	
	Inflammatory myopathy
	Toxic myopathy/acute rhabdomyolysis
	Periodic paralysis
	Hypokalemia
	Hypophosphatemia
	Infections
Disorders of the central nervous system	
	Brainstem stroke
	Brainstem encephalitis
	Acute myelopathy (high cervical)
	Acute anterior poliomyelitis

Table adapted from Vucic et al. [49].

Electrophysiology

Electrophysiology plays an important role in the diagnosis of GBS, classification of subtype and in determining prognosis. The electrodiagnostic criteria by Ho et al. regarding AMAN and AIDP were published in 1995 and are widely used [6]. Minor modifications of these criteria were proposed by Hadden et al. in 1998 [25]. Table 3 provides the electrodiagnostic criteria proposed by Hadden et al. These criteria subdivide AMAN and AIDP. However, it noteworthy that the electrophysiological profile of acute motor sensory axonal neuropathy (AMSAN) is similar to AMAN with the exception that the amplitude of the sensory nerve action potential (SNAP) is either reduced or absent [8].

Table 3. Criteria for electrophysiological classification of Guillain–Barré syndrome

AIDP

At least one of the following in each of at least two nerves, or at least two of the following in one nerve if all others inexcitable and dCMAP ≥10% of LLN.

- MCV <90% of LLN (85% if dCMAP <50% of LLN)
- DML >110% of ULN (120% if dCMAP <100% of LLN)
- pCMAP/dCMAP ratio <0.5 and dCMAP ≥20% of LLN
- F-response latency >120% of ULN

AMAN

None of above features of AIDP in any nerve (except one demyelinating feature allowed in one nerve if dCMAP <10% of LLN) and dCMAP <80% of LLN in at least two nerves.

AMSAN

Results of motor nerve conduction studies indicate AMAN and SNAP amplitude <50% of LLN in at least two nerves

Inexcitable

dCMAP absent in all nerves (or present in only one nerve with dCMAP <10% of LLN)

Equivocal

Does not fit criteria for any other group

AIDP = acute inflammatory demyelinating polyneuropathy; AMAN = acute motor axonal neuropathy; AMSAN = acute motor axonal neuropathy; DML = distal motor latency; ULN = upper limit of normal; LLN = lower limit of normal; MCV = motor conduction velocity; dCMAP = compound muscle action potential amplitude after distal stimulation; pCMAP = compound muscle action potential amplitude after distal stimulation; SNAP = sensory nerve action potential.

AIDP, AMAN, inexcitable, and equivocal criteria from Hadden et al. [25]. Hadden's criteria did not classify AMSAN; so, AMSAN criteria are from Rees et al. [8] and Capasso et al. [64].

AIDP

AIDP is characterized by prolonged distal motor latencies as well as increased duration and temporal dispersion of the compound muscle action potentials (CMAP). All of these suggest demyelination in the locations where the blood-nerve barrier is relatively deficient; the distal axons and the nerve roots [58]. Nerve root involvement may be inferred on the basis of prolonged or absent late responses; F waves and H reflexes. Involvement of the intermediate nerve segments is rare in the early phase of the disease. For example, median and ulnar motor nerve conduction velocities in the forearm segments are usually normal or only slightly decreased [30]. In serial electrodiagnostic studies, motor nerve conduction abnormalities initially predominate, with the nadir of these abnormalities occurring in week 3 [59].

Sensory nerve conduction studies in AIDP frequently reveal a particular pattern of nerve conduction abnormalities. Sensory nerve action potentials (SNAPs) in the median nerve are frequently reduced in amplitude or absent, whereas sural SNAP amplitudes are preserved [60-62]. This is known as an abnormal median-normal sural (AMNS) sensory response [60, 63]. This finding may be due to nerve conduction study methodologies as the median SNAPs are recorded near their axonal terminals whereas sural nerve studies examine the intermediate nerve segments. The AMNS sensory responses are has been reported in 40%–50% of patients with AIDP [30].

AMAN

AMAN is associated with decreased CMAP amplitudes associated with normal sensory nerve conduction studies. This finding may be due to motor axon loss or decreased excitability of the motor fibers. Electrophysiological patterns of simple axonal degeneration and early-reversible conduction block are frequently seen in patients with AMAN, both of which may be related to axonal dysfunction [39]. Reports describing detailed serial electrodiagnostic findings in patients with AMAN suggest there are three patterns of nerve conduction abnormalities in axonal GBS in early disease stage; simple axonal degeneration (48% of patients), transient conduction block/slowing in motor nerve terminals (20%) and absent F-waves as an isolated conduction abnormality (12%) [46]. In addition to simple axonal degeneration, patients with axonal GBS may manifest transient conduction slowing/conduction block in the distal or proximal nerve segments, mimicking demyelination.

As AMAN is very rarely associated with sensory nerve involvement, abnormal sensory nerve conduction studies are usually indicative of AIDP [62]. Studies of serial sensory nerve testing in AMAN indicated normal sensory nerves both at initial and during subsequent studies [46, 62]. In contrast, a recent serial sensory nerve conduction study of 13 patients with AMAN from Italy reported that AMAN patients without sensory symptoms often manifest subclinical sensory nerve involvement [64].

According to the electrodiagnostic criteria for AIDP and AMAN proposed by Ho et al. [6], electrodiagnostic studies are based on motor nerve conduction studies undertaken during the first two weeks of the illness. Other authors report that the electrophysiological profile of a considerable number of patients with GBS, particularly those are anti-ganglioside positive, demonstrate electrophysiological changes during the first 4 weeks, and even as early as within the first two weeks [12, 46, 65]. Therefore, the electrophysiological classification of GBS might be considered on the basis of sequential studies rather than on a single measurement during the first two weeks.

Cerebrospinal Fluid Findings and Other Testing

CSF testing is a traditional method that is almost always appropriate. Elevated CSF protein concentration occurs in approximately 80% of patients with GBS, but is likely to be normal during the initial stages of the illness [33]. Examination of CSF protein concentration may be helpful in confirming the diagnosis in clinically difficult cases. An assay of serum anti-ganglioside antibody may also be helpful. Other investigations may be needed to exclude other causes of acute flaccid paralysis (see differential diagnosis, Table 2). Stool cultures investigating *C. jejuni* culture, serum cytomegalovirus or Epstein–Barr virus titers may be help determine the preceding infection that resulted in GBS.

Table 4. Comparison between the two forms of Guillain–Barré syndrome

	AMAN	AIDP
Antecedent infection	Campylobacter jejuni Haemophilus influenza	Cytomegalovirus Epstein–Barr virus
Epidemics	Summer in northern China	None
High-frequency region	North China, Japan	Western countries
Respiratory failure	Common	Common
Weakness pattern	Frequently distally predominant	Frequently proximally predominant
Cranial palsies	Infrequent	Frequent
Tendon reflexes	Usually absent, occasionally preserved or exaggerated	Absent
Sensory symptoms	Rare	Common
Autonomic dysfunction	Infrequent	Frequent
Urinary disturbance	Infrequent	Frequent
Electrophysiology	Axonal degeneration/ reversible conduction block/slowing	Demyelination
Anti-ganglioside antibodies	GM1, GM1b, GD1a and GalNAc-GD1a	None
Time to nadir	Earlier	Later
Recovery pattern	Rapid or prolonged	Uniform

AMAN = acute motor axonal neuropathy; AIDP = acute inflammatory demyelinating polyneuropathy;

Clinical Features

The typical clinical features of GBS include acute onset of progressive weakness of the four extremities with areflexia or decreased tendon reflexes. Associated sensory signs such as pain or paresthesias are also commonly observed. Cranial nerve involvement or autonomic dysfunction may also be present. AIDP and AMAN appear to have different immunopathogeneses directed against different target molecules that may account for the difference in clinical features observed between these two forms. This section outlines the clinical features of GBS with a specific focus on the differences between AMAN and AIDP as summarized in Table 4.

Weakness

Lower limb weakness and an ascending symmetrical paralysis of all extremities are typical in GBS, but the degree of weakness and dominancy (i.e. distal vs. proximal, lower limb vs. upper limb) vary from patient to patient.

In AMAN, the observed weakness patterns are typically distally predominant [4, 7, 11, 27]. In contrast, AIDP is frequently characterized by proximally predominant weakness [27]. Some anti-ganglioside antibodies such as GM1b [44], GalNac-GD1a [42, 66] and GM1 [14, 67], which are strongly associated with AMAN, are also reported to be associated with distal-dominant weakness. A recent Brazilian study reported that 66.6% of individuals with AMAN had distally predominant weakness whereas only 3.7% had proximally predominant weakness. In contrast, in patients with AIDP, 78.6% had proximally predominant weakness and only 6.5% had distally predominant weakness [27]. An Argentinian childhood GBS study published that 78% of individuals with AMAN had distally predominant weakness and none had proximally predominant weakness. In contrast, individuals with AIDP manifested distally predominant weakness in 33% of cases and proximally predominant weakness in 26% [11]. In addition to limb weakness, neck muscle weakness can occur in GBS and is particularly common in patients with anti-GT1a antibodies [68, 69]. Muscle atrophy, reflecting severe axonal damage, has been observed in severely disabled patients with GBS but its frequency has not been systematically investigated. Nonetheless, patients with significant muscle atrophy tend to have a longer and less complete recovery.

Sensory Symptoms

Sensory symptoms, such as paresthesias and objective sensory disturbances, are often observed in GBS, particularly in AIDP. AIDP commonly presents with signs and symptoms of sensory nerve dysfunction with an estimated occurrence of 58%–86% of cases [9, 11, 27, 70]. In contrast with AIDP, AMAN is considered a purely motor syndrome. When sensory fibers are also affected, it is designated AMSAN [71]. In AMSAN, sensory symptoms may be the sole initial manifestation [71]. Although AMAN is considered a purely motor syndrome, some patients may report mild sensory symptoms such as paresthesias. Previous studies of

AMAN patients published that between 2% and19% of patients report paresthesias in the hands and feet [4, 6].

Pain

Pain is frequently observed in GBS and has been reported in up to 89% of cases [72-76]. It may also be the initial manifesting symptom [9, 72]. Notwithstanding, pain in GBS is often overlooked or under-recognized because most providers focus on the progression of weakness [75]. Types of pain occurring in GBS include paresthesias/dysesthesias, backache/root pain, meningismus, myalgias, arthralgias, and visceral pain [77].

A prospective study of 29 patients with GBS reported that 55% developed myalgias early in the illness. Pain was typically located in the thighs, buttocks and lower back [72]. Another study of 55 patients with GBS noted that 89% had pain with 47% grading it as severe. Pain usually presented as either deep aching back and leg pain or dysesthetic extremity pain [73]. Similar findings were observed in the GBS Research about Pain and Heterogeneity study conducted in the Netherlands published that 66% of patients with GBS reported pain. Myalgias were most common followed by painful paresthesias/dysesthesias and radicular pain [75].

Pain has been reported in the AMSAN variant, which has been hypothesized to reflect sensory nerve injury [78]. As AMAN usually presents as a purely motor syndrome without sensory nerve involvement, pain was thought to be a minor symptom in AMAN. However, a childhood GBS study reported that 56% of individuals with AMAN and 79% of those with AIDP had pain [11]. Similarly, a Brazilian study published that 62.9% of individuals with AMAN and 63.1% of those with AIDP had associated pain [27]. A third study reported that 49% of patients with AMAN experienced pain [79]. Thus, these studies indicate that pain is not uncommon in AMAN. Neuropathic pain should not be a prominent feature in pure motor GBS because this type of pain results from pathology affecting of sensory fibers. Patients with pure motor GBS who reported pain did not have clinical or electrophysiological evidence of large fiber sensory involvement, which may indicate that that pain reported by patients in the acute phase of "purely motor GBS" is likely to be of small fiber origin, perhaps from the activation of nociceptive pathways by inflammation or inflammatory mediators [79]. Of note, a recent study reported that a reduction in intraepidemermal nerve fiber density may correlate with pain in AMAN [76].

Deep Tendon Reflexes

The presence of 'areflexia' (loss of tendon jerks) or 'distal areflexia with definite hyporeflexia of the biceps and knee jerks' is required for diagnosis of GBS [57]. However, some patients with AMAN manifest hyperreflexia during the recovery phase [4, 80-84]. Chinese patients with AMAN often develop hyperreflexia during the early phase of recovery [4]. A Japanese study observed that hyperreflexia was observed in 26% of patients with AMAN 3–4 weeks after disease onset [81]. These patients often had detectable anti-GM1 antibodies and lesser degrees of disability. Increased motor neuron excitability has been postulated as a possible mechanism of hyperreflexia. A recent study of three hospital cohorts in Japan and Italy [84] reported that of 213 patients diagnosed with GBS, 23 had preserved DTRs and 8 demonstrated normal DTRs throughout the clinical course of the illness. Twelve manifested hyperreflexia, with at least one of the exaggerated reflexes experienced at their nadir. These exaggerated reflexes returned to normal at recovery. The remaining three patients demonstrated hyperreflexia throughout the disease course. When these patients were compared to the 190 patients with GBS manifesting reduced or absent DTRs, the 23 DTR-preserved patients more frequently presented with pure motor limb weakness, were able to walk 5 m independently at nadir, more frequently had antibodies against GM1, GM1b, GD1a or GalNAc-GD1a and were more commonly diagnosed with AMAN than with AIDP. This study demonstrated that DTRs could be normal or hyperexcitable during the entire clinical course in approximately 10% of patients with GBS. It is important to recall that patients with the AMAN variant of GBS may develop hyperreflexia as myelopathy ought to be considered in the differential diagnosis of acute motor weakness.

Cranial Nerve Palsy

Patients with GBS may manifest one or more cranial palsies including facial motor weakness, oculomotor weakness or lower cranial nerve (bulbar) weakness. Facial palsy is the most common whereas ptosis and oculomotor weakness is far less common. Specific anti-ganglioside antibodies that are frequently detected with associated cranial nerve palsies include ophthalmoplegia with anti-GQ1b antibody [35, 85, 86] and bulbar palsy with anti-GT1a antibody [68, 69, 85]. Although cranial nerves are affected bilaterally in typical cases, unilateral involvement in a patient with AMAN has also been reported [87].

Cranial nerve palsy is relatively infrequent in AMAN as compared with AIDP [6, 9, 88]. Cranial nerve palsy was reported in 47%–57% of patients with AMAN and 75%–100% of patients with AIDP in northern Chinese reports [6, 88]. However, an Indian study noted that cranial nerve involvement was equally frequent in both AIDP (64%) and AMAN (64%) [16].A Taiwanese study reported that facial palsy was seen in 49% of patients with AIDP and 17% of patients with AMAN, bulbar palsy in 52% of patients with AIDP and 17% of patients with AMAN and oculomotor palsy in 17% of patients with AIDP and 17 % of patients with AMAN [9]. A Brazilian study noted facial palsy in 33.3% of patients with AMAN and 66.9% of patients with AIDP, bulbar palsy in 55.5% of patients with AMAN and 65.5% of patients with AIDP and oculomotor palsy in 3.7% of patients with AMAN and 3.3% of patients with AIDP [27]. An Argentinian study of childhood GBS reported facial palsy in 44% of patients with AIDP and 39% of patients with AMAN, bulbar palsy in 28% of patients with AIDP and 39% of patients with AMAN and oculomotor palsy in 16% of patients with AIDP and 17 % of patients with AMAN [11].

Loss of taste was reported in patients with GBS as an uncommon symptom [89, 90]. However, this may be the initial symptom of GBS [91]. A recent prospective study reported that 60% of patients with GBS had taste impairment symptoms that resolved concomitantly with recovery of motor function [92]. Electrogustometric examinations during hospitalization demonstrated abnormal thresholds in all six patients. This study indicated that taste perturbation may be more frequently involved in patients with GBS than previously thought.

Respiratory Failure

Neuromuscular respiratory failure requiring mechanical ventilation has been shown to occur in between 13% and 43% of patients with GBS [93-98]. Among a group of Chinese patients, 22%–38% of those with AMAN required respiratory assistance compared with 25%–44% of those with AIDP [4, 6, 86]. In a Japanese study, 9% of patients with AMAN and 30% of patients with AIDP required mechanical ventilation at their nadir [99] In contrast, a Pakistani study reported that mechanical ventilation was required in 16% of patients with AIDP and 29% of patients with AMAN [15]. A Taiwanese study reported as many as 32% of patients with AIDP and 17% of patients with AMAN required ventilator assistance [9], However, an Indian study noted that 23% of patients with AIDP and 14% of patients with AMAN required mechanical ventilation [16]. A recent Brazilian study observed that 29.6% of patients with AMAN and 34.4% of patients with AIDP had respiratory failure [27]. Other reports indicated that patients with AIDP often needed mechanical ventilation [93, 96, and 100]. In a report of a Miller Fisher/Guillain–Barré overlap syndrome, more often associated with AMAN than with AIDP, a significant number of patients required mechanical ventilation [86]. An Argentinian childhood GBS study reported contrary findings in that 7% of patients with AIDP and 28% of patients with AMAN had respiratory failure [11]. As such, that the pediatric patients with AMAN had a higher incidence of respiratory failure than those with AIDP. In patients with AMSAN, respiratory failure commonly occurs, reflecting severe axonal loss [71]. In summary, these findings indicate that the incidence of respiratory failure in adult AIDP occurs as frequently and perhaps more frequently than in AMAN.

Autonomic Disturbance

In addition to motor and sensory deficits, GBS may be associated with a variety of autonomic abnormalities, including cardiovascular, vasomotor and sudomotor dysfunction. Thus, GBS may affect both the sympathetic and parasympathetic systems [101, 102]. Although the incidence of autonomic disturbance in GBS varies, some reports have indicated that disturbance of autonomic function is observed in over 60% of patients and is more commonly observed in ventilated patients [101-104]. Moreover, autonomic dysfunction may be the presenting feature of GBS [105]. Some GBS patients manifest excessive sympathetic hyperactivity (e.g. hypertension and hyperhidrosis), whereas others express sympathetic hypoactivity (e.g. hypotension and anhidrosis) or parasympathetic dysfunction (e.g. arrhythmias). Bladder disturbance, bowel dysfunction, pupillary abnormalities and sexual dysfunction have also been reported in GBS [101-103, 106]. Minor cardiovascular complications of GBS include sinus tachycardia, postural hypotension and subclinical electrocardiography changes. More serious cardiac complications include sustained or episodic hypertension, episodic hypotension, and sensitivity to vasoactive drugs. These effects have been attributed to denervation hypersensitivity. Other serious autonomic complications manifest as bradyarrhythmias including asystole that may require a pacemaker [102]. Myocarditis, neurogenic stunned myocardium, heart failure and acute coronary syndrome have also been reported [104]. While AIDP is frequently associated with autonomic disturbances, involvement of the autonomic nervous system is less frequent and less severe in AMAN [9, 26, 106]. On autonomic function tests, patients with AMAN usually demonstrated normal cardiovascular autonomic function, although some expressed sudomotor or skin vasomotor hypoactivity. However, patients with more severe AMAN may manifest generalized hypohidrosis [106].

According to the diagnostic criteria for GBS, the presence of bladder or bowel dysfunction raises uncertainty in diagnosis [57]. This is presumably because patients with GBS should be clearly differentiated from those with acute myelopathy in which urinary retention is common. However, urinary symptoms and bowel dysfunction are not uncommon in GBS. Urinary symptoms (voiding difficulty, retention and urgency) were found to be more common among patients with AIDP (39%) than among patients with AMAN (19%). A Japanese study reported that urinary retention occurred nearly as often among patients with AMAN (7%) as among patients with AIDP (11%) [107]. Urinary dysfunction appears to involve both hypoactive and hyperactive lumbosacral nerves [107, 108]. More recently, an Indian urodynamics study of 38 patients with GBS reported that 15% of patients with AIDP and 32% of patients with axonal GBS (AMAN or AMSAN) manifested urinary symptoms. In contrast, 30.7% of patients with AIDP and 76% of patients with axonal GBS manifested urodynamic abnormalities, which was statistically significant [109]. Constipation, which may be severe, was present in 18% of patients with AIDP and 8% of patients with AMAN patients [107].

Fatigue

Patients often experience fatigue at the onset of GBS, which may persist for many years, even after the total recovery of muscle weakness [110]. Several studies confirm the high prevalence of fatigue in GBS, with a reported range between 38% and 60% [74, 110, 111]. Age was positively correlated with fatigue severity but was not significantly correlated with the degree of residual neurological deficits [110, 112].

The Syndrome of Inappropriate Secretion of Antidiuretic Hormone

The syndrome of inappropriate secretion of antidiuretic hormone (SIADH) is one of the most common causes of hyponatremia in the neuro-intensive care unit. It is a common and important electrolyte disorder encountered in GBS. SIADH associated with GBS may be overlooked despite its being well described. One prospective study reported that in 50 patients with GBS, SIADH was detected in 48% at some stage of the illness (median, 8.8 days after GBS onset) [113]. Of these 50 patients, six of them had mild SIADH, 12 patients had moderate SIADH and six patients had severe SIADH. Of all the patients, nine of 18 patients with AMAN had SIADH, eight of 15 patients with AMSAN had SIADH and seven of 17 patients with AIDP had SIADH. These results imply that there is no difference in SIADH incidence between AMAN and AIDP. SIADH is positively correlated with the severity of GBS and generally portends a poor prognosis. While it may be symptomatic, most patients with SIADH are asymptomatic. The pathogenesis of SIADH in GBS is incompletely understood.

Miller Fisher Syndrome

Miller Fisher syndrome (MFS) is characterized by a clinical triad of ophthalmoplegia, ataxia and areflexia. Diplopia tends to be the first symptom. It is considered a variant of GBS [114]. Such patients frequently test positive for serum anti-GQ1b antibody [115]. In addition to the characteristic triad, ptosis (60%), bulbar palsy (40%) and pupillary abnormalities such as mydriasis (38%), facial palsy (36%) and dysesthesias (29%) are often observed in MFS [116]. Patients with MFS usually have a good recovery [116, 117].

Disease Progression and Severity at Nadir

In GBS, signs and symptoms of motor weakness tend to progress in the initial phase of illness but plateau by the fourth week. AMAN has an earlier nadir than AIDP [7, 27, 100, and 118]. In Chinese patients with AMAN (children or young adults), the mean onset to nadir was 5.9 days [4]. In a Japanese study, the average period between onset and nadir was longer in patients with AMAN (18.0 days) than in those with AIDP (11.5 days) [118]. Most patients with AMAN had reached the nadir at the time of their first examination. In the subgroup of those with mild disability who were able to walk independently at the first neurologic examination, 88% of patients with AMAN versus 65% of patients with AIDP had reached their nadir. The remaining 35% of the patients with AIDP progressed to their nadir over the next 1–2 weeks and were unable to walk at that time [118].

The reported difference in peak disability between patients with AMAN and patients with AIDP varies between studies. In northern China, 66% of patients with AMAN were reported to be bedridden at nadir compared with 88% of patients with AIDP [88]. In Japan, the Hughes functional grading scale at nadir in AMAN and AIDP were similar [99, 118]; 50 % of patients with AMAN and 45% of patients with AIDP were bedridden at nadir whereas 41% of patients with AMAN were able to walk without assistance at nadir. In a Pakistani study, weakness of both the arms and legs was significantly more severe in patients with AMAN than in patients with AIDP [15]. A recent Brazilian study reported that 70.3% of patients with AMAN and 90% of patients with AIDP were bedridden at nadir [27]. Similar findings were reported in an Indian study in which 78.6% of patients with AMAN and 68.4% of patients with AIDP were bedridden at their nadir [16].

While AMAN often produces severe disability, a considerable number of patients manifest only mild disability. Certain antecedent infections correlate with disease severity at nadir in AMAN. *Haemophilus influenzae* has been recognized as the second most frequent preceding pathogen in AMAN. *H. influenzae*-related GBS has been reported to be associated with milder disease and faster recoveries as compared with *C. jejuni*-related GBS [119].

Recovery and Prognosis

In randomized trials of GBS, neither PEX nor IVIg improved mortality, which ranged from 2.4% to 6.3% [120]. When six trials were combined for a total of 649 patients with GBS who were treated with either PEX or supportive care, 4.7% of PEX patients and 5.5% of supportive care only patients expired. Furthermore, 10.9% of PEX patients and 16.8% of supportive care only patients died or had severe disability after one year [120]. In a multicenter trial of 383 patients with GBS, 4.1% of PEX, 4.6% of IVIg and 6.3% of PEX + IVIg patients died [121]. Mortality and severe residual disability rates in the trials ranged between 9% and 17 % and approximately 20% of patients remained unable to walk unaided after 6 months [35, 120]. A recent prospective literature review of PEX or IVIg-treated GBS reported that GBS results in severe persistent disability in 14% of patients at one year. Loss of full strength, persistent pain and disability requiring an employment change occurred in about 40%. Moreover, mortality is 4.4% within the first year [98]. The patterns of recovery and prognosis are somewhat different between AMAN and AIDP. In this section, recovery pattern and prognosis focus on the difference between AMAN and AIDP.

Difference in Recovery Patterns between AMAN and AIDP

Autopsy studies of patients with AMAN have detected extensive Wallerian-type degeneration in the ventral roots [5]. Electrophysiological evidence of axonal degeneration is thought to be an indicator of poor prognosis [10, 29, 122-126]. However, recovery in patients with AMAN is often rapid [88, 99, 127-129]. One Chinese study reported that AMAN patients recovered rapidly [4]. In another report of 32 patients with AMAN and 8 patients with AIDP in northern China [88], some patients with AMAN recovered rapidly, with the recovery time of patients with AIDP and patients with AMAN being similar. In a Japanese study, the AMAN group had a higher percentage of patients with slow recovery (unable to walk independently at 6 months) as well as a higher percentage of patients with a more rapid recovery, (improvement by two Hughes functional grades or more during the first 4 weeks), than the AIDP group [99]. This Japanese study concluded that AMAN patients demonstrate bimodal recovery patterns, rapid and prolonged, whereas patients with AIDP tended to have a more homogenous recovery pattern. These two recovery patterns were also noted in an earlier study of patients with GBS with anti-GM1 antibodies, most of whom had AMAN [127]. The high potential for recovery from AMAN indicates that extensive axonal degeneration is not always the underlying pathophysiology despite the "axonal" patterns typically observed on nerve conduction studies. The rapid recovery of some individuals with AMAN may be explained by early resolution of physiological conduction failure at the nodes of Ranvier in the motor fibers [39, 88, 130]. Alternatively, this may result from collateral sprouting of surviving axons [128]. In contrast, delayed and incomplete recovery of patients with AMAN is more likely to be explained by severe axonal degeneration.

Long-term Prognosis of Severely Disabling AMAN

In the first description of the five cases of axonal GBS reported by Feasby et al., one patient died and 75% of survivors showed poor recovery. Only one of these patients could walk without assistance one year after onset [3]. These authors postulated that this axonal GBS form had a worse prognosis than the demyelinating forms of the disease and that recovery might require axonal regeneration along the entire length of the nerve [131]. Subsequently, it has become apparent that recovery from axonal GBS is not always poor.

In a multicenter study of 369 patients with GBS in 11 Western countries [25], axonal GBS accounted for only 3% of cases. Notably, 10% of those with the axonal form and 17% with the demyelinating form could not walk or were deceased 48 weeks after disease onset. The numbers of patients unable to walk or who died did not differ significantly between the axonal and demyelinating forms. Of 32 patients with AMAN and 8 patients with AIDP in a Northern Chinese study [88], more than 90% of the patients with AMAN and all of those with AIDP could ambulate 5 m with a walker or other support. However, the Chinese patients with AMAN were significantly younger (median age of 10 years) than the patients with AIDP (median age of 42 years). Therefore, it is difficult to quantify the prognosis for patients with AMAN versus those patients with AIDP. A recent Brazilian study reported that 48.1% of patients with AMAN and 5.74% of patients with AIDP were unable to walk 5 m independently at three months [27]. In a Japanese study, long-term prognosis did not differ between patients with AMAN and patients with AIDP [99]. In that study, 8 of the 97 patients with GBS, (six AMAN and two AIDP), could not walk independently 6 months after onset. Four of the six patients with AMAN could walk independently one year after onset. The remaining two patients could walk independently at a later time; one at 28 months, the other 57 months after onset. It was once believed that no additional recovery from GBS could be expected after 2–3 years [132]. However, a Dutch study reported that 21% of patients with GBS continued to improve after 2.5–6.5 years [133]. A Japanese study noted that the most severely disabled patients with AMAN could walk independently within a few years [99]. The mechanism of improvement in severely disabled patients with AMAN several years after onset is not clear, although axonal regeneration along the long course of the nerves or collateral sprouting may be responsible. AIDP may be accompanied by secondary axonal degeneration in severe cases. AMAN might also be associated with functional conduction block as well as axonal degeneration [39]. This might explain why long-term prognoses in AMAN and AIDP appear to be similar.

Prediction of Prognosis in GBS

The results of several studies suggest possible indicators of poor outcome, including increased age, more severe weakness, requirements for mechanical ventilation during the acute phase, shorter latency of the nadir, initial rapid progression, preceding diarrhea, specific antecedent infections (*C. jejuni* or cytomegalovirus), electrophysiological evidence of axonal degeneration, reduced or absent CMAPs and peroneal nerve conduction block [8, 10, 13, 17, 18, 29, 96-98, 122, 124-126, 134-137]. Factors associated with respiratory insufficiency include cranial nerve involvement such as bulbar palsy [95, 96, 138], severe disability on admission [96, 138], inability to cough [94], tongue weakness [139], time from onset to admission of <7 days [94], decreased vital capacity [96, 140], demyelination on nerve conduction studies [93, 96], conduction block of common peroneal nerve [96], prolonged distal latency or decreased CMAP amplitude on phrenic nerve conduction studies [141], serum anti GQ1b antibodies [95] and liver dysfunction [94, 96]. One report published that factors associated with progression to respiratory failure included vital capacity of <20 mL/kg, maximal inspiratory pressure of <30 cm H_2O, maximal expiratory pressure of < 40cm H_2O or a reduction of >30% in vital capacity, maximal inspiratory pressure or maximal expiratory pressure [140]. Nonetheless, the clinical course of GBS in individual patients is highly variable and difficult to predict. The best models for predicting outcome in GBS tend to focus on patients in the acute phase of this illness.

The Erasmus GBS Outcome Score (EGOS) is a prognostic model based on age, presence of diarrhea and GBS disability score two weeks after hospital admission. The EGOS accurately predicts the chance of being able to walk independently at 6 months [142]. On the basis of the EGOS, the predicted chance of independent walking after 6 months ranges from 1% to 83%. The EGOS is a simple and accurate scoring system to predict outcome at 6 months. However, it is not well suited for treatment assessments because a two week delay is required to predict outcomes. A slightly modified EGOS (mEGOS) model based on Medical Research Council sum score, age and preceding diarrhea that can calculate the prognosis only 1 week after hospital admission is currently being developed [97]. The mEGOS predicts reaching independent walking or improving on the GBS disability score at 4 weeks as well as long-term GBS disability scores. In contrast to the EGOS, the mEGOS model may be applied during the first week of admission, when treatment is considered to be most effective. A Dutch group also constructed the Erasmus GBS Respiratory Insufficiency Score (EGRIS) [138]. The EGRIS is a prognostic model based on days between onset of weakness and hospital admission, facial and/or bulbar weakness and Medical Research Council sum score at hospital admission. The EGRIS, which may be accurately calculated upon hospital admission, predicts the probability of respiratory insufficiency during the first week of hospitalization in individual patients with GBS, ranging from 1% to almost 90%.

Treatments

Treatments for GBS are subdivided into supportive care and immunomodulating treatments [30]. Supportive case is necessary for paralyzed patients requiring intensive care and ventilatory support. Immunomodulating treatments, such as PEX and IVIg, are indicated for patients who are unable to walk independently [120]. Results of international randomized trials have shown equivalent efficacy of both PEX and IVIg, while corticosteroids have been shown to be ineffective and possibly harmful [120].

Supportive Care

Sixty percent of patients with GBS admitted to the intensive care unit develop major complications including tracheobronchitis/ pneumonia, bacteremia/sepsis, gastrointestinal hemorrhage and deep venous thrombosis [143]. Deaths in severe GBS most commonly result from ventilator-associated pneumonia [144]. Therefore, proper supportive care is essential for minimizing mortality risk for patients with GBS.

Based on observational studies and expert opinion, supportive care consensus guidelines were published in 2005 [145]. In the acute phase among bedridden adult patients with GBS, the use of subcutaneous heparin and support stockings are recommended to prevent deep vein thrombosis or pulmonary embolus. Monitoring of pulse and blood pressure is recommended in patients who are severely affected by GBS. Respiratory function should also be monitored, with the timely initiation of artificial ventilation and percutaneous tracheostomy if needed.

Bladder catheterization is often needed for severely affected patients. Pain management is difficult, although small randomized controlled trials support the use of gabapentin or carbamazepine in the intensive care unit for the treatment of pain in the acute phase of GBS [145]. Appropriate narcotic analgesics may be used but require careful monitoring of adverse effects in the setting of autonomic dysfunction. Disabled patients with GBS should be treated by a multidisciplinary rehabilitation team and receive an assistive exercise program. Persistent fatigue may be lessened by an exercise program.

Corticosteroids

Corticosteroids alone do not significantly hasten recovery from GBS or affect long-term outcomes. This was based on six trials with 587 participants; four trials of oral steroids with a total of 120 participants and two trials of intravenous steroids with a total of 467 participants. [120, 146]. Two additional studies reported that oral corticosteroids may delay recovery but these data were not from Class I or Class II trials [120, 146]. It is unclear why corticosteroids are ineffective in this illness although it is suggested that they might have harmful effects on denervated muscle or inhibit macrophage repair processes [120]. One additional study reported that the combination of IVIg and intravenous methylprednisolone (MP) was no more effective than IVIg alone [147].

PEX

The proposed autoimmune etiology of GBS and the failure of randomized trials of corticosteroid treatments for GBS led to the introduction of plasma exchange in 1978 [148]. PEX offers significant benefit in GBS, as reported in a randomized trial published in 1985 [149]. This effect was subsequently confirmed by a large French trial [150]. In four trials with a total of 585 severely affected adult participants, those treated using PEX had a statistically significant improvement four weeks after randomization as compared with those who were not treated with PEX [120].

Most PEX studies used an arbitrary protocol in which five single plasma volume exchanges were performed over two weeks [120]. Although PEX is usually well tolerated, hemodynamic instability, coagulopathies, hypocalcemia and allergic reactions can occur. Thus, significant cardiac disease or a coagulopathy are contraindications for PEX [151].

Intravenous Immunoglobulin

In 1988, the first findings regarding IVIg treatment for GBS were published. The investigators observed a beneficial effect as a result of IVIg treatments in some of a group of eight patients with severe GBS [152]. The first randomized controlled trial comparing IVIg and PEX was published in 1992 in which both treatments demonstrated equivalent efficacy [18]. IVIg has replaced PEX as the preferred treatment for GBS in many centers because of its convenience and availability [120, 153]. In five trials with a total of 582 participants, improvement on the disability grade scale using IVIg were similar to those treated with PEX. No significant difference between IVIg and PEX treatment was found for a variety of outcome measures [120]. The combination of PEX followed by IVIg was not superior to either PEX or IVIg alone [121].

The usual IVIg regimen is 0.4g/kg body weight per day for five consecutive days [120]. IVIg is usually well tolerated and has only mild infusion-related adverse effects. Rarely, serious adverse events may occur such as anaphylaxis, thromboembolic events or renal failure [151].

IVIg has been proven to be an effective treatment for GBS. However, not all patients have an acceptable outcome following standard IVIg treatment [154]. Approximately 8%–16% of patients with GBS treated using standard-dose IVIg deteriorate after initial improvement or stabilization; a treatment related fluctuation [154]. The results of one small study reported that a repeated dose of IVIg may be effective in severe, unresponsive patients with GBS [155]. An ongoing randomized placebo-controlled trial conducted in the Netherlands is evaluating a second IVIg dose versus placebo one week after a standard IVIg treatment in patients with GBS assessed as having a poor prognosis [151].

Immune Treatment for Mild GBS

Because IVIg and PEX are indicated for patients who are unable to walk independently [120], the effect of IVIg and PE on patients with mild GBS who are able to walk independently has not been clearly established. In one trial, individuals with mild GBS who were able to walk unaided at randomization received either two sessions of PEX in 3 days or supportive care [156]. The number of patients with one or more functional grades of improvement at 1 month was significantly greater in the treated group as compared to the control group.

It appears that a considerable proportion of patients with mild GBS still have residual disability after six months [157]. Moreover, a significant number of patients with mild GBS may subsequently progress [118]. Therefore, investigations assessing the effectiveness of immune treatments for mild GBS are required.

Other Pharmacological Treatments

Several small studies have reported pharmacological treatments for GBS other than corticosteroids, IVIg and PEX.

Mycophenolate mofetil (MM) is an immunosuppressive agent that affects the function of B and T lymphocytes such that it may be effective in treating immune-mediated neurological conditions. A Dutch GBS study group conducted an open label pilot study to assess the value added benefit of MM when simultaneously administered with IVIg and MP. This combination of IVIg-MP-MM was found to be safe but demonstrated no statistically significant effect on outcome when compared to the historical control group from the Dutch IVIg-MP trial [158].

Brain-derived neurotrophic factor (BDNF) has the potential to protect neurons from axonal degeneration. A randomized controlled trial of 10 patients was conducted, with six patients receiving subcutaneous BDNF daily compared with four patients receiving a placebo. The rate and extent of recovery were similar in the BDNF and placebo groups, although no serious adverse events were attributed to BDNF treatment [159]. This trial was discontinued after only 10 patients had been randomized because a preliminary analysis of a phase three study failed to show any significant benefit of BDNF in amyotrophic lateral sclerosis.

Two case reports are reported of patients with GBS showing rapid recovery after interferon β-1a treatments [160, 161]. Thereafter, an investigator-led, double blind, randomized, placebo-controlled pilot safety trial of interferon β-1a (Rebif) was conducted in 19 non-ambulatory patients with GBS in the United Kingdom [162]. Participants received subcutaneous interferon β-1a or placebo in addition to IVIg. No significant differences in outcomes were observed between these groups.

In a prospective, controlled clinical trial, 37 patients with acute GBS were randomized to receive either CSF filtration or PEX [163]. These authors reported that the treatment using with CSF filtration is at least as effective as that using PEX. CSF filtration may function by removing inflammatory mediators, autoantibodies or other factors from the CSF.

Potential Treatments (Evidence from Animal Studies)

Other agents have been reported as effective treatments in animal models of GBS. Histological studies of both patients with AMAN and patients with AIDP have indicated that complement activation at the nerve membrane is strongly associated with nerve damage in GBS [50, 164]. A study using an animal model of AMAN reported a complement-mediated immune attack on motor nerve fibers [55]. Novel GBS treatments are being assessed that interfere with this complement system. Some drugs with anti-complement activity have been shown to be effective in an animal model of GBS [151]. Another drug, flecainide, a sodium channel-blocking agent, protects axons from degeneration in EAN [165]. A recent study indicates a beneficial effect of the agent fasudil, a Rho-kinase inhibitor, in EAN as well [166]. Their efficacy in human GBS will require confirmation in clinical trials..

Future Studies

Since the 1990s, many studies investigating anti-ganglioside antibodies and their relationship to GBS have reported clinical variants or atypical cases of the disease. Patients with electrodiagnostically confirmed AMAN have demonstrated preserved or exaggerated DTRs or severe sphincter dysfunction. The authors recommend that the clinical criteria for GBS should be expanded to include atypical clinical presentations and laboratory data including anti-ganglioside antibodies. Moreover, more reliable electrodiagnostic criteria should be devised to distinguish AMAN and AIDP subtypes of GBS, in which AMAN's reversible conduction failure pattern is taken into consideration [167]. It is also important to elucidate whether molecular mimicry exists not only in AMAN but also in AIDP. The development of novel treatments is most important because IVIg and PEX treatments do not appear to significantly decrease mortality in GBS [120]. The development of novel treatments and further improvements in supportive care are also necessary in order to reduce the morbidity and mortality of this syndrome.

References

[1] Guillain G, Barre J, Strohl A. Sur un syndrome de radiculo-nevrite avec hyperalbuminose du liquide cephalorachidien sans reaction cellulaire. Remarques sur les caracteres cliniques et graphiques des reflexes tendineux. *Bull. Soc. Med. Hop. Paris* 1916; 28:1462–1470.

[2] Landry O. Note sur la paralysie ascendante aigue. *Gazette Hebdomadaire Med. Chir* 1859; 6: 472–74, 486–488.

[3] Feasby TE, Gilbert JJ, Brown WF, Bolton CF, Hahn AF, Koopman WF, Zochodne DW. An acute axonal form of Guillain–Barré polyneuropathy. *Brain* 1986;109:1115-1126.

[4] McKhann GM, Cornblath DR, Griffin JW, Ho TW, Li CY, Jiang Z, Wu HS, Zhaori G, Liu Y, Jou LP, Liu TC, Gao CY, Mao JY, Blaser MJ, Mishu B, Asbury AK. Acute motor axonal neuropathy: a frequent cause of acute flaccid paralysis in China. *Ann. Neurol.* 1993;33:333-342.

[5] Griffin JW, Li CY, Ho TW, Xue P, Macko C, Gao CY, Yang C, Tian M, Mishu B, Cornblath DR. Guillain–Barré syndrome in northern China: the spectrum of neuropathological changes in clinically defined cases. *Brain* 1995;118:577-595.

[6] Ho TW, Mishu B, Li CY, Gao CY, Cornblath DR, Griffin JW, Asbury AK, Blaser MJ, McKhann GM. Guillain–Barré syndrome in northern China: relationship to *Campylobacter jejuni* infection and anti-glycolipid antibodies. *Brain* 1995;118:597-605.

[7] Visser LH, van der Meché FGA, van Doorn PA, Meulstee J, Jacobs BC, Oomes PG, Kleyweg RP, Meulstee J. Guillain–Barré syndrome without sensory loss (acute motor neuropathy): a subgroup with specific clinical, electrodiagnostic and laboratory features. *Brain* 1995;118:841-847.

[8] Rees JH, Soudain SE, Gregson NA, Hughes RAC. *Campylobacter jejuni* infection and Guillain–Barré syndrome. *N. Engl. J. Med.* 1995;333:1374-1379.

[9] Lyu R-K, Tang L-M, Cheng S-Y, Hsu W-C, Chen S-T. Guillain–Barré syndrome in Taiwan: a clinical study of 167 patients. *J. Neurol. Neurosurg. Psychiatry* 1997;63:494-500.

[10] Emilia-Romagna Study Group on Clinical and Epidemiological Problems in Neurology. A prospective study on the incidence and prognosis of Guillain–Barré syndrome in Emilia-Romagna region, Italy (1992-1993). *Neurology* 1997;48:214-221.

[11] Paradiso G, Tripoli J, Galicchio S, Fejerman N. Epidemiological, clinical, and electrodiagnostic findings in childhood Guillain–Barré syndrome: a reappraisal. *Ann. Neurol.* 1999;46:701-707.

[12] Ogawara K, Kuwabara S, Mori M, Hattori T, Koga M, Yuki N. Axonal Guillain–Barré syndrome: relation to anti-ganglioside antibodies and *Campylobacter jejuni* infection in Japan. *Ann. Neurol.* 2000;48:624-631.

[13] Chiò A, Cocito D, Leone M, Giordana MT, Mora G, Mutani R, Piemonte and Valle d'Aosta Register for Guillain-Barré Syndrome. Guillain–Barré syndrome: a prospective, population-based incidence and outcome survey. *Neurology* 2003;60:1146-1150.

[14] Dourado ME, Duarte RC, Ferreira LC, Queiroz JW, Illa I, Perez-Perez G, Guerrant RL, Jerônimo SM. Anti-ganglioside antibodies and clinical outcome of patients with Guillain–Barré syndrome in northeast Brazil. *Acta Neurol. Scand.* 2003;108:102-108.

[15] Shafqat S, Khealani BA, Awan F, Abedin SE. Guillain–Barré syndrome in Pakistan: similarity of demyelinating and axonal variants. *Eur. J. Neurol.* 2006 ;13:662-665.

[16] Gupta D, Nair M, Baheti NN, Sarma PS, Kuruvilla A; Diplomate-American Board. Electrodiagnostic and clinical aspects of Guillain–Barré syndrome: an analysis of 142 cases. *J. Clin. Neuromuscul. Dis.* 2008 ;10:42-51.

[17] Islam Z, Jacobs BC, van Belkum A, Mohammad QD, Islam MB, Herbrink P, Diorditsa S, Luby SP, Talukder KA, Endtz HP. Axonal variant of Guillain–Barré syndrome associated with *Campylobacter* infection in Bangladesh. *Neurology* 2010 16;74:581-587.

[18] van der Meché FG, Schmitz PI, Dutch Guillain–Barré Study Group. A randomized trial comparing intravenous immune globulin and plasma exchange in Guillain–Barré syndrome. *N. Engl. J. Med.* 1992;326:1123–1129.

[19] McGrogan A, Madle GC, Seaman HE, de Vries CS. The epidemiology of Guillain–Barré syndrome worldwide: a systematic literature review. *Neuroepidemiology* 2009;32(2):150-163.

[20] Willison HJ. The immunobiology of Guillain–Barré syndromes. *J. Peripher. Nerv. Syst.* 2005;10:94-112.

[21] Burns TM. Guillain–Barré syndrome. *Semin. Neurol.* 2008;28:152-167.

[22] Sejvar JJ, Baughman AL, Wise M, Morgan OW. Population incidence of Guillain–Barré syndrome: a systematic review and meta-analysis. *Neuroepidemiology* 2011;36:123-133.

[23] Hughes RAC, Rees JH. Clinical and epidemiologic features of Guillain–Barré syndrome. *J. Infect. Dis.* 1997;176 (Suppl 2):S92-S98.

[24] Ree JH, Gregson NA, Hughes RAC. Anti-ganglioside GM_1 antibodies in Guillain–Barré syndrome and their relationship to *Campylobacter jejuni* infection. *Ann. Neurol.* 1995;38:809-816.

[25] Hadden RDM, Cornblath DR, Hughes RAC, Zielasek J, Hartung HP, Toyka KV, Swan AV. Electrophysiological classification of Guillain–Barré syndrome: clinical associations and outcome. *Ann. Neurol.* 1998 ;44:780-788.

[26] Kuwabara S. Guillain–Barré syndrome: epidemiology, pathophysiology and management. *Drugs* 2004;64:597-610.

[27] Dourado ME, Félix RH, da Silva WK, Queiroz JW, Jeronimo SM. Clinical characteristics of Guillain–Barré syndrome in a tropical country: a Brazilian experience. *Acta Neurol. Scand.* 2012;125:47-53.

[28] Jacobs BC, Rothbarth PH, van der Meché FG, Herbrink P, Schmitz PI, de Klerk MA, van Doorn PA. The spectrum of antecedent infections in Guillain–Barré syndrome: a case-control study. *Neurology* 1998 ;51:1110-1115.

[29] Hadden RDM, Karch H, Hartung H-P, Hadden RD, Karch H, Hartung HP, Zielasek J, Weissbrich B, Schubert J, Weishaupt A, Cornblath DR, Swan AV, Hughes RAC, Toyka KV, Plasma Exchange/Sandoglobulin Guillain-Barré Syndrome Trial Group.

Preceding infections, immune factors, and outcome in Guillain–Barré syndrome. *Neurology* 2001;56:758-765.
[30] Kuwabara S. Guillain–Barré syndrome. *Curr. Neurol. Neurosci. Rep.* 2007;7:57-62.
[31] Schonberger LB, Bregman DJ, Sullivan-Bolyai JZ, Keenlyside RA, Ziegler DW, Retailliau HF, Eddins DL, Bryan JA. Guillain–Barré syndrome following vaccination in the National Influenza Immunization Program, United States, 1976-1977. *Am. J. Epidemiol.* 1979;110:105-123.
[32] Lehmann HC, Hartung HP, Kieseier BC, Hughes RAC. Guillain–Barré syndrome after exposure to influenza virus. *Lancet Infect. Dis.* 2010;10:643-651.
[33] Hughes RAC, Cornblath DR. Guillain–Barré syndrome. *Lancet* 2005;366:1653-1666.
[34] Souayah N, Nasar A, Suri MF, Qureshi AI. Guillain–Barré syndrome after vaccination in United States: data from the Centers for Disease Control and Prevention/Food and Drug Administration Vaccine Adverse Event Reporting System (1990-2005). *J. Clin. Neuromuscul. Dis.* 2009;11:1-6.
[35] van Doorn PA, Ruts L, Jacobs BC. Clinical features, pathogenesis, and treatment of Guillain–Barré syndrome. *Lancet Neurol.* 2008;7:939-950.
[36] Pithadia AB, Kakadia N. Guillain–Barré syndrome (GBS). *Pharmacol. Rep.* 2010; 62:220-232.
[37] Gensicke H, Datta AN, Dill P, Schindler C, Fischer D. Increased incidence of Guillain–Barré syndrome after surgery. *Eur. J. Neurol.* 2012;19:1239-1244.
[38] Kusunoki S, Chiba A, Kon K, Ando S, Arisawa K, Tate A, Kanazawa I. N-acetylgalactosaminyl GD1a is a target molecule for serum antibody in Guillain–Barré syndrome. *Ann. Neurol.* 1994;35:570-576.
[39] Kuwabara S, Yuki N, Koga M, Hattori T, Matsuura D, Miyake M, Noda M. IgG anti-GM1 antibody is associated with reversible conduction failure and axonal degeneration in Guillain–Barré syndrome. *Ann. Neurol.* 1998;44: 202-208.
[40] Ho TW, Willison HJ, Nachamkin I, Li CY, Veitch J, Ung H, Wang GR, Liu RC, Cornblath DR, Asbury AK, Griffin JW, McKhann GM. Anti-GD1a antibody is associated with axonal but not demyelinating forms of Guillain–Barré syndrome. *Ann. Neurol.* 1999;45:168-173.
[41] Yuki N, Ho TW, Tagawa Y, Koga M, Li CY, Hirata K, Griffin JW. Autoantibodies to GM1b and GalNAc-GD1a: relationship to *Campylobacter jejuni* infection and acute motor axonal neuropathy in China. *J. Neurol. Sci.* 1999;164:134-138.
[42] Kaida K, Kusunoki S, Kamakura K, Motoyoshi K, Kanazawa I. Guillain–Barré syndrome with antibody to a ganglioside, N-acetylgalactosaminyl GD1a. *Brain* 2000;123:116-124.
[43] Kuwabara S, Ogawara K, Mizobuchi K, Koga M, Mori M, Hattori T, Yuki N. Isolated absence of F waves and proximal axonal dysfunction in Guillain–Barré syndrome with antiganglioside antibodies. *J. Neurol. Neurosurg. Psychiatry* 2000;68:191-195.
[44] Yuki N, Ang CW, Koga M, Jacobs BC, van Doorn PA, Hirata K, van der Meché FG. Clinical features and response to treatment in Guillain–Barré syndrome associated with antibodies to GM1b ganglioside. *Ann. Neurol.* 2000;47:314-321.
[45] Ogawara K, Kuwabara S, Koga M, Mori M, Yuki N, Hattori T. Anti-GM1b IgG antibody is associated with acute motor axonal neuropathy and *Campylobacter jejuni* infection. *J. Neurol. Sci.* 2003;15;210:41-45.

[46] Hiraga A, Kuwabara S, Ogawara K, Misawa S, Kanesaka T, Koga M, Yuki N, Hattori T, Mori M. Patterns and serial changes in electrodiagnostic abnormalities of axonal Guillain–Barré syndrome. *Neurology* 2005;64:856-860.

[47] Yuki N, Kuwabara S. Axonal Guillain–Barré syndrome: carbohydrate mimicry and pathophysiology. *J. Peripher. Nerv. Syst.* 2007;12:238-249.

[48] Prineas JW. Pathology of the Guillain–Barré syndrome. *Ann. Neurol.* 1981;9 (Suppl):S6–S19.

[49] Vucic S, Kiernan MC, Cornblath DR. Guillain–Barré syndrome: an update. *J. Clin. Neurosci.* 2009;16:733-741.

[50] Hafer-Macko C, Hsieh ST, Li CY, Ho TW, Sheikh K, Cornblath DR, McKhann GM, Asbury AK, Griffin JW. Acute motor axonal neuropathy: an antibody-mediated attack on axolemma. *Ann. Neurol.* 1996;40:635-644.

[51] Kuwabara S, Ogawara K, Misawa S, Koga M, Mori M, Hiraga A, Kanesaka T, Hattori T, Yuki N. Does *Campylobacter jejuni* infection elicit "demyelinating" Guillain–Barré syndrome? *Neurology* 2004; 63:529–533.

[52] Yuki N, Susuki K, Koga M, Nishimoto Y, Odaka M, Hirata K, Taguchi K, Miyatake T, Furukawa K, Kobata T, Yamada M. Carbohydrate mimicry between human ganglioside GM1 and *Campylobacter jejuni* lipooligosaccharide causes Guillain–Barré syndrome. *Proc. Natl. Acad. Sci. USA* 2004;101:11404–11409.

[53] Yuki N, Yamada M, Koga M, Odaka M, Susuki K, Tagawa Y, Ueda S, Kasama T, Ohnishi A, Hayashi S, Takahashi H, Kamijo M, Hirata K. Animal model of axonal Guillain–Barré syndrome induced by sensitization with GM1 ganglioside. *Ann. Neurol.* 2001;49:712–720.

[54] Susuki K, Nishimoto Y, Yamada M, Baba M, Ueda S, Hirata K, Yuki N. Acute motor axonal neuropathy rabbit model: immune attack on nerve root axons. *Ann. Neurol.* 2003;54:383–388.

[55] Susuki K, Rasband MN, Tohyama K, Koibuchi K, Okamoto S, Funakoshi K, Hirata K, Baba H, Yuki N. Anti-GM1 antibodies cause complement-mediated disruption of sodium channel clusters in peripheral motor nerve fibers. *J. Neurosci.* 2007;27:3956–3967.

[56] Koga M, Takahashi M, Masuda M, Hirata K, Yuki N. Campylobacter gene polymorphism as a determinant of clinical features of Guillain–Barré syndrome. *Neurology* 2005;65:1376–1381.

[57] Asbury AK, Cornblath DR. Assessment of current diagnostic criteria for Guillain–Barré syndrome. *Ann. Neurol.* 1990;27(Suppl):S21-24.

[58] Olsson Y. Microenvironment of the peripheral nervous system under normal and pathological conditions. *Crit. Rev. Neurobiol.* 1990;5:265–311.

[59] Albers JW, Donofrio PD, McGonagle TK. Sequential electrodiagnostic abnormalities in acute inflammatory demyelinating polyradiculoneuropathy. *Muscle Nerve* 1985;8:528-539.

[60] Bromberg M, Albers JW: Patterns of sensory nerve conduction abnormalities in demyelinating and axonal peripheral nerve disorders. *Muscle Nerve* 1993;16:262–266.

[61] Bansal R, Kalita J, Misra UK. Pattern of sensory conduction in Guillain–Barré Syndrome. *Electromyogr. Clin. Neurophysiol.* 2001;41:433-437.

[62] Kuwabara S, Ogawara K, Misawa S, Mizobuchi K, Sung JY, Kitano Y, Mori M, Hattori T. Sensory nerve conduction in demyelinating and axonal Guillain–Barré syndromes. *Eur. Neurol.* 2004;51:196-198.

[63] Taly AB, Veerendrakumar M, Das KB, Gupta SK, Suresh TG, Rao S, Nagaraja D, Swamy HS. Sensory dysfunction in GB syndrome: a clinical and electrophysiological study of 100 patients. *Electromyogr. Clin. Neurophysiol.* 1997 ;37:49-54.

[64] Capasso M, Notturno F, Manzoli C, Uncini A. Involvement of sensory fibres in axonal subtypes of Guillain–Barré syndrome. *J. Neurol. Neurosurg. Psychiatry* 2011 ;82:664-670.

[65] Sekiguchi Y, Uncini A, Yuki N, Misawa S, Notturno F, Nasu S, Kanai K, Noto Y, Fujimaki Y, Shibuya K, Ohmori S, Sato Y, Kuwabara S. Antiganglioside antibodies are associated with axonal Guillain–Barré syndrome: a Japanese-Italian collaborative study. *J. Neurol. Neurosurg. Psychiatry* 2012;83:23-28.

[66] Hao Q, Saida T, Yoshino H, Kuroki S, Nukina M, Saida K. Anti-GalNAc-GD1a antibody-associated Guillain–Barré syndrome with a predominantly distal weakness without cranial nerve impairment and sensory disturbance. *Ann. Neurol.* 1999;45:758-768.

[67] Jacobs BC, van Doorn PA, Schmitz PI, Tio-Gillen AP, Herbrink P, Visser LH, Hooijkass H, van der Meché FG. *Campylobacter jejuni* infections and anti-GM1 antibodies in Guillain–Barré syndrome. *Ann. Neurol.* 1996 ;40:181-187.

[68] Koga M, Yoshino H, Morimatsu M, Yuki N. Anti-GT1a IgG in Guillain–Barré syndrome. *J. Neurol. Neurosurg. Psychiatry* 2002 ;72:767-771.

[69] Nagashima T, Koga M, Odaka M, Hirata K, Yuki N. Clinical correlates of serum anti-GT1a IgG antibodies. *J. Neurol. Sci.* 2004 ;219:139-145.

[70] Gupta SK, Taly AB, Suresh TG, Rao S, Nagaraja D. Acute idiopathic axonal neuropathy (AIAN): a clinical and electrophysiological observation. *Acta Neurol. Scand.* 1994;89:220-224.

[71] Griffin JW, Li CY, Ho TW, Tian M, Gao CY, Xue P, Mishu B, Cornblath DR, Macko C, McKhann GM, Asbury AK. Pathology of the motor-sensory axonal Guillain–Barré syndrome. *Ann. Neurol.* 1996;39:17-28.

[72] Ropper AH, Shahani BT. Pain in Guillain–Barré syndrome. *Arch. Neurol. 1984;*41: 511-514.

[73] Moulin DE, Hagen N, Feasby TE, Amireh R, Hahn A. Pain in Guillain–Barré syndrome. *Neurology* 1997;48:328-331.

[74] Rekand T, Gramstad A, Vedeler CA. Fatigue, pain and muscle weakness are frequent after Guillain–Barré syndrome and poliomyelitis. *J. Neurol.* 2009;256:349–354.

[75] Ruts L, Drenthen J, Jongen JL, Hop WC, Visser GH, Jacobs BC, van Doorn PA, Dutch GBS Study Group. Pain in Guillain–Barré syndrome: a long-term follow-up study. *Neurology* 2010:75;1439–1447.

[76] Ruts L, van Doorn PA, Lombardi R, Haasdijk ED, Penza P, Tulen JH, Hempel RJ, van den Meiracker AH, Lauria G. Unmyelinated and myelinated skin nerve damage in Guillain–Barré syndrome: correlation with pain and recovery. *Pain* 2012;153:399-409.

[77] Pentland B, Donald SM. Pain in the Guillain–Barré syndrome: a clinical review. *Pain* 1994;59:159-164.

[78] Rostásy KM, Huppke P, Beckers B, Brockmann K, Degenhardt V, Wesche B, König F, Gärtner J. Acute motor and sensory axonal neuropathy (AMSAN) in a 15-year-old boy

presenting with severe pain and distal muscle weakness. *Neuropediatrics* 2005 ;36:260-264.

[79] Ruts L, Rico R, van Koningsveld R, Botero JD, Meulstee J, Gerstenbluth I, Merkies IS, van Doorn PA. Pain accompanies pure motor Guillain–Barré syndrome. *J. Peripher. Nerv. Syst.* 2008;13:305-306.

[80] Yuki N, Hirata K. Preserved tendon reflexes in *Campylobacter* neuropathy. *Ann. Neurol.* 1998;43:546-547.

[81] Kuwabara S, Ogawara K, Koga M, Mori M, Hattori T, Yuki N. Hyperreflexia in Guillain–Barré syndrome: relation with acute motor axonal neuropathy and anti-GM1 antibody. *J. Neurol. Neurosurg. Psychiatry* 1999;67:180-184.

[82] Podnar S, Vodusek DB. Hyperreflexia in a patient with motor axonal Guillain–Barré syndrome. *Eur. J. Neurol.* 2000 ;7:727-730.

[83] Kuwabara S, Nakata M, Sung JY, Mori M, Kato N, Hattori T, Koga M, Yuki N. Hyperreflexia in axonal Guillain–Barré syndrome subsequent to *Campylobacter jejuni* enteritis. *J. Neurol. Sci.* 2002;199:89-92.

[84] Yuki N, Kokubun N, Kuwabara S, Sekiguchi Y, Ito M, Odaka M, Hirata K, Notturno F, Uncini A. Guillain–Barré syndrome associated with normal or exaggerated tendon reflexes. *J. Neurol.* 2012; 259:1181-1190.

[85] Yoshino H, Harukawa H, Asano A. IgG antiganglioside antibodies in Guillain–Barré syndrome with bulbar palsy. *J. Neuroimmunol.* 2000;105:195-201.

[86] Funakoshi K, Kuwabara S, Odaka M, Hirata K, Yuki N. Clinical predictors of mechanical ventilation in Fisher/ Guillain–Barré overlap syndrome. *J. Neurol. Neurosurg. Psychiatry* 2009 ;80:60-64.

[87] Sakakibara Y, Mori M, Kuwabara S, Katayama K, Hattori T, Koga M, Yuki N. Unilateral cranial and phrenic nerve involvement in axonal Guillain–Barré syndrome. *Muscle Nerve* 2002 ;25:297-299.

[88] Ho TW, Li CY, Cornblath DR, Gao CY, Asbury AK, Griffin JW, McKhann GM. Patterns of recovery in the Guillain–Barré syndromes. *Neurology* 1997;48:695-700.

[89] Soria ED, Candaras MM, Truax BT. Impairment of taste in the Guillain–Barré syndrome. *Clin. Neurol. Neurosurg.* 1990; 92:75-79.

[90] Odaka M, Yuki N, Nishimoto Y, Hirata K. Guillain–Barré syndrome presenting with loss of taste. *Neurology* 2002; 58:1437-1438.

[91] Combarros O, Pascual J, de Pablos C, Ortega F, Berciano J. Taste loss as an initial symptom of Guillain–Barré syndrome. *Neurology* 1996;47:1604-1605.

[92] Nishijima H, Tomiyama M, Suzuki C, Kon T, Funamizu Y, Ueno T, Haga R, Miki Y, Arai A, Baba M, Kimura T. Taste impairment in Guillain–Barré syndrome: more frequent than thought? *J. Peripher. Nerv. Syst.* 2011; 16:270-271.

[93] Durand MC, Lofaso F, Lefaucheur JP, Chevret S, Gajdos P, Raphaël JC, Sharshar T. Electrophysiology to predict mechanical ventilation in Guillain–Barré syndrome. *Eur. J. Neurol.* 2003;10:39–44.

[94] Sharshar T, Chevret S, Bourdain F, Raphaël JC, French Cooperative Group on Plasma Exchange in Guillain–Barré Syndrome. Early predictors of mechanical ventilation in Guillain-Barré syndrome. *Crit. Care Med.* 2003;31:278-283.

[95] Kaida K, Kusunoki S, Kanzaki M, Kamakura K, Motoyoshi K, Kanazawa I. Anti-GQ1b antibody as a factor predictive of mechanical ventilation in Guillain–Barré syndrome. *Neurology* 2004; 62:821-824.

[96] Durand MC, Porcher R, Orlikowski D, Aboab J, Devaux C, Clair B, Annane D, Gaillard JL, Lofaso F, Raphael JC, Sharshar T. Clinical and electrophysiological predictors of respiratory failure in Guillain–Barré syndrome: a prospective study. *Lancet Neurol.* 2006; 5:1021-1028.

[97] Walgaard C, Lingsma HF, Ruts L, van Doorn PA, Steyerberg EW, Jacobs BC. Early recognition of poor prognosis in Guillain–Barré syndrome. *Neurology* 2011; 76:968-975.

[98] Rajabally YA, Uncini A. Outcome and its predictors in Guillain–Barré syndrome. *J. Neurol. Neurosurg. Psychiatry* 2012; 83:711-718.

[99] Hiraga A, Mori M, Ogawara K, Kojima S, Kanesaka T, Misawa S, Hattori T, Kuwabara S. Recovery patterns and long term prognosis for axonal Guillain–Barré syndrome. *J. Neurol. Neurosurg. Psychiatry* 2005; 76:719-722.

[100] Kokubun N, Nishibayashi M, Uncini A, Odaka M, Hirata K, Yuki N. Conduction block in acute motor axonal neuropathy. *Brain* 2010;133:2897-2908.

[101] Lichtenfeld P. Autonomic dysfunction in the Guillain–Barré syndrome. *Am. J. Med.* 1971; 50:772-780.

[102] Zochodne DW. Autonomic involvement in Guillain–Barré syndrome: a review. *Muscle Nerve* 1994 ;17:1145-1155.

[103] Singh NK, Jaiswal AK, Misra S, Srivastava PK. Assessment of autonomic dysfunction in Guillain–Barré syndrome and its prognostic implications. *Acta Neurol. Scand.* 1987;75:101-105.

[104] Mukerji S, Aloka F, Farooq MU, Kassab MY, Abela GS. Cardiovascular complications of the Guillain–Barré syndrome. *Am. J. Cardiol.* 2009;104:1452-1455.

[105] Ferraro-Herrera AS, Kern HB, Nagler W. Autonomic dysfunction as the presenting feature of Guillain–Barré syndrome. *Arch. Phys. Med. Rehabil.* 1997;78:777-779.

[106] Asahina M, Kuwabara S, Suzuki A, Hattori T. Autonomic function in demyelinating and axonal subtypes of Guillain–Barré syndrome. *Acta Neurol. Scand.* 2002;105:44-50.

[107] Sakakibara R, Uchiyama T, Kuwabara S, Mori M, Ito T, Yamamoto T, Awa Y, Yamaguchi C, Yuki N, Vernino S, Kishi M, Shirai K. Prevalence and mechanism of bladder dysfunction in Guillain–Barré Syndrome. *Neurourol Urodyn* 2009;28:432-437.

[108] Sakakibara R, Uchiyama T, Tamura N, Kuwabara S, Asahina M, Hattori T. Urinary retention and sympathetic sphincter obstruction in axonal Guillain–Barré syndrome. *Muscle Nerve* 2007 ;35:111-115.

[109] Naphade PU, Verma R, Garg RK, Singh M, Malhotra HS, Shankwar SN. Prevalence of bladder dysfunction, urodynamic findings, and their correlation with outcome in Guillain–Barré syndrome. *Neurourol. Urodyn.* 2012; 31:1135-1140.

[110] Garssen MP, Van KR, Van Doorn PA. Residual fatigue is independent of antecedent events and disease severity in Guillain-Barré syndrome. *J. Neurol.* 2006;253:1143-1146.

[111] Forsberg A, Press R, Einarsson U, de Pedro-Cuesta J, Widén Holmqvist L, Swedish Epidemiological Study Group. Impairment in Guillain–Barré syndrome during the first 2 years after onset: a prospective study. *J. Neurol. Sci.* 2004;227:131-138.

[112] Merkies IS, Schmitz PI, Samijn JP, van der Meché FG, van Doorn PA, European Inflammatory Neuropathy Cause and Treatment (INCAT) Group. Fatigue in immune-mediated polyneuropathies. *Neurology* 1999;53:1648–1654.

[113] Saifudheen K, Jose J, Gafoor VA, Musthafa M. Guillain–Barré e syndrome and SIADH. *Neurology* 2011;76:701-704.
[114] Fisher CM. An unusual variant of acute idiopathic polyneuritis (syndrome of ophthalmoplegia, ataxia, and areflexia). *N. Engl. J. Med.* 1956;255:57-65.
[115] Chiba A, Kusunoki S, Shimizu T, Kanazawa I. Serum IgG antibody to ganglioside GQ1b is a possible marker of Miller Fisher syndrome. *Ann. Neurol.* 1992; 31:677-679.
[116] Mori M, Kuwabara S, Yuki N. Fisher syndrome: clinical features, immunopathogenesis and management. *Expert Rev. Neurother.* 2012;12:39-51.
[117] Mori M, Kuwabara S, Fukutake T, Yuki N, Hattori T. Clinical features and prognosis of Miller Fisher syndrome. *Neurology* 2001;56:1104-1106.
[118] Hiraga A, Mori M, Ogawara K, Hattori T, Kuwabara S. Differences in patterns of progression in demyelinating and axonal Guillain–Barré syndromes. *Neurology* 2003; 61:471-474.
[119] Mori M, Kuwabara S, Miyake M, Noda M, Kuroki H, Kanno H, Ogawara K, Hattori T. *Haemophilus influenzae* infection and Guillain–Barré syndrome. *Brain* 2000; 123:2171-2178.
[120] Hughes RAC, Swan AV, Raphaël JC, Annane D, van Koningsveld R, van Doorn PA. Immunotherapy for Guillain–Barré syndrome: a systematic review. *Brain* 2007; 130:2245-2257.
[121] Plasma Exchange/Sandoglobulin Guillain–Barré Syndrome Trial Group. Randomised trial of plasma exchange, intravenous immunoglobulin, and combined treatments in Guillain–Barré syndrome. *Lancet* 1997; 349:225–230.
[122] McKhann GM, Griffin JW, Cornblath DR, Mellits ED, Fisher RS, Quaskey SA. Plasmapheresis and Guillain–Barré syndrome: analysis of prognostic factors and the effect of plasmapheresis. *Ann. Neurol.* 1988; 23:347-353.
[123] Winer JB, Hughes RAC, Osmond C. A prospective study of acute idiopathic neuropathy. I : clinical features and their prognostic value. *J. Neurol. Neurosurg. Psychiatry* 1988; 51:605-612.
[124] Cornblath DR, Mellits ED, Griffin JW, Cornblath DR, Mellits ED, Griffin JW, McKhann GM, Albers JW, Miller RG, Feasby TE, Quaskey SA. Motor conduction studies in Guillain–Barré syndrome: description and prognostic value. *Ann. Neurol.* 1988; 23:354-359.
[125] The Italian Guillain–Barré Study Group. The prognosis and main prognostic indicators of Guillain–Barré syndrome: a multicentre prospective study of 297 patients. *Brain* 1996; 119:2053-2061.
[126] Visser LH, Schmitz PIM, Meulstee J, van Doorn PA, van der Meché FGA, Dutch Guillain–Barré Study Group. Prognostic factors of Guillain–Barré syndrome after intravenous immunoglobulin or plasma exchange. *Neurology* 1999; 53:598-604.
[127] Kuwabara S, Asahina M, Koga M, Mori M, Yuki N, Hattori T. Two patterns of clinical recovery in Guillain–Barré syndrome with IgG anti-GM1 antibody. *Neurology* 1998; 51:1656-1660.
[128] Kuwabara S, Ogawara K, Mizobuchi K, Mori M, Hattori T. Mechanisms of early and late recovery in acute motor axonal neuropathy. *Muscle Nerve* 2001; 24:288-291.

[129] Kuwabara S, Mori M, Ogawara K, Hattori T, Yuki N. Indicators of rapid clinical recovery in Guillain–Barré syndrome. *J. Neurol. Neurosurg. Psychiatry* 2001; 70:560-562.

[130] Ho TW, Hsieh S-T, Nachamkin I, Willison HJ, Sheikh K, Kiehlbauch J, Flanigan K, McArthur JC, Cornblath DR, McKhann GM, Griffin JW. Motor nerve terminal degeneration provides a potential mechanism for rapid recovery in acute motor axonal neuropathy after *Campylobacter* infection. *Neurology* 1997; 48:717-724.

[131] Gabriel CM. Prognosis in the acute motor axonal form of Guillain–Barré syndrome. *J. Neurol. Neurosurg. Psychiatry* 2005; 76:622.

[132] Ropper AH. Severe acute Guillain–Barré syndrome. *Neurology* 1986; 36:429-432.

[133] Bernsen RAJAM, de Jager AEJ, Schmitz PIM, van der Meché FGA. Long-term impact on work and private life after Guillain–Barré syndrome. *J. Neurol. Sci.* 2002; 201:13-17.

[134] Visser LH, van der Meché FG, Meulstee J, Rothbarth PP, Jacobs BC, Schmitz PI, van Doorn PA, Dutch Guillain–Barré Study Group. Cytomegalovirus infection and Guillain-Barré syndrome: the clinical, electrophysiologic, and prognostic features. *Neurology* 1996; 47:668-673.

[135] Vedeler CA, Wik E, Nyland H. The long-term prognosis of Guillain–Barré syndrome: evaluation of prognostic factors including plasma exchange. *Acta Neurol. Scand.* 1997; 95:298-302.

[136] Rees JH, Thompson RD, Smeeton NC, Hughes RAC. Epidemiological study of Guillain–Barré syndrome in south east England. *J. Neurol. Neurosurg. Psychiatry* 1998; 64:74-77.

[137] Fletcher DD, Lawn ND, Wolter TD, Wijdicks EF. Long-term outcome in patients with Guillain–Barré syndrome requiring mechanical ventilation. *Neurology* 2000; 54:2311-2315.

[138] Walgaard C, Lingsma HF, Ruts L, Drenthen J, van Koningsveld R, Garssen MJ, van Doorn PA, Steyerberg EW, Jacobs BC. Prediction of respiratory insufficiency in Guillain–Barré syndrome. *Ann. Neurol.* 2010;67:781-787.

[139] Orlikowski D, Terzi N, Blumen M, Sharshar T, Raphael JC, Annane D, Lofaso F. Tongue weakness is associated with respiratory failure in patients with severe Guillain–Barré syndrome. *Acta Neuro. Scand.* 2009 ;119:364-370.

[140] Lawn ND, Fletcher DD, Henderson RD, Wolter TD, Wijdicks EF. Anticipating mechanical ventilation in Guillain–Barré syndrome. *Arch. Neurol.* 2001; 58:893-898.

[141] Ito H, Ito H, Fujita K, Kinoshita Y, Takanashi Y, Kusaka H. Phrenic nerve conduction in the early stage of Guillain–Barré syndrome might predict the respiratory failure. *Acta Neurol. Scand.* 2007;116:255-258.

[142] van Koningsveld R, Steyerberg EW, Hughes RAC, Swan AV, van Doorn PA, Jacobs BC. A clinical prognostic scoring system for Guillain–Barré syndrome. *Lancet Neurol.* 2007 ;6:589-594.

[143] Henderson RD, Lawn ND, Fletcher DD, McClelland RL, Wijdicks EF. The morbidity of Guillain–Barré syndrome admitted to the intensive care unit. *Neurology* 2003; 60:17-21.

[144] Lawn ND, Wijdicks EF. Fatal Guillain–Barré syndrome. *Neurology* 1999;52:635-638.

[145] Hughes RAC, Wijdicks EF, Benson E, Cornblath DR, Hahn AF, Meythaler JM, Sladky JT, Barohn RJ, Stevens JC, Multidisciplinary Consensus Group. Supportive care for patients with Guillain–Barré syndrome. *Arch. Neurol.* 2005;62:1194-1198.
[146] Hughes RAC, Swan AV, van Doorn PA. Corticosteroids for Guillain–Barré syndrome. *Cochrane Database Syst. Rev.* 2010; CD001446.
[147] van Koningsveld R, Schmitz PI, Meché FG, Visser LH, Meulstee J, van Doorn PA. Effect of methylprednisolone when added to standard treatment with intravenous immunoglobulin for Guillain–Barré syndrome: randomised trial. *Lancet* 2004; 363:192-196.
[148] Brettle RP, Gross M, Legg NJ, Lockwood M, Pallis C. Treatment of acute polyneuropathy by plasma exchange. *Lancet* 1978; 2:1100.
[149] The Guillain-Barre syndrome Study Group. Plasmapheresis and acute Guillain-Barre syndrome. *Neurology* 1985; 35:1096-1104.
[150] French Cooperative Group on Plasma Exchange in Guillain-Barre syndrome. Efficiency of plasma exchange in Guillain–Barré syndrome: role of replacement fluids. *Ann. Neurol.* 1987;22:753-761.
[151] Walgaard C, Jacobs BC, van Doorn PA. Emerging drugs for Guillain–Barré syndrome. *Expert Opin. Emerg. Drugs* 2011; 16:105-120.
[152] Kleyweg RP, van der Meche FGA, Meulstee J. Treatment of Guillain–Barré syndrome with high-dose gammaglobulin. *Neurology* 1988; 38:1639-1641.
[153] Hughes RAC, Swan AV, van Doorn PA. Intravenous immunoglobulin for Guillain–Barré syndrome. *Cochrane Database Syst. Rev.* 2010; CD002063.
[154] van Doorn PA, Kuitwaard K, Walgaard C, van Koningsveld R, Ruts L, Jacobs BC. IVIG treatment and prognosis in Guillain–Barré syndrome. *J. Clin. Immunol.* 2010; 30 (Suppl 1):S74-S78.
[155] Farcas P, Avnun L, Frisher S, Herishanu YO, Wirguin I. Efficacy of repeated intravenous immunoglobulin in severe unresponsive Guillain–Barré syndrome. *Lancet* 1997; 350:1747.
[156] French Cooperative Group on Plasma Exchange in Guillain- Barré Syndrome. Appropriate number of plasma exchanges in Guillain–Barré syndrome. *Ann. Neurol.* 1997; 41: 298-306.
[157] van Koningsveld R, Schmitz PI, Ang CW, Groen J, Osterhaus AD, Van der Meché FG, Van Doorn PA. Infections and course of disease in mild forms of Guillain–Barré syndrome. *Neurology* 2002;58:610-614.
[158] Garssen MP, van Koningsveld R, van Doorn PA, Merkies IS, Scheltens-de Boer M, van Leusden JA, van Schaik IN, Linssen WH, Visscher F, Boon AM, Faber CG, Meulstee J, Prick MJ, van den Berg LH, Franssen H, Hiel JA, van den Bergh PY, Sindic CJ. Treatment of Guillain–Barré syndrome with mycophenolate mofetil: a pilot study. *J. Neurol. Neurosurg. Psychiatry* 2007;78:1012-1013.
[159] Bensa S, Hadden RD, Hahn A, Hughes RAC, Willison HJ. Randomized controlled trial of brain-derived neurotrophic factor in Guillain–Barré syndrome: a pilot study. *Eur. J. Neurol.* 2000;7:423-426.
[160] Créange A, Lerat H, Meyrignac C, Degos JD, Gherardi RK, Cesaro P. Treatment of Guillain–Barré syndrome with interferon-beta. *Lancet* 1998;352:368-369.

[161] Schaller B, Radziwill AJ, Steck AJ. Successful treatment of Guillain–Barré syndrome with combined administration of interferon-beta-1a and intravenous immunoglobulin. *Eur. Neurol.* 2001;46:167-168.

[162] Pritchard J, Gray IA, Idrissova ZR, Lecky BR, Sutton IJ, Swan AV, Willison HJ, Winer JB, Hughes RAC. A randomized controlled trial of recombinant interferon-beta 1a in Guillain–Barré syndrome. *Neurology* 2003;61:1282-1284.

[163] Wollinsky KH, Hülser PJ, Brinkmeier H, Aulkemeyer P, Bössenecker W, Huber-Hartmann KH, Rohrbach P, Schreiber H, Weber F, Kron M, Büchele G, Mehrkens HH, Ludolph AC, Rüdel R. CSF filtration is an effective treatment of Guillain–Barré syndrome: a randomized clinical trial. *Neurology* 2001; 57:774-780.

[164] Hafer-Macko CE, Sheikh KA, Li CY, Ho TW, Cornblath DR, McKhann GM, Asbury AK, Griffin JW. Immune attack on the Schwann cell surface in acute inflammatory demyelinating polyneuropathy. *Ann. Neurol.* 1996;39:625-635.

[165] Bechtold DA, Yue X, Evans RM, Davies M, Gregson NA, Smith KJ. Axonal protection in experimental autoimmune neuritis by the sodium channel blocking agent flecainide. *Brain* 2005; 128:18-28.

[166] Pineda AA, Minohara M, Kawamura N, Matsushita T, Yamasaki R, Sun X, Piao H, Shimokawa H, Kira J. Preventive and therapeutic effects of the selective Rho-kinase inhibitor fasudil on experimental autoimmune neuritis. *J. Neurol. Sci.* 2011; 306:115-120.

[167] Uncini A, Kuwabara S. Electrodiagnostic criteria for Guillain–Barré syndrome: a critical revision and the need for an update. *Clin. Neurophysiol.* 2012; 123:1487-1495.

In: Contemporary Issues in Peripheral Neuropathy
Editor: Daniel L. Menkes
ISBN: 978-1-62948-681-9

Chapter V

Evolving Concepts in the Pathogenesis of Chronic Inflammatory Demyelinating Polyradiculoneuropathy (CIDP)

Paolo Ripellino*[*], *Thomas Fleetwood, Roberto Cantello and Cristoforo Comi
Department of Translational Medicine, Section of Neurology
and Interdisciplinary Research Centre of Autoimmune Diseases (IRCAD),
Amedeo Avogadro University, Novara, Italy

Abstract

Strong evidence supports the role of autoimmunity in the pathogenesis of chronic inflammatory demyelinating polyradiculoneuropathy (CIDP). This chapter focuses on several aspects of CIDP including genetic factors, disease development, factors associated with progression and the role of antecedent infections. Thereafter, an analysis of the complex interactions between cellular and humoral immune responses in its pathogenesis is provided. This is followed by a discussion of potential biomarkers for diagnosis, prognosis and treatment. Finally, this chapter discusses the current and potential treatments for CIDP.

Introduction

Chronic inflammatory demyelinating polyradiculoneuropathy (CIDP), a term used synonymously with chronic inflammatory demyelinating polyneuropathy, is an immune-mediated disease of the peripheral nervous system that results from a synergistic interaction of cell-mediated and humoral immune responses [1-3]. The target antigens of the aberrant

[*] E-mail: pao.ripe@hotmail.it.

immune response still remain elusive [4]. Nonetheless, it is likely that "molecular mimicry" plays a role in the process, as demonstrated in the inflammatory variant of Guillain-Barré syndrome (GBS), which shares several pathogenetic aspects with CIDP.

The candidate myelin protein auto-antigens evaluated to date include P2, P0 and PMP22 because each can induce Experimental Autoimmune Neuritis (EAN) in rodent models [5]. Currently, the strongest evidence points to P0, as autoantibodies to P0 have been identified in 20% of CIDP cases [6].

Additional evidence of "molecular mimicry" is suggested by a small subset of CIDP patients who display concomitant peripheral and central nervous system demyelination. These patients present with a clinical picture that combines features of CIDP and multiple sclerosis, such that a common myelin antigen is suspected to induce this autoimmunity. Nonetheless, this observation should be tempered by the fact that there is marked clinical heterogeneity observed in CIDP, which may correspond to differences in target antigens. Nevertheless, several observations suggest the presence of a common inflammatory-autoimmune background. Nerve biopsies of CIDP patients demonstrate infiltration of immune cells along with deposition of immunoglobulins and complement [7]. These immune cells include macrophages, lymphocytes and dendritic cells.

Table 1. Clinical diagnostic criteria for CIDP

Investigation	Typical findings
Neurological examination	Progressive or Relapsing-Remitting course (>8 weeks). Disproportionate large fiber sensory impairment (glove and stocking distribution), loss of vibration or joint position sense. Motor weakness out of proportion to the degree of atrophy (proximal+distal) , reduction of reflexes or areflexia
Electrophysiological study	Evidence of demyelination that may include : -distal motor latency prolongation (at least 2 nerves); -reduction of motor conduction velocity (at least 2 nerves); -prolongation of F-wave minimum latency or absence of F-waves (at least 2 nerves); -partial motor conduction block (at least 2 nerves); -abnormal temporal dispersion (at least 2 nerves); -increase of distal CMAP duration (at least 1 nerve)
Cerebrospinal fluid examination	Protein increase (>45mg/dl) with a paucity of white blood cells (<10/mm^3). Note: Patients recently infected with HIV may have up to 50 cells/mm^3
Spinal cord MRI	Gadolinium-enhancement of the spinal nerve roots, brachial or lumbosacral plexus
Nerve biopsy	Inflammatory infiltrates of T cells and macrophages; clusters of macrophages around vessels; signs of concomitant demyelination and remyelination (onion bulbs)
(Immunomodulatory treatment)	Objective clinical improvement after administration of an immunomodulatory agent

(Adapted from EFNS 2010 guidelines)

Finally, the strongest evidence for an inflammatory mechanism derives from the clinical improvement noted with immune modulation. Intravenous immunoglobulin (IVIg), plasma exchange (PE) and steroids are all effective in CIDP. Each of these treatments addresses different aspects of the inflammatory response.

To date, no sensitive or specific biomarker has been identified for this disorder. Therefore, the diagnosis must still be made on the basis of clinical, electrophysiological and cerebrospinal fluid findings [31; Table 1].

Genetic Predisposition

Studies on common autoimmune diseases clearly support the role of a genetic predisposition associated with HLA genes as well as the interleukins [8]. Thus, it is possible that CIDP may have similar associations. However, the rarity of this disease has limited the number of genetic studies, as association analysis requires a large patient population. Given these limitations, some authors focused on a candidate gene approach in which they targeted genes involved in specific immune system functions. The CD1 antigen-presenting molecules are transmembrane glycoproteins that capture and present a variety of microbial and self-glycolipids to antigen-specific T cells. There are five CD1 genes in the human genome located on chromosome 1(q22-23), which are designated CD1A, B, C, D, and E [9]. Caporale and colleagues investigated the possible role of CD1 gene polymorphisms in the susceptibility to GBS by comparing 65 patients with 100 controls. Their results suggested that the polymorphisms of the CD1 genes might have a role in the complex scenario of GBS pathogenesis [10]. Subsequently, these authors investigated polymorphisms of CD1A and CD1E genes in CIDP and multifocal motor neuropathy but no similar association was found [11]. Notwithstanding, other authors reported an association with SH2D2A, a gene involved in autoreactive T cell activation [12, 13]. SH2D2A is a gene located on chromosome 1q23.1 in a region conferring susceptibility to developing chronic allergic encephalomyelitis. It codes for a T-cell-specific adapter (TSAd) protein, which is expressed in activated T cells [14]. A low expression of TSAd in T cells may result in defective clearance of autoreactive T cells. This may lead to a higher risk of developing CIDP with a chronic, progressive course.

Weak associations between CIDP and HLA-8, CW7 and DR3 were reported in three small studies [15, 16] but were not confirmed in two other studies [17, 18]. More recently, other authors described gender related HLA associations in both GBS and CIDP [19].

In order to overcome sample size limitations, larger studies with international collaboration are required. This is even more relevant as CIDP heterogeneity may require sample stratification for clinical variants.

DNA microarray analysis provides a powerful tool for investigating the genetic component of CIDP by evaluating the gene expression patterns within tissues obtained by nerve or skin biopsies. DNA microarray analysis allows for a rapid comparison of gene products expressed in normal and diseased tissues such that it is possible to search for a gene differentially expressed in CIDP as compared to other diseases. Using microarray technology and confirmative Real Time-Polymerase Chain Reaction (RT-PCR), Renaud et al. identified different gene expression patterns in sural nerve biopsies from three different patient groups; controls, CIDP and vasculitis [20, 21]. Significant changes were detected for Tachykinin precursor 1 (TAC1), stearoyl-CoA desaturase and Allograft Inflammatory Factor 1 (AIF-1) [20].

CIDP patients demonstrated that the TAC1 gene expression was upregulated at a 27.8-fold increase as compared to the controls. The tachykinins are a family of amidated neuropeptides. TAC1 gene encodes for a precursor containing both substance P and neurokinin A. Tachykinins are excitatory neurotransmitters that are required to produce moderate to intense pain [22]. Stearoyl-CoA desaturase has also been reported to be upregulated in CIDP as compared to normal nerve [20]. This enzyme is involved in the biosynthesis of monounsaturated fatty acids that are present in myelin sheaths such that it may be involved in the remyelination process [23]. Finally, AIF-1 exerts an immunomodulatory function during macrophage activation. Its role is not specific, as this gene is generally upregulated during inflammatory conditions such as vasculitis. It is noteworthy that Lee at al. detected upregulation of AIF-1 in a study of skin punch biopsies that compared CIDP patients to controls [24]. In summary, there is a body of literature that supports the concept of autoimmunity due to molecular mimicry in CIDP but the precise mechanisms have yet to be elucidated.

Role of Preceding Infections

Some authors have investigated the potential role of preceding infections in triggering CIDP, similarly to what was demonstrated in GBS. The hypothesis of "molecular mimicry" proposes that the host's immune response is directed against an infectious agent that shares epitopes with the host's affected tissue. In the case of CIDP, the host's immune system mistakes peripheral nerve myelin antigens as foreign tissue such that an inflammatory response against peripheral nerve myelin results in myelin dysfunction and secondary axon loss. Most of the evidence supporting "molecular mimicry" in GBS was obtained from patients with an antecedent Campylobacter jejuni infection [25, 26]. Nonetheless, there is little evidence-based-medicine that correlates antecedent infections with CIDP. The authors found a single manuscript that reported that 35% of 92 CIDP patients had a history of a preceding infection [27]. It is possible that as yet unidentified infective agents may trigger clinical exacerbations in CIDP patients. The family of herpes viruses, such as EBV, have been assessed in untreated CIDP patients and compared to controls. One report suggested that the behavior and regulation of mature B cells alter the state of EBV persistence thus leading to increased viral replication and antiviral immune responses [28]. This may be a potential mechanism by which inflammation may persist in CIDP as opposed to the monophasic illness usually noted in the inflammatory variant of GBS.

Role of Cellular and Humoral Immune Responses

Peripheral nerve injury results from a synergistic interaction of cell-mediated and humoral immune responses directed against peripheral nerve antigens that have not been completely characterized [29].

Nerve biopsies demonstrate inflammatory cell infiltrates of T cells and macrophages [7, 30]. On paraffin sections, mononuclear cell infiltrates may be observed as scattered cells surrounding vessels. While these infiltrates may be viewed with conventional microscopy in the endoneurium, and to a lesser extent in the perineurium as well as in the epineurium, they are best defined with ultrastructural examination. However, the presence of these small clusters of inflammatory cells in nerve biopsy samples is not mandatory for the diagnosis of CIDP [31]. Macrophages suggest a diagnosis of CIDP when they are present as small perivascular clusters in the endoneurium [32]. Nonetheless, demyelination and remyelination are the pathological hallmarks of CIDP. Remyelinating lesions evident on electron microscopy are characterized by disproportionately thin myelin sheaths as compared to axon diameter associated with onion-bulb proliferations.

Nerve-biopsy specimens and animal models have demonstrated that activated T lymphocytes can invade peripheral-nerve tissue. The T-cell populations belong to both the CD4 and CD8 subgroups. In order to generate inflammatory lesions within the nerves, activated T cells must cross the blood-nerve barrier. Once within the peripheral nervous system, CD8+ T cells may undergo clonal expansion after encountering an antigen presented in the context of appropriate MHC molecules and co-stimulatory signals [33]. T cells subsequently activate resident or passenger macrophages, which then discharge an array of neurotoxic molecules. Macrophages may also act as antigen presenting cells in CIDP. As such, macrophages play a fundamental role in the inflammatory cascade as both initiators and facilitators [34]. Finally, specialized subpopulations of T cells may terminate the acute inflammatory process by secreting down-regulatory cytokines [35, 36].

The development of a spontaneous autoimmune polyneuropathy in B7-2 knockout Non-Obese Diabetic (NOD) mice underlines the role of co-stimulatory molecules in controlling the balance between detrimental and regulatory T cells (T regs) in inflammatory neuropathies. In this model, pathogenic T cells are directed against myelin protein zero (P0); the most prominent peripheral myelin protein that is a member of immunoglobulin gene superfamily [37]. Hu et al. demonstrated that mRNA upregulation of the inducible costimulator (ICOS) and its ligand (ICOS-L) in biopsy specimens of CIDP patients compared to controls. These observations underline the role of ICOS pathway in inducing and maintaining inflammation in CIDP [38]. We previously reported that ICOS pathway dysfunction, both at gene and cytokine production levels, is involved in MS pathogenesis [39].

T-cell-dependent inflammation may also be terminated by a programmed cell death mechanism involving Fas [40]. In peripheral nerve autoimmunity, the Fas-mediated elimination of T cells leads to the clinical recovery seen in GBS. In contrast, defective T cell apoptosis is responsible for a chronic disease evolution [41, 42]. In GBS, the pattern of T cell apoptosis may help to differentiate patients with a self limiting disease from those who are destined to develop a chronic disease such as CIDP [43].

Some authors recently investigated the distribution of Th17 cells and Th1 cells in the peripheral blood and cerebrospinal fluid (CSF) of CIDP patients. They reported that the percentage of Th17 cells correlated with the severity of inflammation within the spinal roots [44]. The mRNA transcripts associated with macrophage activation are upregulated in the nerves and skin of CIDP Patients. Macrophages can mediate demyelination through antibody and complement or Fas–FasL receptor interactions [45]. It is possible that macrophages play a fundamental role not only in the last step of the inflammatory process, which is demyelination, but also in the early steps, by acting as antigen presenting cells. Moreover, macrophages as well as neutrophils express Fc receptors on their membrane. Recruitment and activation of innate immune effector cells through cellular Fc receptors recognizing the constant fragment of IgG is the dominant pathway responsible for tissue inflammation. Animals lacking all activating Fcγ receptors are protected from the development of autoimmune disease [46].

Fcγ receptors (FcγR) are a family of receptors that can be distinguished on the basis of their affinity for IgG. Fcγ RI has the highest affinity as it can recognize monomeric IgG. Therefore, it is saturated if expressed on blood circulating cells such as monocytes. All the other receptors (Fcγ RIIA, Fcγ RIIB and Fcγ RIII) have a lower affinity and only bind IgG if present in the form of multimeric immune complexes [46]. Moreover, Fcγ RI, Fcγ RIIA and Fcγ RIIIA initiate activating signaling pathways via immunoreceptor tyrosine based activation motifs, whereas Fcγ RIIB is linked to an inhibitory signal. The inhibitory Fcγ RIIB is crucial in the regulation of the immune system because it is co-expressed with activating FcγRs on innate immune effector cells (mast cells, neutrophils and eosinophils). When immune complexes bind to these cells, both activating and inhibitory signaling pathways are triggered. Thus, the Fcγ RIIB system could be important for the activation threshold of innate effector cells. In contrast, B cells only express the inhibitory Fcγ RIIB. This pathway is triggered by the B-cell receptor and serves as a late checkpoint in the humoral immune system to prevent the expansion of autoreactive plasma cells.

The anti-inflammatory activity of IVIg therapy seems to be related to Fcγ RIIB expression. In CIDP the inhibitory Fcγ RIIB is impaired, but it can be partially restored with IVIg treatment [47, 48].

The role of autoantibodies in CIDP was suggested more than 20 years ago on the basis of immunoglobulin and complement deposition on myelinated nerve fibers and the presence of oligoclonal IgG bands in the CSF. Sera and immunoglobulin G (IgG) antibodies from patients with CIDP induce peripheral demyelination in host animals [49]. They can increase the permeability of the blood-nerve barrier [48] and adversely affect nerve conduction in various models of peripheral neuropathies [50]. The mechanism of antibody-induced damage involves several sequential steps. The first is the induction of the antibody-dependent cellular cytotoxicity upon binding to the Fc receptor of macrophages. This is followed by promotion of phagocytosis of target structures by opsonization. Subsequently, activation of the classic complement pathway upon binding to the antigenic epitopes results in pore formation allowing calcium influx, which triggers myelin-integral proteases that degrade the myelin sheath. In addition to mediating structural damage, antibodies may alter nerve impulse propagation and neuromuscular transmission when they bind near the nodes of Ranvier or the motor axon terminals. The removal of humoral immune mediators is the rationale of plasma exchange (PE), an effective treatment for CIDP.

Antibody Testing

Specific autoantibodies have been identified in a number of chronic neuropathic syndromes (e.g. anti-GM-1 in MMN), whereas this is not the case with CIDP. However, the presence and relevance of such antibodies in CIDP is implied given the beneficial effect of PE. The low frequency of specific antibodies that is observed in patients with CIDP suggests that various antibodies and separate mechanisms are involved in individual patients. This may explain why investigations seeking to identify antibodies to myelin antigens in CIDP have been unsuccessful [1].

The earliest studies attempted to identify antibodies to myelin by immunofluorescence but found that no more than 20% of CIDP patients had such autoantibodies [51, 52].

Antibodies to P0 and other myelin proteins, including PMP22 and P2, have been found in a small number of CIDP patients, but as an inconsistent finding [6].

The search for anti-galactocerebroside (the major target of complement-fixing anti-myelin antibodies in animals that have been immunized with myelin) antibodies in CIDP has been uniformly negative. The search for antibodies to gangliosides has been more rewarding in other forms of inflammatory neuropathy than in any other class of molecules. The associations between antibodies to ganglioside GM1 and axonal forms of GBS and between antibodies to ganglioside GQ1b and Miller Fisher syndrome are well known [53]. Antibodies to ganglioside GM1 are found in 30–80% of patients with multifocal motor neuropathy, but are hardly ever present in symmetrical sensorimotor CIDP [54]. Antibodies to sulfatides have not been consistently found more often in CIDP than in control subjects [54].

Animal models have clarified the pathogenesis of many autoimmune diseases, including GBS and other inflammatory neuropathies, but not in the case of CIDP [55].

Rationale for Immunomodulatory Treatments

Currently available treatments for CIDP are corticosteroids, immunoglobulin (IVIg), PE and chronic immunosuppressive agents [50, 56, 57; Table 2].

Corticosteroids should be considered as the first-line therapy in CIDP as they are effective in nearly 60% of patients [58, 59].

The first reported use of corticosteroids in CIDP dates from 1958 [60]. Their efficacy has been confirmed by subsequent reports [61, 62].

Their pleiotropic mechanism of action is not fully understood but it seems likely that they facilitate apoptosis of autoreactive T cells directed against the peripheral nerves [63, 64]. A similar anti-inflammatory effect may be involved in multiple sclerosis [65].

Intravenous methylprednisolone, dexamethasone [66] and oral prednisone and prednisolone [67] are all validated treatments. Clinical improvement or long-term remission may be achieved in approximately one-quarter of patients with CIDP after 1 or 2 courses of pulsed dexamethasone or 8 months of daily prednisolone [68].

There is no evidence-based-medicine or consensus whether it is best to use daily or alternate day prednisolone or prednisone or intermittent high-dose monthly intravenous methylprednisolone. The most common daily dose of prednisolone is 60 mg/day (or 1mg/kg/day) for the induction phase followed by maintenance therapy that is slowly tapered over months or years. In our experience, when corticosteroids are chosen as a first-line treatment, intravenous pulsed therapy leads to more rapid improvement, slightly longer remission, relatively fewer relapses and fewer adverse events when compared to continuous prednisolone treatment, especially if the therapy lasts more than 6 months [69, 70]. A controlled study reported that a 6-week course of 60 mg daily oral prednisolone with rapid tapering is as effective as one course of IVIg at the standard dose of 2 g/kg [67].

Table 2. Common treatments in CIDP

Drug	Suggested starting dose	Site of administration	Duration of treatment	Possible side effects	Assessments
Methylprednisolone (MP)	500 mg/day for 4 days	iv	At least 6 months, then re-evaluation	Cushing, cataracts, glaucoma, diabetes, hypertension, weight gain, osteonecrosis, gastrointestinal ulcer, psychiatric disorders, edema, hypokalemia, myopathy; increased risk of infection	Blood sugar; K^+, Na^+, Ca^{2+}; blood pressure; bone density; gastric ulcer; psychiatric disorders
Prednisone	60 mg/day (or 1 mg/kg/day)	oral	4 weeks every day; then the dose should be tapered in 3-6 months. To reduce side effects, the every other day treatment is strongly suggested	Same as MP	Same as MP
Prednisolone	60 mg/day (or 1 mg/kg/day)	oral	Same as prednisone	Same as MP	Same as MP
Polyclonal intravenous immunoglobulin (IVIg)	Starting dose: 0.4 g/kg/day for 5 days. Maintenance dose: 1g/kg/month (tailor-made)	iv	Months-years	Headache; skin rash; anaphylaxis; kidney or heart failure (rare); stroke	IgA level (before starting the treatment); kidney function
Plasma exchange (PE)	Induction: 3-5 PE/week for 2 weeks Maintenance: 1 PE every 1-3 weeks (tailor-made)	iv	Weeks	Electrolyte imbalance with hypocalcemia or alterations of acid-basis system; depletion of coagulation factors (bleeding) and IgG (increased risk of bleeding and infections); pneumothorax, thrombosis, septicemia related to the central venous access; hypotension or fluid overload; myocardial infarction	Consult a hematologist, pathologist or nephrologist
Azathioprine	Test dose: 50 mg/day. Maintenance dose: 2 mg/kg/daily divided in 2 or 3 doses; the dose should be tailored according to the number of lymphocytes (800-1200/μl, with total WBC >4000)	oral	Years	Allergic reaction; nausea; vomiting; hepatotoxicity; increased risk of malignancy (lymphoma) after years of treatment; increased risk of infections; infertility and teratogenity. Avoid allopurinol concomitant therapy (or reduce the dose of AZA at 30% as usual)	Perform the following studies every 2 weeks for the first 3 weeks, then every month: -WBC count: if <3500/μl, modify the dose; if <3000/μl, interrupt it immediately; -MCV; -AST, ALT, γGT

Drug	**Suggested starting dose**	**Site of administration**	**Duration of treatment**	**Possible side effects**	**Assessments**
Cyclophosphamide	0.5-1g/m^2 body surface pulse therapy every 4-6 weeks; or 1-2mg/kg/day (oral)	Iv oral	6 months	Bone-marrow suppression; increased risk of malignancy; increased risk of infections; alopecia; nausea; infertility; hemorrhagic cystitis, stomatitis, cardiomyopathy; infertility and teratogenity. Antiemetic and uroprotective agents are essential	Blood count; kidney function
Cyclosporine A (Cyc A)	Starting dose: 5 mg/kg divided in two doses, i.e. 100-150 mg twice daily (200-300 mg/day, trough concentration 70-100 µg/L Maintenance dose: 2.5mg/kg	oral	Years	Hirsutism; nephrotoxicity; hypertension; hyperlipidemia; tremor; weight gain; increased risk of malignancy, increased risk of infections; infertility and teratogenity	-Creatinine: if increased >50% than baseline or more than 1.5 mg/dl the dose of Cyc A should be adjusted; -blood pressure; -blood lipids; -Cyc A blood concentration (12 hours after the last dose)
Mycophenolate mofetil (MMF)	1g twice daily (2 g/day); blood concentration of 1-2 mg/L	oral	Years	Bone marrow suppression (leukopenia); diarrhea, lymphoma, hepatotoxicity, increased risk of infections (especially virus), gastrointestinal bleeding headache; infertility and teratogenity	Blood count; MMF blood concentration
Rituximab	375 mg/m^2 weekly; speed of infusion 50 mg/h for the first time, then up to 100 mg/h	iv	4 weeks	Hypotension, leukopenia, neutropenia, thrombocytopenia, bronchospasm, kidney failure; cytokine release syndrome	Blood count; creatinine

As second line treatments, two alternative but equally effective approaches are currently used: PE and IVIg [71, 72].

If a patient does not respond to one of these first-line therapies, it is advisable to switch to the other [31].

PE results in the rapid removal of antibodies, cytokines, immune complexes and immune cells [73]. The main limitation of PE is that it is a short-term treatment. The amount of autoantibodies removed by PE is likely outnumbered by the continuous synthesis of replacement autoantibodies with repeated antigenic stimulation. A sudden decline in autoantibody levels may even result in an increased antibody production after cessation of treatment. Furthermore, PE removes large molecular weight substances primarily from the intravascular space rather than from the extravascular space. The removal of these autoantibodies from the intravascular space may result in a rapid shift into the extravascular space, especially in conditions when the diffusion is facilitated by a leaky blood-tissue barrier. Therefore, repeated treatments are usually required. The optimal number of plasma exchange treatments in GBS has been reported in one large multicenter study [74]; 2 PE are recommended for mild GBS, whereas 4 PE should be reserved for patients with moderate to severe forms.

Polyclonal human immunoglobulin infusion is a highly effective treatment that results in a clinical response in 50% of patients who do not respond to corticosteroids and has a cost comparable (or lower) to that of PE [75]. As IVIg tends to have has fewer side effects than PE, IVIg should be used as maintenance therapy [76].

The anti-inflammatory activity of IVIg cannot be attributed to one specific mechanism of action, but is hypothesized to result from a variety of different mechanisms. These include anti-idiotype antibody production, inhibition of the complement pathway, Fc receptor modulation on macrophages and other effector cells, suppression of pathogenic cytokines, effects on cell migration by modulation of adhesion molecules and T-cell modulation [77-80].

Various antibodies against myelin components have been implicated in CIDP. IVIg contains IgG with a wide range of idiotypic and anti-idiotypic specificities, which may neutralize pathogenic autoantibodies such as anti-DNA, anti-AChR, anti-thyroglobulin and anti-GM1.

The IgG antibodies are capable of binding through their Fc region to Fcγ receptors on macrophages. This binding triggers an intracellular signalling, which interferes with macrophage-mediated demyelination [81]. The inhibitory Fcγ RIIB, expressed on myeloid and B cells, has a critical role in the balance of tolerance and auto-immunity. Nimmerjahn and colleagues reported that treatment-naive CIDP patients have an impaired expression of Fcγ IIB levels on naive B cells and fail to upregulate Fcγ IIB, as B cells mature from to memory B cells [48]. Of note, this impaired expression of Fcγ RIIB seems to be partially restored by IVIg treatment [48].

The balance between inhibition and activation of Fcγ receptors determines the final outcome. Activation of phagocytosis occurs when Fcγ RI and Fcγ RIII are overexpressed whereas inhibition of phagocytosis and interference with antibody dependent cell-mediated cytotoxicity occurs when Fcγ RII is overexpressed [46].

IVIg treatment can upregulate the inhibitory Fcγ RII receptors and modulate the Fcγ RII/Fcγ RIII ratio on macrophages [82]. An increase in the number of monocytes bearing the Fcγ RII inhibitory receptors and an increase in the Fcγ RII/ Fcγ RIII ratio on monocytes has been noted just one week after IVIg in patients with CIDP who started to improve [82]. This data suggests that such inhibitory signalling may be clinically relevant.

Various cytokines, chemokines and adhesion and co-stimulatory molecules are also upregulated in CIDP and may play a role in enhancing antigen presentation [83]. *In vitro* and *in vivo* studies have reported that IVIg causes a dose-dependent downregulation of tissue expression or reduction in the circulating levels of cytokines and adhesion molecules such as IL-1, TNF-α, IL-1β, TGF-α and TGF-α mRNA, MHC-I and ICAM-I on the endothelial cells [84]. Although the infused IVIg freely enters the endoneurial parenchyma via the end plate region and the dorsal roots, a site where there is a relative paucity of the blood-nerve barrier, the exact mechanism of action remains unknown [29].

Long-term Treatment Strategy

Although IVIg has been proven to be an effective treatment for CIDP [76; 85-87], it is uncertain if the profile of IVIg is favorable enough to outweigh the higher costs associated with its long-term use. An observational prospective study (TEPORE) is currently being conducted in Italy in order to address this issue.

The initial dose is usually 0.4 g/kg/day for 5 days, whereas the second infusion of IVIg should be administered after a 6 week interval [31]. During the follow-up visits, the neurologist should establish a schedule for maintenance infusions. The standard maintenance dose is 0.5 g/kg/day for 2 consecutive days (1g/kg/month), but the dose has to be tailored according to the principle of the "lowest effective maintenance dose".

The maximal clinical response to IVIg should be evident 3 weeks after the infusion [88]. Recently Eduardo Nobile-Orazio et al. compared IVIg and IV Methylprednisolone (IVMP) in a small RCT [89]. This trial reported evidence that the efficacy of MP is comparable to that of IVIg, that IVMP has a more sustained effect, that approximately 50% of patients in these two groups did not require any further infusions after the first year and that chronic treatment with steroids is associated with a higher rate of side effects. These results suggest that IVMP could be considered as first line treatment with IVIg being reserved for patients who do not respond or who develop side effects with IVMP therapy.

However, it should be mentioned that the inclusion of non-treatment-naïve patients might limit the extent to which the results can be generalized to previously untreated patients. Restated, these results are applicable to treatment of patients in an active or stationary phase of their disease with significant disability who have no contraindication to corticosteroids or IVIg and who have not failed to respond to one of the treatments.

About 50% of non-responders to first-line therapy become responders when switched to an alternative treatment [56]. However, this proportion is higher if the treatments are combined. Lack of response to one treatment does not preclude a response to another. It is mandatory to reconsider the diagnosis if the patient does not respond to first-line treatment or before initiating an immunosuppressive drug.

Hughes at al. recently concluded that there is insufficient evidence to support the use of immunosuppressive drugs in CIDP [90]. Nonetheless, there are case reports and small case series in the medical literature that these agents may be beneficial in some refractory patients with CIDP [56, 76, 91].

Azathioprine is an immunosuppressive drug that inhibits proliferating immunocompetent cells and is often used as steroid-sparing agent. An open-label, randomized, controlled trial of 27 patients with CIDP compared the relative efficacy of azathioprine combined with prednisone to prednisone alone and reported no significant difference between treatments [92]. However, it should be noted that the sample size was small and the treatment period of 9 months may have been insufficient as azathioprine may take up to 6 months to reach its maximum efficacy [93]. Azathioprine has been widely used in open label trials after initial PE or IVIG and corticosteroid treatment in order to maintain remission [94, 95].

Cyclosporine A is a calcineurin inhibitor that inhibits the production of cytokines and is mainly used in patients who have undergone organ transplantation. The most serious adverse effects of cyclosporine are dose-dependent nephrotoxicity and hypertension. Cyclosporine has been used in refractory patients with variables results [96-98].

Mycophenolate mofetil inhibits the proliferation of T and B lymphocytes and is generally well tolerated and relatively safe to use. Its side effects include mild bone marrow suppression. The most reported adverse effects are diarrhea, leukopenia, thrombocytopenia, neutropenia, lymphoma, gastrointestinal bleeding and headache. There are only few reports on its use in CIDP [99-101].

Cyclophosphamide depletes T and B lymphocytes [102]. Two small series of 15 [103] and 5 patients [104] treated with intravenous pulse cyclophosphamide reported positive results.

Neutropenic infections and transient renal insufficiency as well as other mild adverse effects have been reported. Cyclophosphamide's most common adverse effects include hemorrhagic cystitis, stomatitis, leukopenia, thrombocytopenia, malignancy and cardiomyopathy. Therefore, cyclophosphamide should only be considered for patients with a severe form of CIDP who have been refractory to other treatments.

Rituximab is a new promising agent that has been reported to be effective in CIDP associated with hematological disorders such as monoclonal gammopathy of undetermined significance associated with anti-MAG [105, 106] and multiple myeloma [107]. The most frequently reported adverse effects of rituximab are hypotension, leukopenia, neutropenia, thrombocytopenia, bronchospasm and kidney failure. Many immunosuppressive agents including cyclophosphamide and rituximab have been associated with instances of progressive multifocal leukoencephalopathy; a condition with a high fatality rate [108, 109]. It is unclear if testing for JC virus antibodies will permit risk stratification [108]. For all these reasons, patients who do not respond to corticosteroids, PE or IVIg should be counseled regarding this risk before immunosuppressant medications are prescribed [108].

Biomarkers for Diagnosis/Prognosis or Treatment Evaluation

There is no evidence of any biomarker that is either specific or sensitive for diagnosing CIDP such that the diagnosis must be made on the basis of clinical, electrodiagnostic and cerebrospinal fluid parameters [110, 31].

In 2010 a panel of experts reviewed potential diagnostic and prognostic biomarkers in CIDP, and assessed the most relevant findings on genetics, immunology and neurobiology of this disorder [111]. Reliable *in situ* biomarkers, such as the disposition of macrophages [32] or the Fc expression on B cells, are promising approaches for diagnostic purposes [112].

The Fcγ RIIB on B-cells transduces inhibitory signals and prevents their transformation into IgG-producing plasma cells. Patients with CIDP were found to have lower Fcγ RIIB on naive B-cells and failed to upregulate or maintain Fcγ RIIB as the disease progressed. Notably, Fcγ RIIB protein expression was up-regulated on monocytes and B-cells after clinically effective IVIg therapy, suggesting that the effect of IVIg on Fcγ RIIB may be a factor predicting those patients who will be more likely to respond to IVIg.

Additional data were provided by studies on skin and nerve biopsies [24]. The Würzburg group assessed the presence of inflammatory cells, particularly macrophages in nerve biopsies from patients with diabetes and from patients with both CIDP and diabetes. While no significant difference was found in the number of inflammatory cells between these two groups, the CIDP-diabetic population's endothelial cells demonstrated a higher expression of matrix metalloproteinase 9 [113].

Another promising approach would involve genome-wide screening for relevant candidate genes that encode for proteins associated with inflammation, demyelination and axonal degeneration, before and after therapies.

At present, epidemiological data are the best outcome predictors. Younger age, female gender, more acute presentation, short disease duration and a short interval of time before treatment initiation are characteristic of CIDP responders. Greater disability has been associated with a chronic progressive course likely on the basis of secondary axonal degeneration.

Clinical experience indicates that some patients only respond to steroids, whereas others, especially those with pure motor CIDP, not only fail to respond but may even worsen with steroids [114]. There is increasing evidence that CIDP is not a single disease entity but consists of several variants with different responses to the various therapies [115]. Such heterogeneity highlights the need for biomarkers able to predict clinical response such that patients can be appropriately treated at the time of diagnosis.

Some patients with CIDP may need at least two IVIg courses before signs of clinical improvement are evident [88]. At present, this clinical response is the only indicator used to adjust the IVIg dose and interval during maintenance treatment. Biomarkers reflecting disease activity or IVIg pharmacokinetics might help to define dosage and frequency of IVIg treatments in each patient.

Recently, the pharmacokinetics of IVIg in relation to clinical outcome was examined in 174 patients with GBS treated with IVIg [116]. Patients with a lower increase in serum IgG recovered significantly more slowly and even fewer regained the ability to walk unaided at 6 months.

Factors that tend to be associated with a better response to IVIg include: disease duration < 1 year; progression of weakness before treatment; absence of discrepancy in weakness between arms and legs; areflexia of the arms; and slowing of motor conduction velocities in the median nerve. Of note, these are all indicative of recent onset, generalized, and progressive demyelination. The probability of a favorable response to immunotherapy approaches 90% if all the above five parameters are met [117]. It is also our experience that patients with severe axonal damage are less likely to manifest clinical improvement.

An overlooked action of IVIg is its effect on gene modulation in the respective targeted tissues. IVIg modulates a large number of genes associated with adhesion molecules, tissue remodeling and inflammation.

Sobue et al. compared the frequency of singlc nucleotide polymorphisms (SNPs) of Transient Axonal Glycoprotein-1 (TAG-1) gene in IVIg responders and non-responders. They reported that haplotype G-G-T was more frequent in non-responders [118]. TAG-1 is a nerve-specific adhesion molecule in the immunoglobulin superfamily that is distributed not only on the axon but also on the myelin sheath at the juxtaparanode [119]. Knockout of TAG-1 can induce the disruption of juxtaparanodal molecules, such as Caspr2 and Kv channels, eventually decreasing the number of Kv1.1 and 1.2 channels in the actual axonal region [118]. Therefore, it is has been hypothesized that TAG-1 subserves a role in inducing the proper distribution of potassium channels on the juxtaparanode thereby maintaining axonal function in the peripheral nervous system with the presence of Schwann cells or myelin sheath [120]. Iijima et al. suggested that the clinical response to IVIg may be genetically determined [118]. However, a recent work by Pang et al. that analyzed the same SNP in 24 CIDP patients failed to replicate their findings [121].

Conclusion

In the last years significant steps towards the understanding of CIDP pathogenesis have been made. As no biomarker has been identified as being sensitive or specific for this disorder, the diagnosis must still be rendered on the basis of clinical, electrophysiological and cerebrospinal fluid data [31; tab 1]. Corticosteroids are the first recommended treatment as approximately 60% of patients will respond. IVIg and PE should be considered if there is a high index of suspicion for CIDP and corticosteroids prove ineffective. On general principles, the best outcomes occur when the patients are treated earlier in the course of their disease as there tends to be a lesser degree of secondary axon loss. The efficacy of other immunosuppressive agents has not yet been established on an evidence-based level. Future research should be directed towards identifying a biomarker for CIDP, elucidating the underlying pathogenesis and developing novel therapies that address these mechanisms.

References

[1] Hughes RA, Allen D, Makowska A, Gregson NA. Pathogenesis of chronic inflammatory demyelinating polyradiculoneuropathy. *J. Peripher. Nerv. Syst.* 2006; 11:30-46.

[2] Köller H, Kieseier BC, Jander S, Hartung HP. Chronic inflammatory demyelinating polyneuropathy. *N. Engl. J. Med.* 2005; 352:1343-56.

[3] Kieseier BC, Kiefer R, Gold R, Hemmer B, Willison HJ, Hartung HP. Advances in understanding and treatment of immune-mediated disorders of the peripheral nervous system. *Muscle Nerve.* 2004; 30:131-56.

[4] Quattrini A, Previtali SC, Kieseier BC, Kiefer R, Comi G, Hartung HP. Autoimmunity in the peripheral nervous system. *Crit. Rev. Neurobiol.* 2003; 15:1-39.

[5] Soliven B. Autoimmune neuropathies: insights from animal models. *J. Peripher. Nerv. Syst.* 2012; 17 Suppl 2:28-33.

[6] Allen D, Giannopoulos K, Gray I, Gregson N, Makowska A, Pritchard J, Hughes RA. Antibodies to peripheral nerve myelin proteins in chronic inflammatory demyelinating polyradiculoneuropathy. *J. Peripher. Nerv. Syst.* 2005; 10:174-80.

[7] Vital C, Vital A, Lagueny A, Ferrer X, Fontan D, Barat M, Gbikpi-Benissan G, Orgogozo JM, Henry P, Brechenmacher C, Bredin A, Desbordes P, Ribière-Bachelier C, Latinville D, Julien J, Pétry KG. Chronic inflammatory demyelinating polyneuropathy: immunopathological and ultrastructural study of peripheral nerve biopsy in 42 cases. *Ultrastruct. Pathol.* 2000; 24:363-9.

[8] Sadovnick AD. Genetic background of multiple sclerosis. *Autoimmun. Rev.* 2012; 11:163-6.

[9] Porcelli SA, Modlin RL. The CD1 system: antigen-presenting molecules for T cell recognition of lipids and glycolipids. *Annu. Rev. Immunol.* 1999; 17:297-329.

[10] Caporale CM, Papola F, Fioroni MA, Aureli A, Giovannini A, Notturno F, Adorno D, Caporale V, Uncini A. Susceptibility to Guillain-Barré syndrome is associated to polymorphisms of CD1 genes. *J. Neuroimmunol.* 2006; 177:112-8.

[11] De Angelis MV, Notturno F, Caporale CM, Pace M, Uncini A. Polymorphisms of CD1 genes in chronic dysimmune neuropathies. *J. Neuroimmunol.* 2007; 186:161-3.

[12] Notturno F, Pace M, De Angelis MV, Caporale CM, Giovannini A, Uncini A. Susceptibility to chronic inflammatory demyelinating polyradiculoneuropathy is associated to polymorphic GA repeat in the SH2D2A gene. *J. Neuroimmunol.* 2008; 197:124-7.

[13] Uncini A, Notturno F, Pace M, Caporale CM. Polymorphism of CD1 and SH2D2A genes in inflammatory neuropathies. *J. Peripher. Nerv. Syst.* 2011;S1:48-51.

[14] Sundvall M, Jirholt J, Yang HT, Jansson L, Engström A, Pettersson U, Holmdahl R. Identification of murine loci associated with susceptibility to chronic experimental autoimmune encephalomyelitis. *Nat. Genet.* 1995; 10:313-7.

[15] Stewart GJ, Pollard JD, McLeod JG, Wolnizer CM. HLA antigens in the Landry-Guillain-Barré syndrome and chronic relapsing polyneuritis. *Ann. Neurol.* 1978; 4:285-9.

[16] Vaughan RW, Adam AM, Gray IA, Hughes RA, Sanders EA, van Dam M, Welsh KI. Major histocompatibility complex class I and class II polymorphism in chronic idiopathic demyelinating polyradiculoneuropathy. *J. Neuroimmunol.* 1990; 27:149-53.

[17] Feeney DJ, Pollard JD, McLeod JG, Stewart GJ, Doran TJ. HLA antigens in chronic inflammatory demyelinating polyneuropathy. *J. Neurol. Neurosurg. Psychiatry.* 1990; 53:170-2.

[18] van Doorn PA, Schreuder GM, Vermeulen M, d'Amaro J, Brand A. HLA antigens in patients with chronic inflammatory demyelinating polyneuropathy. *J. Neuroimmunol.* 1991;32:133-9.

[19] McCombe PA, Csurhes PA, Greer JM. Studies of HLA associations in male and female patients with Guillain-Barré syndrome (GBS) and chronic inflammatory demyelinating polyradiculoneuropathy (CIDP). *J. Neuroimmunol.* 2006; 180:172-7.

[20] Renaud S, Hays AP, Brannagan TH 3rd, Sander HW, Edgar M, Weimer LH, Olarte MR, Dalakas MC, Xiang Z, Danon MJ, Latov N. Gene expression profiling in chronic inflammatory demyelinating polyneuropathy. *J. Neuroimmunol.* 2005; 159:203-14.

[21] Steck AJ, Kinter J, Renaud S. Differential gene expression in nerve biopsies of inflammatory neuropathies. *J. Peripher. Nerv. Syst.* 2011; S1:30-3.

[22] Pennefather JN, Lecci A, Candenas ML, Patak E, Pinto FM, Maggi CA. Tachykinins and tachykinin receptors: a growing family. *Life Sci.* 2004; 74:1445-63.

[23] Miyazaki M, Ntambi JM. Role of stearoyl-coenzyme A desaturase in lipid metabolism. *Prostaglandins Leukot Essent Fatty Acids*. 2003; 68:113-21.

[24] Lee G, Xiang Z, Brannagan TH 3rd, Chin RL, Latov N. Differential gene expression in chronic inflammatory demyelinating polyneuropathy (CIDP) skin biopsies. *J. Neurol. Sci.* 2010; 290:115-22.

[25] Enders U, Karch H, Toyka KV, Michels M, Zielasek J, Pette M, Heesemann J, Hartung HP. The spectrum of immune responses to Campylobacter jejuni and glycoconjugates in Guillain-Barré syndrome and in other neuroimmunological disorders. *Ann. Neurol.* 1993; 34:136-44.

[26] Yuki N. Carbohydrate mimicry: a new paradigm of autoimmune diseases. *Curr. Opin. Immunol.* 2005; 17:577-82.

[27] McCombe PA, Pollard JD, McLeod JG. Chronic inflammatory demyelinating polyradiculoneuropathy. A clinical and electrophysiological study of 92 cases. *Brain.* 1987; 110:1617-30.

[28] Lünemann JD, Tackenberg B, Stein A, Wandinger KP, Oertel WH, Wagner HJ, Münz C, Meisel H, Sommer N, Zipp F. Dysregulated Epstein-Barr virus infection in patients with CIDP. *J. Neuroimmunol.* 2010; 218:107-11.

[29] Kieseier BC, Dalakas MC, Hartung HP. Immune mechanisms in chronic inflammatory demyelinating neuropathy. *Neurology*. 2002; 59:S7-12.

[30] Bosboom WM, van den Berg LH, Franssen H, Giesbergen PC, Flach HZ, van Putten AM, Veldman H, Wokke JH. Diagnostic value of sural nerve demyelination in chronic inflammatory demyelinating polyneuropathy. *Brain*. 2001; 124:2427-38.

[31] Van den Bergh PY, Hadden RD, Bouche P, Cornblath DR, Hahn A, Illa I, Koski CL, Léger JM, Nobile-Orazio E, Pollard J, Sommer C, van Doorn PA, van Schaik IN; European Federation of Neurological Societies; Peripheral Nerve Society. European Federation of Neurological Societies/Peripheral Nerve Society guideline on management of chronic inflammatory demyelinating polyradiculoneuropathy: report of a joint task force of the European Federation of Neurological Societies and the Peripheral Nerve Society - first revision. *Eur. J. Neurol.* 2010; 17:356-63.

[32] Sommer C, Koch S, Lammens M, Gabreels-Festen A, Stoll G, Toyka KV. Macrophage clustering as a diagnostic marker in sural nerve biopsies of patients with CIDP. *Neurology*. 2005; 65:1924-9.

[33] Schneider-Hohendorf T, Schwab N, Uçeyler N, Göbel K, Sommer C, Wiendl H. CD8+ T-cell immunity in chronic inflammatory demyelinating polyradiculoneuropathy. *Neurology*. 2012; 78:402-8.

[34] Kiefer R, Kieseier BC, Stoll G, Hartung HP. The role of macrophages in immune-mediated damage to the peripheral nervous system. *Prog. Neurobiol.* 2001; 64:109-27.

[35] Jander S, Pohl J, Gillen C, Stoll G. Differential expression of interleukin-10 mRNA in Wallerian degeneration and immune-mediated inflammation of the rat peripheral nervous system. *J. Neurosci. Res.* 1996; 43:254-9.

[36] Kiefer R, Funa K, Schweitzer T, Jung S, Bourde O, Toyka KV, Hartung HP. Transforming growth factor-beta 1 in experimental autoimmune neuritis. Cellular localization and time course. *Am. J. Pathol.* 1996; 148:211-23.
[37] Soliven B. Immune mechanisms in spontaneously occurring CIDP in NOD mice. *J. Peripher. Nerv. Syst.* 2011; S1:56-9.
[38] Hu W, Janke A, Ortler S, Hartung HP, Leder C, Kieseier BC, Wiendl H. Expression of CD28-related costimulatory molecule and its ligand in inflammatory neuropathies. *Neurology*. 2007; 68:277-82.
[39] Castelli L, Comi C, Chiocchetti A, Nicola S, Mesturini R, Giordano M, D'Alfonso S, Cerutti E, Galimberti D, Fenoglio C, Tesser F, Yagi J, Rojo JM, Perla F, Leone M, Scarpini E, Monaco F, Dianzani U. ICOS gene haplotypes correlate with IL10 secretion and multiple sclerosis evolution. *J. Neuroimmunol.* 2007; 186:193-8.
[40] Comi C, Fleetwood T, Dianzani U. The role of T cell apoptosis in nervous system autoimmunity. *Autoimmun. Rev.* 2012;12:150-6.
[41] Comi C, Gaviani P, Leone M, Ferretti M, Castelli L, Mesturini R, Ubezio G, Chiocchetti A, Osio M, Muscia F, Bogliun G, Corso G, Gavazzi A, Mariani C, Cantello R, Monaco F, Dianzani U. Fas-mediated T-cell apoptosis is impaired in patients with chronic inflammatory demyelinating polyneuropathy. *J. Peripher. Nerv. Syst.* 2006; 11:53-60.
[42] Comi C. Fas-mediated T-cell apoptosis in chronic inflammatory demyelinating polyneuropathy. *J. Peripher. Nerv. Syst.* 2011; S1:45-7.
[43] Comi C, Osio M, Ferretti M, Mesturini R, Cappellano G, Chiocchetti A, Carecchio M, Nascimbene C, Varrasi C, Cantello R, Mariani C, Monaco F, Dianzani U. Defective Fas-mediated T-cell apoptosis predicts acute onset CIDP. *J. Peripher. Nerv. Syst.* 2009; 14:101-6.
[44] Chi LJ, Xu WH, Zhang ZW, Huang HT, Zhang LM, Zhou J. Distribution of Th17 cells and Th1 cells in peripheral blood and cerebrospinal fluid in chronic inflammatory demyelinating polyradiculoneuropathy. *J. Peripher. Nerv. Syst.* 2010; 15:345-56.
[45] Dace DS, Khan AA, Stark JL, Kelly J, Cross AH, Apte RS. Interleukin-10 overexpression promotes Fas-ligand-dependent chronic macrophage-mediated demyelinating polyneuropathy. *PLoS One*. 2009; 4:e7121.
[46] Nimmerjahn F, Ravetch JV. Fc gamma receptors as regulators of immune responses. *Nat. Rev. Immunol.* 2008 ;8:34-47.
[47] Samuelsson A, Towers TL, Ravetch JV. Anti-inflammatory activity of IVIG mediated through the inhibitory Fc receptor. *Science*. 2001; 291:484-6.
[48] Nimmerjahn F, Lünemann JD. Expression and function of the inhibitory Fcγ-receptor in CIDP. *J. Peripher. Nerv. Syst.* 2011; S1:41-4.
[49] Yan WX, Taylor J, Andrias-Kauba S, Pollard JD. Passive transfer of demyelination by serum or IgG from chronic inflammatory demyelinating polyneuropathy patients. *Ann. Neurol.* 2000 ; 47:765-75.
[50] Meyer zu Hörste G, Hartung HP, Kieseier BC. From bench to bedside--experimental rationale for immune-specific therapies in the inflamed peripheral nerve. *Nat. Clin. Pract. Neurol.* 2007; 3:198-211.
[51] Latov N, Gross RB, Kastelman J, Flanagan T, Lamme S, Alkaitis DA, Olarte MR, Sherman WH, Chess L, Penn AS. Complement-fixing antiperipheral nerve myelin

antibodies in patients with inflammatory polyneuritis and with polyneuropathy and paraproteinemia. Neurology. 1981; 31:1530-4.

[52] McCombe PA, Pollard JD, McLeod JG. Absence of antimyelin antibodies and serum demyelinating factors in most patients with chronic inflammatory demyelinating polyradiculoneuropathy. *Clin. Exp. Neurol.* 1988; 25:53-60.

[53] Willison HJ, Yuki N. Peripheral neuropathies and anti-glycolipid antibodies. *Brain.* 2002; 125:2591-625.

[54] Nobile-Orazio E, Giannotta C. Testing for anti-glycolipid IgM antibodies in chronic immune-mediated demyelinating neuropathies. *J. Peripher. Nerv. Syst.* 2011; S1:18-23.

[55] Willison HJ. Biomarkers in experimental models of antibody-mediated neuropathies. *J. Peripher. Nerv. Syst.* 2011; S1:60-2.

[56] Cocito D, Paolasso I, Antonini G, Benedetti L, Briani C, Comi C, Fazio R, Jann S, Matà S, Mazzeo A, Sabatelli M, Nobile-Orazio E; Italian Network for CIDP Register. A nationwide retrospective analysis on the effect of immune therapies in patients with chronic inflammatory demyelinating polyradiculoneuropathy. *Eur. J. Neurol.* 2010; 17:289-94.

[57] Toyka KV, Gold R. The pathogenesis of CIDP: rationale for treatment with immunomodulatory agents. *Neurology.* 2003; 60:S2-7.

[58] Mehndiratta MM, Hughes RA. Corticosteroids for chronic inflammatory demyelinating polyradiculoneuropathy. Cochrane Database Syst Rev. 2002; (1):CD002062.

[59] Nobile-Orazio E. Treatment of dys-immune neuropathies. *J. Neurol.* 2005; 252:385-95.

[60] Austin JH. Recurrent polyneuropathies and their corticosteroid treatment; with five-year observations of a placebo-controlled case treated with corticotrophin, cortisone and prednisone. *Brain* 1958;81:157–92

[61] Dyck PJ, O'Brien PC, Oviatt KF, Dinapoli RP, Daube JR, Bartleson JD, Mokri B, Swift T, Low PA, Windebank AJ. Prednisone improves chronic inflammatory demyelinating polyradiculoneuropathy more than no treatment. *Ann. Neurol.* 1982; 11:136-41.

[62] Gorson KC, Allam G, Ropper AH. Chronic inflammatory demyelinating polyneuropathy: clinical features and response to treatment in 67 consecutive patients with and without a monoclonal gammopathy. *Neurology.* 1997; 48:321-8.

[63] Gold R, Hartung HP, Lassmann H. T-cell apoptosis in autoimmune diseases: termination of inflammation in the nervous system and other sites with specialized immune-defense mechanisms. *Trends Neurosci.* 1997; 20:399-404.

[64] Flammer JR, Rogatsky I. Minireview: Glucocorticoids in autoimmunity: unexpected targets and mechanisms. *Mol. Endocrinol.* 2011; 25:1075-86.

[65] Schweingruber N, Reichardt SD, Lühder F, Reichardt HM. Mechanisms of glucocorticoids in the control of neuroinflammation. *J. Neuroendocrinol.* 2012; 24:174-82.

[66] Muley SA, Kelkar P, Parry GJ. Treatment of chronic inflammatory demyelinating polyneuropathy with pulsed oral steroids. *Arch. Neurol.* 2008; 65:1460-4.

[67] Hughes R, Bensa S, Willison H, Van den Bergh P, Comi G, Illa I, Nobile-Orazio E, van Doorn P, Dalakas M, Bojar M, Swan A; Inflammatory Neuropathy Cause and Treatment (INCAT) Group. Randomized controlled trial of intravenous immunoglobulin versus oral prednisolone in chronic inflammatory demyelinating polyradiculoneuropathy. *Ann. Neurol.* 2001; 50:195-201.

[68] Eftimov F, Vermeulen M, van Doorn PA, Brusse E, van Schaik IN; PREDICT. Long-term remission of CIDP after pulsed dexamethasone or short-term prednisolone treatment. *Neurology*. 2012; 78:1079-84.
[69] Lopate G, Pestronk A, Al-Lozi M. Treatment of chronic inflammatory demyelinating polyneuropathy with high-dose intermittent intravenous methylprednisolone. *Arch. Neurol.* 2005; 62:249-54.
[70] van Schaik IN, Eftimov F, van Doorn PA, Brusse E, van den Berg LH, van der Pol WL, Faber CG, van Oostrom JC, Vogels OJ, Hadden RD, Kleine BU, van Norden AG, Verschuuren JJ, Dijkgraaf MG, Vermeulen M. Pulsed high-dose dexamethasone versus standard prednisolone treatment for chronic inflammatory demyelinating polyradiculoneuropathy (PREDICT study): a double-blind, randomised, controlled trial. *Lancet Neurol.* 2010; 9:245-53.
[71] Lehmann HC, Hartung HP. Plasma exchange and intravenous immunoglobulins: mechanism of action in immune-mediated neuropathies. *J. Neuroimmunol.* 2011; 231:61-9.
[72] Mehndiratta MM, Hughes RA, Agarwal P. Plasma exchange for chronic inflammatory demyelinating polyradiculoneuropathy. *Cochrane Database Syst. Rev.* 2004; (3):CD003906.
[73] Lehmann HC, Hartung HP, Hetzel GR, Stüve O, Kieseier BC. Plasma exchange in neuroimmunological disorders: part 2. Treatment of neuromuscular disorders. *Arch. Neurol.* 2006; 63:1066-71.
[74] The French Cooperative Group on Plasma Exchange in Guillain-Barré Syndrome. Appropriate number of plasma exchanges in Guillain-Barré syndrome. *Ann. Neurol.* 1997;41:298-306.
[75] Tsai CP, Wang KC, Liu CY, Sheng WY, Lee TC. Pharmacoeconomics of therapy for Guillain-Barré syndrome: plasma exchange and intravenous immunoglobulin. *J. Clin. Neurosci.* 2007; 14:625-9.
[76] Eftimov F, Winer JB, Vermeulen M, de Haan R, van Schaik IN. Intravenous immunoglobulin for chronic inflammatory demyelinating polyradiculoneuropathy. *Cochrane Database Syst. Rev.* 2009 Jan 21; (1):CD001797.
[77] Dalakas MC. The use of intravenous immunoglobulin in the treatment of autoimmune neuromuscular diseases: evidence-based indications and safety profile. *Pharmacol. Ther.* 2004; 102:177-93.
[78] Dalakas MC. Mechanisms of action of IVIg and therapeutic considerations in the treatment of acute and chronic demyelinating neuropathies. *Neurology*. 2002; 59: S13-21.
[79] Jacob S, Rajabally YA. Current proposed mechanisms of action of intravenous immunoglobulins in inflammatory neuropathies. *Curr. Neuropharmacol.* 2009; 7: 337-42.
[80] Weishaupt A, Kuhlmann T, Schönrock LM, Toyka KV, Brück W, Gold R. Effects of intravenous immunoglobulins on T cell and oligodendrocyte apoptosis in high-dose antigen therapy in experimental autoimmune encephalomyelitis. *Acta Neuropathol.* 2002; 104:385-90.
[81] Nimmerjahn F, Ravetch JV. Anti-inflammatory actions of intravenous immunoglobulin. *Annu. Rev. Immunol.* 2008; 26:513-33.

[82] Créange A, Gregson NA, Hughes RA. Intravenous immunoglobulin modulates lymphocyte CD54 and monocyte Fc gamma RII expression in patients with chronic inflammatory neuropathies. *J. Neuroimmunol.* 2003; 135:91-5.

[83] Kaveri SV, Lacroix-Desmazes S, Bayry J. The antiinflammatory IgG. *N. Engl. J. Med.* 2008; 359:307-9.

[84] Anthony RM, Nimmerjahn F, Ashline DJ, Reinhold VN, Paulson JC, Ravetch JV. Recapitulation of IVIG anti-inflammatory activity with a recombinant IgG Fc. *Science.* 2008; 320:373-6.

[85] Hughes RA, Donofrio P, Bril V, Dalakas MC, Deng C, Hanna K, Hartung HP, Latov N, Merkies IS, van Doorn PA; ICE Study Group. Intravenous immune globulin (10% caprylate-chromatography purified) for the treatment of chronic inflammatory demyelinating polyradiculoneuropathy (ICE study): a randomised placebo-controlled trial. *Lancet Neurol.* 2008; 7:136-44.

[86] Merkies IS, Bril V, Dalakas MC, Deng C, Donofrio P, Hanna K, Hartung HP, Hughes RA, Latov N, van Doorn PA; ICE Study Group. Health-related quality-of-life improvements in CIDP with immune globulin IV 10%: the ICE Study. *Neurology.* 2009; 72:1337-44.

[87] Nobile-Orazio E. Evidence for long-term IVIg treatment of chronic inflammatory demyelinating polyradiculoneuropathy. *Nat. Clin. Pract. Neurol.* 2008; 4:352-3.

[88] Latov N, Deng C, Dalakas MC, Bril V, Donofrio P, Hanna K, Hartung HP, Hughes RA, Merkies IS, van Doorn PA; IGIV-C CIDP Efficacy (ICE) Study Group. Timing and course of clinical response to intravenous immunoglobulin in chronic inflammatory demyelinating polyradiculoneuropathy. *Arch. Neurol.* 2010; 67:802-7.

[89] Nobile-Orazio E, Cocito D, Jann S, Uncini A, Beghi E, Messina P, Antonini G, Fazio R, Gallia F, Schenone A, Francia A, Pareyson D, Santoro L, Tamburin S, Macchia R, Cavaletti G, Giannini F, Sabatelli M; IMC Trial Group. Intravenous immunoglobulin versus intravenous methylprednisolone for chronic inflammatory demyelinating polyradiculoneuropathy: a randomised controlled trial. *Lancet Neurol.* 2012; 11:493-502.

[90] Hughes RA, Swan AV, van Doorn PA. Cytotoxic drugs and interferons for chronic inflammatory demyelinating polyradiculoneuropathy. *Cochrane Database Syst. Rev.* 2004 Oct 18; (4):CD003280.

[91] Gold R, Dalakas MC, Toyka KV. Immunotherapy in autoimmune neuromuscular disorders. *Lancet Neurol.* 2003; 2:22-32.

[92] Dyck PJ, O'Brien P, Swanson C, Low P, Daube J. Combined azathioprine and prednisone in chronic inflammatory-demyelinating polyneuropathy. *Neurology.* 1985; 35:1173-6.

[93] Gilman A, Brunton LL, LS Goodman, Chabner BA, Knollmann BC. Goodman and Gilman's. The pharmacological basis of therapeutics. Chapter 35-Immunosuppressants, tolerogens, and immunostimulants. 12th edition (2011). McGraw-Hill.

[94] Dalakas MC, Engel WK. Chronic relapsing (dysimmune) polyneuropathy: pathogenesis and treatment. *Ann. Neurol.* 1981; 9 Suppl:134-45.

[95] Walker GL. Progressive polyradiculoneuropathy: treatment with Azathioprine. *Aust. N. Z. J. Med.* 1979; 9:184-7.

[96] Barnett MH, Pollard JD, Davies L, McLeod JG. Cyclosporin A in resistant chronic inflammatory demyelinating polyradiculoneuropathy. *Muscle Nerve.* 1998; 21:454-60.

[97] Matsuda M, Hoshi K, Gono T, Morita H, Ikeda S. Cyclosporin A in treatment of refractory patients with chronic inflammatory demyelinating polyradiculoneuropathy. *J. Neurol. Sci.* 2004; 224:29-35.

[98] Hodgkinson SJ, Pollard JD, McLeod JG. Cyclosporin A in the treatment of chronic demyelinating polyradiculoneuropathy. *J. Neurol. Neurosurg. Psychiatry*. 1990; 53:327-30.

[99] Gorson KC, Amato AA, Ropper AH. Efficacy of mycophenolate mofetil in patients with chronic immune demyelinating polyneuropathy. *Neurology*. 2004; 63:715-7.

[100] Benedetti L, Grandis M, Nobbio L, Beronio A, Ghiglione E, Manzino M, Primavera A, Mancardi G, Schenone A. Mycophenolate mofetil in dysimmune neuropathies: a preliminary study. *Muscle Nerve*. 2004; 29:748-9.

[101] Umapathi T, Hughes R. Mycophenolate in treatment-resistant inflammatory neuropathies. *Eur. J. Neurol.* 2002; 9:683-5.

[102] Brannagan TH 3rd, Pradhan A, Heiman-Patterson T, Winkelman AC, Styler MJ, Topolsky DL, Crilley PA, Schwartzman RJ, Brodsky I, Gladstone DE. High-dose cyclophosphamide without stem-cell rescue for refractory CIDP. *Neurology*. 2002; 58:1856-8.

[103] Good JL, Chehrenama M, Mayer RF, Koski CL. Pulse cyclophosphamide therapy in chronic inflammatory demyelinating polyneuropathy. *Neurology*. 1998; 5:1735-8.

[104] Gladstone DE, Prestrud AA, Brannagan TH 3rd. High-dose cyclophosphamide results in long-term disease remission with restoration of a normal quality of life in patients with severe refractory chronic inflammatory demyelinating polyneuropathy. *J. Peripher. Nerv. Syst.* 2005; 10:11-6.

[105] Pestronk A, Florence J, Miller T, Choksi R, Al-Lozi MT, Levine TD. Treatment of IgM antibody associated polyneuropathies using rituximab. *J. Neurol. Neurosurg. Psychiatry.* 2003; 74:485-9.

[106] Renaud S, Fuhr P, Gregor M, Schweikert K, Lorenz D, Daniels C, Deuschl G, Gratwohl A, Steck AJ. High-dose rituximab and anti-MAG-associated polyneuropathy. *Neurology*. 2006; 66:742-4.

[107] Benedetti L, Briani C, Franciotta D, Fazio R, Paolasso I, Comi C, Luigetti M, Sabatelli M, Giannini F, Mancardi GL, Schenone A, Nobile-Orazio E, Cocito D. Rituximab in patients with chronic inflammatory demyelinating polyradiculoneuropathy: a report of 13 cases and review of the literature. *J. Neurol. Neurosurg. Psychiatry*. 2011; 82:306-8.

[108] Palazzo E, Yahia SA. Progressive multifocal leukoencephalopathy in autoimmune diseases. *Joint Bone Spine.* 2012; 79:351-5.

[109] Ripellino P, Comi C, Mula M, Varrasi C, Conconi A, Stecco A, Brustia D, Nasuelli N, Savio K, De Paoli L, Cantello R, Gaidano G, Monaco F. Progressive multifocal leucoencephalopathy after autologous bone marrow transplantation: a treatment option. *BMJ Case Rep*. 2011. doi:10.1136/bcr.11.2010.3549.

[110] Brannagan TH 3rd. Current diagnosis of CIDP: the need for biomarkers. *J. Peripher. Nerv. Syst.* 2011; S1:3-13.

[111] Latov N, Dalakas M, Vallat JM, Donofrio P, Hartung HP, Toyka KV. Biomarkers in the diagnosis and therapy of CIDP: Proceedings of the Biomarkers Faculty Meeting; June 8-9, 2010, Athens, Greece. *J. Peripher. Nerv. Syst.* 2011; S1:1-2.

[112] Tackenberg B, Jelcic I, Baerenwaldt A, Oertel WH, Sommer N, Nimmerjahn F, Lünemann JD. Impaired inhibitory Fc gamma receptor IIB expression on B cells in

chronic inflammatory demyelinating polyneuropathy. *Proc. Natl. Acad. Sci. U. S. A.* 2009; 106:4788-92.

[113] Jann S, Bramerio MA, Beretta S, Koch S, Defanti CA, Toyka KV, Sommer C. Diagnostic value of sural nerve matrix metalloproteinase-9 in diabetic patients with CIDP. *Neurology*. 2003; 61:1607-10.

[114] Donaghy M, Mills KR, Boniface SJ, Simmons J, Wright I, Gregson N, Jacobs J. Pure motor demyelinating neuropathy: deterioration after steroid treatment and improvement with intravenous immunoglobulin. *J. Neurol. Neurosurg. Psychiatry*. 1994; 57:778-83.

[115] Dalakas MC. Potential biomarkers for monitoring therapeutic response in patients with CIDP. *J. Peripher. Nerv. Syst.* 2011 Jun; S1:63-7.

[116] van Doorn PA, Kuitwaard K, Walgaard C, van Koningsveld R, Ruts L, Jacobs BC. IVIG treatment and prognosis in Guillain-Barré syndrome. *J. Clin. Immunol.* 2010;30:S74-8.

[117] Chan YC, Wilder-Smith E. Predicting treatment response in chronic, acquired demyelinating neuropathies. *Expert Rev. Neurother*. 2006; 6:1545-53.

[118] Iijima M, Koike H, Katsuno M, Sobue G. Polymorphism of transient axonal glycoprotein-1 in chronic inflammatory demyelinating polyneuropathy. *J. Peripher. Nerv. Syst.* 2011; S1:52-5.

[119] Traka M, Goutebroze L, Denisenko N, Bessa M, Nifli A, Havaki S, Iwakura Y, Fukamauchi F, Watanabe K, Soliven B, Girault JA, Karagogeos D. Association of TAG-1 with Caspr2 is essential for the molecular organization of juxtaparanodal regions of myelinated fibers. *J. Cell Biol.* 2003; 162:1161-72.

[120] Lonigro A, Devaux JJ. Disruption of neurofascin and gliomedin at nodes of Ranvier precedes demyelination in experimental allergic neuritis. *Brain* 2009; 132:260-73.

[121] Pang SY, Chan KH, Mak WW, Kung MH, Lee CN, Tsoi TH, Yip EK, Ho SL. Single-nucleotide polymorphism of transient axonal glycoprotein-1 and its correlation with clinical features and prognosis in chronic inflammatory demyelinating polyneuropathy. *J. Peripher. Nerv. Syst.* 2012; 17:72-5.

In: Contemporary Issues in Peripheral Neuropathy
Editor: Daniel L. Menkes
ISBN: 978-1-62948-681-9

Chapter VI

Chronic Inflammatory Demyelinating Polyneuropathy in Children: A Pediatric Neurologist's Perspective

*Christian Ionita**
Connecticut Children's Medical Center/
University of Connecticut Health Center, US

Abstract

Childhood chronic inflammatory demyelinating polyradiculoneuropathy (CIDP) is a rare, treatable, immune-mediated disease of the peripheral nervous system. It is characterized by primary demyelination of the peripheral nerves with secondary axonal loss. Although observed more frequently in adults, CIDP may occur at any age including infancy. Childhood CIDP often presents with a gait abnormality from muscle weakness with minimal muscle atrophy. CIDP is diagnosed based on specific clinical, electrophysiological and cerebrospinal fluid findings.

Although similar to adult forms, childhood CIDP differs in two significant ways. The first is that the childhood form has a more acute onset, often resembling the Guillain Barre Syndrome. Secondly, it tends to be more treatment responsive resulting in a more favorable prognosis. Nonetheless, some children have significant residual disability. Therefore, it is imperative that the clinicians make a rapid diagnosis in order to initiate treatment in short order.

Introduction

Childhood chronic inflammatory demyelinating polyradiculoneuropathy (CIDP) is a treatment responsive immune-mediated disease of the peripheral nervous system directed at

* E-mail: cionita@ccmckids.org<mailto:cionita@ccmckids.org>.

the myelin sheath that is observed in all age groups. The most common childhood presentation is that of a gait abnormality that results from insidious onset of progressive muscle weakness out of proportion to the degree of muscle atrophy. Deep tendon reflexes are usually depressed or absent. The underlying demyelination of the peripheral nerves is identified by needle electromyography (EMG) and nerve conduction studies (NCS). Investigation of cerebrospinal fluid (CSF) often demonstrates an elevated CSF protein with a relative paucity of leukocytes termed albuminocytologic dissociation. Overall, children tend to have a better outcome than adults. Given the paucity of cases of childhood CIDP, little evidence-based medicine exists to guide treatment such that the authors recommend following adult treatment guidelines. Thus, intravenous immunoglobulin (IVIg), plasma exchange (PEX) and/or corticosteroids are regarded as the first line agents. When these prove ineffective, empiric second-line treatment strategies for refractory disease may be attempted but evidence of their efficacy is sparse and is generally based on anecdotal reports.

Childhood CIDP - Overview

As Childhood CIDP is relatively rare, the author was only able to identify a few small case series and isolated case reports. As of this writing, the author was able to identify approximately 170 cases of Childhood CIDP in the literature.

Prevalence, Incidence

The data extracted from several epidemiological studies suggest that Childhood CIDP prevalence ranges between 0.35/100000 in New South Wales, Australia [1] and 0.57/100000 in Piemonte and Valle d'Aosta, Italy [2]. Both these studies used the more restrictive AHSAAN criteria. [3] When two different sets of diagnostic criteria were applied to the population in Leicestershire and Rutland, UK, the prevalence of Childhood CIDP was 0.42/100000 based on AHSAAN criteria and 1.26/100000 based on PNS [4] criteria. [5] Over a 20 year period, 30 cases of Childhood CIDP were encountered in a large tertiary care center. [6] In contrast to the male predominance observed in the adult population, there is no significant gender difference in the pediatric population. [6] No significant racial differences are apparent either. In a recent epidemiological study from Japan, Childhood CIDP (defined as less than 15 years of age) had a prevalence of 0.23/100000. [7] CIDP has been described in all pediatric age groups. For majority of pediatric series, the mean age at onset is reported to be between 6.3 and 11.5 years. [8, 9] Only a few cases were reported with onset in utero (congenital) or in early infancy suggesting that CIDP is rare in this age group. [10-12] The age of presentation distribution, as compiled from all pediatric case series, is presented in Figure 1. [8, 12-22] Two separate peaks at 3 and 13 years of age were noted in one publication. [20] The paucity of cases in the late teenage years is of unclear significance, although one possibility is that these patients may be under the care of adult neurologists.

Clinical Presentation

Childhood CIDP typically presents with progressive symmetrical muscle weakness that evolves over a period of at least 4 to 8 weeks.

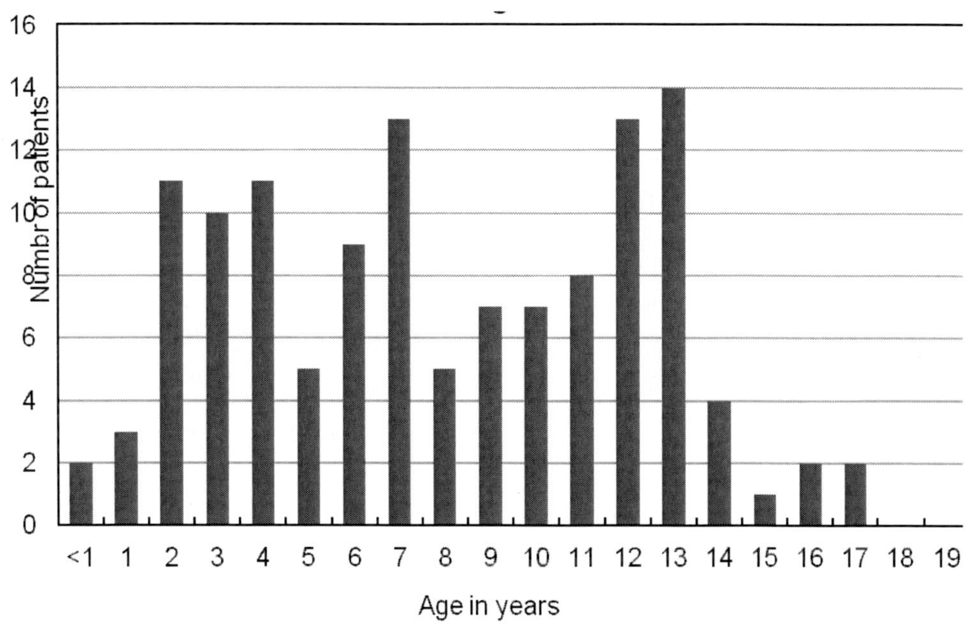

Figure 1. Age at presentation in childhood CIDP compiled from pediatric CIDP series.

The lower extremities are usually much more affected than upper extremities. [16] Nonetheless, a combination of proximal and distal leg weakness is the most common clinical presentation. Deep tendon reflexes are often absent or hypoactive. [6] Significant atrophy is absent. Typically, the affected child develops a gait abnormality manifested by unsteadiness and frequent falls. While a gait abnormality was noted in 29/30 patients at presentation in a large case series, only a minority of patients were non-ambulatory. [6] Respiratory insufficiency and swallowing difficulties are rare. Sensory symptoms such as paresthesias are hardly ever reported. However, this may be due to difficulties in eliciting a comprehensive history in younger children. Back and limb pain can be significant in some patients with the pain preceding clinical weakness by several months. [8] Preceding infections or vaccinations were reported in up to 50% of patients. [8, 14] Notwithstanding, there has been no proven association between vaccination and childhood CIDP.

Childhood CIDP may present with either the more common relapsing-remitting course or with a monophasic course. In a recent review of 143 Childhood CIDP cases, the relapsing-remitting course was observed in 61% and the monophasic course in 39% of patients. [6] The number of relapses, while variable, is usually between 1 and 4 relapses. [6] Patients with more than 10 relapses have been described. [16, 23] While most of the relapses occur within months from discontinuing treatment, some patients relapse after many symptom-free years. [8, 23] Acute and subacute progression of weakness over a period of 4 to 8 weeks is more common in children than in adults. [15, 24,25] In different series, the proportion of cases with acute or subacute onset varied between 30% and 40%. [6, 14] Children who have a monophasic course tend to present with an insidious onset. Nonetheless, either the parents or the child can usually identify the onset.

In addition to the most common presentations, multiple clinical variants are reported in literature in both adults and in children. The widely recognized CIDP variants described in adults, (e.g. MADSAM, DADS, Pure sensory CIDP), are rarely observed in children.

Occasionally, the weakness may predominantly or significantly involve the upper extremities. [8, 13, 14] Hand tremor has being described with upper limb involvement. [13] Although facial weakness is frequently observed, [14] other cranial nerves are hardly ever affected although diplopia is occasionally noted. [16] Bulbar symptoms, dysphagia and dysarthria are rare. Mild respiratory involvement can present in some patients. [8] Rarely, phrenic nerve involvement with significant respiratory failure has being noted. [26] Demyelination of the CNS associated with CIDP was described in children leading to a complex clinical presentation. [27, 28] Rarely, asymmetrical involvement of the limbs is observed. [29] Cases that do not clearly fulfill the diagnostic criteria have also been noted. For these patients, an unequivocal response to immunomodulatory or immunosuppressant treatment may be the only means by which an immune mediated neuropathy can be identified.

Differential Diagnosis

Once the peripheral nervous system involvement is established by the distribution of weakness, presence of areflexia and sensory disturbances, the differential diagnosis is substantially narrowed. In the cases with acute or subacute onset of muscle weakness, the distinction between Guillain Barre Syndrome and Childhood CIDP may be impossible at the time of the initial presentation. This distinction becomes clearer with time. Some authors suggest that markedly slow conduction velocities found early in the course of the Guillain Barre syndrome may suggest a more protracted course, possibly CIDP. [28]

When the child presents with chronic muscle weakness of unclear onset, differentiation between CIDP and much more frequent hereditary neuropathies may be difficult. [17] A positive family history directs the clinician towards a hereditary neuropathy. Parents and siblings should be carefully examined. In the absence of a positive family history, clinical and electrophysiological findings help to establish the diagnosis. The findings of non-uniform, segmental demyelination either on electrophysiological studies or on nerve biopsy favor the diagnosis of an acquired demyelinating polyneuropathy. Of note, Hereditary Neuropathy with liability to Pressure Palsies [HNPP] may present with conduction block at entrapment sites. X-linked CMT due to Connexin-32 mutation may also manifest non-uniform demyelination on nerve conduction studies and temporal dispersion. [30, 31] No improvement with immunotherapy is to be expected in hereditary neuropathies or those due to metabolic derangements.

Notably, some leukodystrophies such as Metachromatic Leukodystrophy [MLD] and Krabbe disease may present with a demyelinating polyneuropathy in isolation and a temporal course compatible with CIDP. Signs and symptoms attributable to CNS involvement (cognitive decline, behavioral problems) follow after a variable period of time. A neuropathy with mixed demyelinating and axonal features has been reported in X-Linked Adrenoleukodystrophy [X-L ALD]. [32] Nerve conduction studies usually reveal evidence of a myelinopathy with uniform slowing. Infrequently, electrophysiological features suggestive of an acquired demyelinating neuropathy (non-uniform slowing, temporal dispersion) are described in patients with MLD, and X-L ALD. [32, 33] Refsum disease should be considered when a patient presents with a demyelinating polyneuropathy with very slow conduction velocities, anosmia, retinitis pigmentosa, ichthyosis and elevated serum phytanic acid. [34]

The temporal course of CIDP is also compatible with peripheral nervous involvement in infectious disorders including Lyme disease, HIV, and diphtheria. Porphyria may present as an acute axonal polyneuropathy whereas certain vasculitides may present as a mononeuritis multiplex, which can be confused with CIDP. Vitamin deficiencies, intoxication with heavy metals and other toxic neuropathies need to be considered in differential diagnosis. Glue sniffing is becoming more prevalent in adolescent population worldwide. The associated glue sniffing neuropathy has both demyelinating and axonal features. [35]

Diagnosis

Diagnostic criteria for Childhood CIDP were last revised in 2002 and are presented in Table 1. [28] The diagnosis of either confirmed or possible CIDP relies on both clinical criteria and supportive laboratory criteria (i.e. electrophysiological, cerebrospinal fluid data and pathology). In addition, one must satisfy a set of exclusionary criteria.

The two mandatory clinical criteria are as follows: 1) Progression of muscle weakness in both proximal and distal muscles of the upper and lower extremities over at least 4 weeks, or alternatively when rapid progression (GBS-like presentation) is followed by relapsing or protracted course for more than 1 year and, 2) Areflexia or hyporeflexia. Progression over more than 4 weeks was accepted in order to better reflect the increased frequency of Childhood CIDP cases with acute and subacute onset when compared to the adult population. The majority of children with CIDP are areflexic at presentation. [6] Preservation of deep tendon reflexes [DTRs] is rare in CIDP and should raise diagnostic doubt. In one series, three patients maintained all their DTRs with reinforcement throughout their illness, while five other patients only maintained DTRs in the upper extremities. [8]

Electrophysiological testing remains essential as the means of establishing the diagnosis of CIDP and excluding other types of neuropathies as well as myopathies or myasthenic syndromes. Presence of conduction block, temporal dispersion and non-uniform slowing of conduction velocities are considered the hallmark of acquired demyelination (e.g. CIDP, AIDP). The Childhood CIDP electrophysiological criteria are adapted from the AAN research criteria. [3] In young children, where nerve segments are short, attention to detail is necessary in order to avoid measurement-associated abnormalities. The study should be extensive and include side-to-side comparisons. Expertise in pediatric electrophysiological studies is recommended.

Lumbar puncture is mandatory if a diagnosis of definite CIDP is to be established. Albuminocytologic dissociation is noted in approximately 90% of patients. [6] Elevated CSF protein was defined as more than 35mg/dl. In one series, CSF protein values ranged between 42-900mg/dl. [8] The WBC count must be less than 10 cells/mm3. It should be recalled that elevated CSF protein levels occur in a number of other hereditary and metabolic demyelinating neuropathies. [36] CSF protein levels tend to remain elevated after treatment, independent of the patient's clinical outcome. [8] Nerve biopsy is neither routinely performed nor is it considered mandatory in order to establish a definitive diagnosis of Childhood CIDP. [28] The nerve biopsy findings in CIDP are relatively inconsistent and highly variable.

Table 1. Diagnostic criteria Childhood CIDP

Mandatory clinical criteria: 1. Progression of muscle weakness in proximal and distal muscles of upper and lower extremities over at least 4 weeks, or alternatively when rapid progression (GBS-like presentation) is followed by relapsing or protracted course. (more than 1 year). 2. Areflexia or hyporeflexia
A.1. Major laboratory features A.1.1. Electrophysiological criteria Must demonstrate at least three of the following four abnormalities in motor nerves (or 2 of the major plus 2 of the supportive criteria): A.1.1.1. Major 1. Conduction block or abnormal temporal dispersion in one or more nerves at sites not prone to compression. (a)Conduction block: at least 50% drop in negative peak area or peak-to-peak amplitude of proximal compound muscle action potential (CMAP) if duration of negative peak of proximal CMAP is <130% of distal CMAP duration. (b)Temporal dispersion: abnormal if duration of negative peak of proximal CMAP is <130% of distal CMAP duration. Recommendations: (a) Conduction block and temporal dispersion can be assessed only in nerves where amplitude of distal CMAP is >1mV. (b) Supramaximal stimulation should always be used. 2. Reduction in conduction velocity (CV) in two or more nerves: <75% of the mean minus 2 standard deviations (SD) CV value for age 3. Prolonged distal latency (DL) in two or more nerves: >130%of the mean + 2 SD DL value for age 4. Absent F waves or prolonged F wave minimal latency (ML) in two or more nerves: >130% of the mean + 2SD F wave ML for age. 5. Recommendation: F wave study should include a minimum of 10 trials. A.1.1.2. Supportive 1. When conduction block is absent, the following abnormal electrophysiological parameters are indicative of non-uniform slowing and thus of an acquired neuropathy: 2. Abnormal median sensory nerve action potential (SNAP) while the sural nerve SNAP is normal. 3. Abnormal minimal latency index (TLI) 4. Differences of >10 m/s in motor CVs between nerves of upper or lower limbs (either different nerves from the same limb for example left median versus left ulnar or the same nerve from different sides for example left versus right ulnar nerves).

A.1.2. Cerebrospinal fluid (CSF studies) CSF protein >35 mg/dl. Cell count < 10 cells/mm^3
A.1.3. Nerve biopsy features Nerve biopsy with predominant features of demyelination A.1.3.1. Exclusion criteria 1. Clinical features or history of a hereditary neuropathy, other diseases or exposure to drugs or toxins that are known to cause peripheral neuropathy 2. Laboratory findings (including nerve biopsy or DNA studies) that show evidence for a different etiology other than CIDP.

Nerve biopsy may demonstrate inflammatory infiltrates containing a mixture of CD4 and CD8 T lymphocytes, segmental demyelination and onion bulb formation. [28] A normal nerve biopsy does not rule out CIDP as the sural nerve segment biopsied may not be affected by the demyelinating process. Earlier pediatric series reported a high frequency of abnormal nerve biopsies with the most common abnormality identified as a reduced density of myelinated fibers. Inflammatory infiltrates were reported in 6/10 in one case series and 6/15 in another. [8, 13]

The role of magnetic resonance evaluation in CIDP has yet to be determined. To date, it has not been part of the diagnostic criteria. Gadolinium enhanced magnetic resonance imaging of the spinal cord often reveals nerve root enhancement. In a recent series, only 8/21 patients (38%) had MRI images that demonstrated enhancement or thickening of the nerve roots. [6] Other series have documented enhancement of lumbosacral roots in children with CIDP as well. [8, 37, 38]

At times, the enhancement can be subtle. [37] Less frequently, nerve root enlargement is noted. [6, 37] Of note, the presence of nerve root enhancement and/or enlargement did not correlate with either the clinical presentation or the clinical course. [6] Although not routinely recommended, gadolinium enhanced MRI of the lumbosacral spine can provide supportive evidence in favor of CIDP. Enlargement of the nerve roots is rarely observed in the dysmyelinating form of Charcot Marie Tooth disease [CMT IA]. [37, 39, 40] Notably, lumbosacral nerve root enhancement is much more frequently seen in pediatric Guillain Barre Syndrome. [41]

Infrequently, one will encounter situations where diagnostic criteria for CIDP are not met, despite careful and exhaustive laboratory evaluations. In these situations, an unequivocal response to intravenous immunoglobulin is considered compelling evidence for acquired demyelination [42]

Pathogenesis of CIDP

No clear evidence exists to suggest that the pathophysiology of Childhood CIDP is in any significant way different than adult CIDP. Evidence in favor of an autoimmune etiology include antecedent infections or vaccinations are reported in a significant proportion of cases, demyelinating findings on electrodiagnostic studies or nerve biopsy and a positive response to immunosuppressive or immunomodulatory treatments. The interactions between the cell-mediated and humoral responses in CIDP have been reviewed by Koller et al. [43] and Dalakas MC [44] Although the antigen or antigens implicated in the autoimmune process have not yet been identified, there are compelling data to suggest that both cell-mediated and humoral immune responses are involved. It is believed that activated T-cells cross the blood-nerve interface, undergo clonal expansion and secrete soluble factors, which stimulate the endoneurial population of macrophages. Macrophages secrete neurotoxic molecules that demonstrate increased phagocytosis and cytotoxic activity against the myelin sheath and Schwann cells. The involvement of the humoral response in pathogenesis of CIDP is suggested by the deposition of immunoglobulin and complement on myelinated fibers. [45] At least in some patients with CIDP, humoral factors seem to be important as demonstrated by the induction of demyelination and conduction block in rat nerves by transfer of serum and purified IgG from patients with CIDP. [46] Both myelin proteins (myelin protein zero, gangliosides) [47-49] and non-myelin Schwann cell antigens have been proposed as potential antigens. [50] Although molecular mimicry may play a role in CIDP [48, 51], it does not fully explain its pathogenesis. While anti-ganglioside GM1 antibodies have being demonstrated in adult CIDP, specific antibodies were not found in children with CIDP.

Management of Childhood CIDP

No prospective trials evaluating the response of Childhood CIDP to different therapies are available. The current recommendations are based on retrospective reviews of generally small series of children and expert opinions. In addition, the few reported series reflect the treatments available at the time of publication. Similar to other pediatric autoimmune neuromuscular conditions, the therapies have been adopted from studies in adult patients.

Immunosuppressant and immunomodulatory therapies are the mainstay of treatment in both adult and childhood CIDP. The three commonly employed first line therapies are IVIG, oral corticosteroids and plasma exchange. Their efficacy has being demonstrated in prospective studies in adults and retrospective studies in children. A treatment algorithm for childhood CIDP has been proposed. IVIG therapy should be considered the first line of treatment for children with CIDP based on the generally positive response and favorable side effect profile. In the adult population, approximately one third of patients will require steroids or IVIG-sparing agents. In contrast, the use of these agents in children is rarely necessary. A thorough initial evaluation is necessary in order to document treatment response such as the use of a disability scale (e.g. modified Rankin scale). A child with minimal symptoms, which do not interfere with daily activities, should not be treated. Before any treatment is prescribed, the author recommends a comprehensive discussion of the risks and benefits with the parents or guardians.

IVIG

The short-term efficacy of IVIG in adult CIDP has being clearly established with randomized placebo-controlled studies. [52-55] Hughes et al. reported that its efficacy is maintained long-term. [55]

Table 2. Response to IVIG monotherapy in Childhood CIDP

Childhood CIDP Series	Total patients reported per series	Patients with initial IVIG monotherapy	Good /Marked response	Unsatisfactory /No response	Patients who needed other therapy than initial IVIG	Patients in remission after IVIG monotherapy[a]	Comments
McMillan et al. 2012[6]	30	25	20	5	5	6	Some patients had limited follow up
Riekhoff et al. 2012[76]	3	3	1	2	3	0	One patient was atypical
Jo et al. 2010[21]	7	6	6	0	1	5	
Teasley 2008[63]	5	5	3	2	1	4	
Rossignol et al. 2007[16]	13	3	3	0	3	0	All responded well initially, but required retreatment or additional therapies for recurrences. No mention on how long IVIG monotherapy was tried before adding other therapy
Ryan et al. 2000[8]	16	4	3	1	1	3	None of the patients received IVIG for more than 5 months
Hattori et al. 1998[13]	10	2	1	1	1	1	
Simmons et al. 1997[9]	12	5	5	0	0	3	
Korinthenberg et al. 1999[20]	21	12	10	2	6	4	
Total	117	65	52 (80%)	13 (20%)		26 (40%)	

[a]Patients in remission after IVIG monotherapy currently on no treatment and with minimal or no disability.

Legend: CIDP-Chronic Inflammatory Demyelinating Polyneuropathy; IVIG-Intravenous immunoglobulin;

When compared to oral corticosteroids and plasma exchange, IVIG was reported to have equal efficacy in adult patients over the short term as well [56, 57]. Which of the multitude of the postulated immunoregulatory mechanisms is important in patients with CIDP remains unclear. IVIG has replaced corticosteroids as the first line of treatment for childhood CIDP in the last decade. Table 2 presents the available retrospective data compiled from a number of pediatric series.

IVIG produces a good response in majority of patients (80%) given that 40% of patients who received IVIG as monotherapy were in remission (receiving no treatment and manifesting few or minimal symptoms) and an additional 15% of children with CIDP entered into long term remission after one or two IVIG courses. [28] In children, as well as in adults, IVIG has been used in a number of autoimmune neurologic and non-neurologic conditions and has been found to be generally safe and well tolerated. [58] The most common side effects are headache, fever, chills and rash, which are thought to be on the basis of an allergic reaction. These usually respond well to premedication with acetaminophen and an antihistamine (e.g. diphenhydramine) and a slow infusion rate. More serious side effects including thromboembolic events, aseptic meningitis, reversible renal insufficiency and severe allergic reactions are very rare in children. IVIG is generally administered over 2 consecutive days at a dose of 1gm/kg/day whereas other authors prefer to administer 0.4gm/kg/day for 5 consecutive days. The improvement is usually rapid even when transient. Repeated courses of 0.4-2gm/kg/course are given at 3-6 weeks intervals depending on the patient's treatment response. Adjustments with respect to the dose and interval of administration are necessary over time. One must remember that a significant proportion of patient will undergo remission such that the need for IVIG ought to be reevaluated at regular intervals in order to avoid unnecessary treatment. Subcutaneous Immunoglobulin (SCIg), which is better suited for home administration, has been used with success in adult patients with CIDP. [59] However, the author was unable to locate any evidence based medicine regarding its use in childhood CIDP. Nonetheless, SCIg has been administered with success in pediatric patients with Primary Immunodeficiencies. [60, 61] As such, SCIg may be an option for patients who require long-term immunoglobulin administration.

Corticosteroids

Responsiveness to corticosteroids is one of the differentiating factors between CIDP and the Guillain Barre Syndrome. Oral steroids, prednisone and prednisolone, have been used as the first line treatment in the previous decades. In the last two decades, steroids have been replaced by IVIG as the treatment of first choice in childhood CIDP. [6] While corticosteroids are less expensive than IvIg, their long-term negative consequences tend to negate any cost savings. A discussion of oral steroids versus IVIG as initial treatment in Childhood CIDP has been reviewed elsewhere. [62, 63] Oral corticosteroids have been reported to have similar efficacy to IVIG in both children [6] and adults. [56] Oral corticosteroids can be used as monotherapy in children. However, a proportion of children will not respond to corticosteroids alone and will require either a change in treatment or the addition of other agents. The usual starting dose of 1-2mg/kg/day (60-80mg/day for older teenagers) is initiated for 4-8 weeks followed by a slow taper over 3-6 months. In one series, the clinical improvement on oral corticosteroids was noted within one month in majority of patients. [8]

In another series, the response was noted within one week in majority of patients. [15] Relapses during the tapering phase were treated with reinstitution of the initial starting dose for 4 weeks followed by another attempt with a slower taper. [8] Alternate day administration of corticosteroids should be considered when long periods of steroid treatment are expected in order to minimize their side effects. These side effects are more common with higher doses and longer treatment duration including weight gain, short stature, poor bone health, behavioral disturbances, immunusuppression, hypertension, cataract formation, hyperglycemia and dyspepsia. Adequate calcium intake and monitoring of the serum Vitamin D level is recommended. Other recommendations include insuring the presence of protective varicella antibody titers and a negative tuberculin test. Intravenous steroids such as methylprednisolone have being employed as a means of achieving rapid improvement in a child with significant weakness.[8]

Plasma Exchange

Plasma exchange [PEX] has been demonstrated to be effective in adults with CIDP. [64, 65] Its efficacy in adult population is similar to that of IVIG and oral steroids. [57, 66] Nonetheless, its beneficial effect is transient and must be repeated when used long-term. In childhood CIDP, its efficacy seems to be significantly lower than in adults. Only 14% of patients had a good response to PEX when it was employed as the initial therapy. [6] The risks of PEX include hypotension, sepsis, pneumothorax, pulmonary embolism and electrolyte imbalance. Vascular access is especially problematic in young children. Although PEX is not considered a first line treatment in children with CIDP, it remains a therapeutic option in refractory cases.

Other Immunosuppressant Agents

A number of immunosuppressants have being reported to be useful in adult CIDP patients including azathioprine, cyclosporine, cyclophosphamide, methotrexate, mycophenolate mofetil, and rituximab. The data available regarding the use of such agents in children is very limited. Azathioprine inhibits purine metabolism and affects rapidly dividing cells, including lymphocytes. It has been used in adults for its steroid-sparing effects. Azathioprine was reported as being beneficial in a number of small case series of adult CIDP. [67, 68] In an open parallel study of oral steroids vs. oral steroids and azathioprine for 9 months, no significant differences between the two treatment groups were noted. Limitations of this study included a small number of patients, the dosage used and the short duration of follow up. [69] Azathioprine is the most used steroid sparing oral immunosuppressant agent in Childhood CIDP. [6, 16, 20] A number of studies report a positive effect when azathioprine is added to corticosteroids. Its use is limited by potential serious side effects and a significant delay in clinical response (3-12 months). The usual initial dose in children is 1 mg/kg/day given in one or two divided doses. This initial dose is increased in 0.5 mg/kg/day increments every 4 weeks up to a maximum of 2.5 mg/kg/day. The duration of treatment has not been clearly established. The maximum dose is maintained for 12-24 months followed by a slow taper. [28] Leukocyte counts and liver function tests need to be monitored every week for the first month and monthly thereafter. Cyclosporine was reported to be of no benefit in a small series of CIDP patients reported by Nevo et al. and Ryan et al. [8, 14] Some improvement with cyclophosphamide was reported in two patients. [8, 16] Given the significant toxicity of cyclophosphamide, its use would be difficult to justify this agent's use in the pediatric population. Methotrexate, a relatively less expensive and better tolerated agent, was reported to be effective in a few pediatric patients. [8, 14] Positive results were reported in adults as well. [70] Rituximab is a chimeric monoclonal antibody against the CD20 antigen on B-cells. It is approved for the treatment of B-cell lymphoma and rheumatoid arthritis. It has been used off- label in refractory cases of pediatric autoimmune myasthenia gravis [71] as well as in few cases of refractory Childhood CIDP with a reported benefit. [16, 72]

However, the adult literature does not clearly support Rituximab as a significant therapeutic modality in CIDP. Mycophenolate mofetil was found to be beneficial in one patient. [6] Its advantages over other immunosuppressants include relatively milder bone marrow suppression and a more rapid onset of action. In adult patients, mycophenolate mofetil allowed for concomitant reduction of oral corticosteroid and IVIG doses. [73, 74] A few adults with severe disease that were not responding to multiple agents underwent stem cell transplantation with positive results. [75] To date, the author has not identified a case report of a child who underwent stem cell transplantation for CIDP.

Table 3. Response to corticosteroids monotherapy in Childhood CIDP

Childhood CIDP Series	Total patients reported per series	Patients with initial corticosteroid monotherapy	Good /Marked response	Unsatisfactory /No response to initial corticosteroid therapy	Patients who needed other therapy than initial corticosteroids	Patients in remission after corticosteroids monotherapy[a]
Rossignol et al. 2007[16]	13	8	8	0	3	4
Rodriquez-Casero et al. 2005[15]	5	4	3	1	1	3
Ryan et al. 2000[8]	16	11	11	0	5	4[b]
Korinthenberg et al. 1999[20]	21	11	8	3	6	2
Hattori et al. 1998[13]	10	6	4	2	2	3[b]
Simmons et al. 1997[9]	12	3	3	0	1	2
Nevo et al. 1996[14]	13	13	13	0	8	3[b]
Uncini et al. 1991[17]	5	4	4	0	0	3[b]
Total	95	60	54 (90%)	6(10%)	26(43%)	24 (40%)

[a]Patients in remission after corticosteroids monotherapy currently on no treatment and with minimal or no disability.

[b]Patients assumed to be in remission off therapy, but not clearly stated in the respective articles.

Legend: CIDP-Chronic Inflammatory Demyelinating Polyneuropathy; IVIG-Intravenous immunoglobulin; nr-not reported.

Outcome in Childhood CIDP

In general, Childhood CIDP has a good prognosis. The rate of spontaneous remission (with no immunosuppressant or immunomodulatory therapy) is probably very low although natural history studies are lacking.

As noted from Tables 2 and 3, the overall rate of remission with monotherapy (either IVIG or corticosteroids) is approximately 40%. The majority of children will respond clinically. Modified Rankin scale [MRS] scores at presentation varied between 4.4 (Hattori et al. [13]) and 2.8 (McMillan et al. [6]). At the last follow up, MRS varied between 0.2 (Simmons et al. [23]) and 1.9 (Hattori et al. [13]). In the McMillan et al. series, of the 23 patients who had long term follow up, 9 were either asymptomatic or minimally symptomatic off treatment. Despite a generally good prognosis, occasional patients may pose significant therapeutic challenges and require multiple therapeutic interventions while remaining severely affected. Others will require long-term treatment with either IVIG or corticosteroids with or without adjunctive therapies.

Conclusion

Childhood CIDP is a rare immune mediated disorder of the peripheral nervous system, which tends to have a good outcome when correctly diagnosed and treated. Electrophysiological testing is essential in reaching the correct diagnosis. Current data supports the use of IVIG and corticosteroids as monotherapy with good results in the majority of patients. Some patients will require long-term treatment. Immunosuppressant drugs other than steroids are rarely necessary.

References

[1] McLeod J. G., Pollard J. D., Macaskill P., Mohamed A., Spring P., Khurana V. Prevalence of chronic inflammatory demyelinating polyneuropathy in New South Wales, Australia. *Ann Neurol.*, 1999; 46:910-913.

[2] Chio A., Cocito D., Bottacchi E., et al. Idiopathic chronic inflammatory demyelinating polyneuropathy: an epidemiological study in Italy. *J Neurol. Neurosurg. Psychiatry*, 2007; 78:1349-1353.

[3] Research criteria for diagnosis of chronic inflammatory demyelinating polyneuropathy (CIDP). Report from an Ad Hoc Subcommittee of the American Academy of Neurology AIDS Task Force. Neurology 1991; 41:617-618.

[4] Van den Bergh P. Y., Hadden R. D., Bouche P., et al. European Federation of Neurological Societies/Peripheral Nerve Society guideline on management of chronic inflammatory demyelinating polyradiculoneuropathy: report of a joint task force of the European Federation of Neurological Societies and the Peripheral Nerve Society - first revision. *Eur. J. Neurol.*, 2010; 17:356-363.

[5] Rajabally Y. A., Simpson B. S., Beri S., Bankart J., Gosalakkal J. A. Epidemiologic variability of chronic inflammatory demyelinating polyneuropathy with different diagnostic criteria: study of a UK population. *Muscle Nerve*, 2009; 39:432-438.
[6] McMillan H. J., Kang P. B., Jones H. R., Darras B. T. Childhood chronic inflammatory demyelinating polyradiculoneuropathy: Combined analysis of a large cohort and eleven published series. *Neuromuscular Disord.*, 2012; 23:103-111.
[7] Iijima M., Koike H., Hattori N., et al. Prevalence and incidence rates of chronic inflammatory demyelinating polyneuropathy in the Japanese population. *J. Neurol. Neurosurg. Psychiatry*, 2008; 79:1040-1043.
[8] Ryan M. M., Grattan-Smith P. J., Procopis P. G., Morgan G., Ouvrier R. A. Childhood chronic inflammatory demyelinating polyneuropathy: clinical course and long-term outcome. *Neuromuscular Disord.*, 2000; 10:398-406.
[9] Simmons Z., Wald J. J., Albers J. W. Chronic inflammatory demyelinating polyradiculoneuropathy in children: I. Presentation, electrodiagnostic studies, and initial clinical course, with comparison to adults. *Muscle Nerve,* 1997; 20:1008-1015.
[10] Majumdar A., Hartley L., Manzur A. Y., King R. H., Orrell R. W., Muntoni F. A case of severe congenital chronic inflammatory demyelinating polyneuropathy with complete spontaneous remission. *Neuromuscular Disord.*, 2004; 14:818-821.
[11] Pasternak J. F., Fulling K., Nelson J., Prensky A. L. An infant with chronic relapsing polyneuropathy responsive to steroids. *Dev. Med. Child Neurol.*, 1982; 24:504-524.
[12] Sladky J. T., Brown M. J., Berman P. H. Chronic inflammatory demyelinating polyneuropathy of infancy: a corticosteroid-responsive disorder. *Ann. Neurol.*, 1986; 20:76-81.
[13] Hattori N., Ichimura M., Aoki S., et al. Clinicopathological features of chronic inflammatory demyelinating polyradiculoneuropathy in childhood. *J. Neurol. Sci.,* 1998; 154:66-71.
[14] Nevo Y., Pestronk A., Kornberg A. J., et al. Childhood chronic inflammatory demyelinating neuropathies: clinical course and long-term follow-up. *Neurology*, 1996; 47:98-102.
[15] Rodriguez-Casero M. V., Shield L. K., Kornberg A. J. Subacute inflammatory demyelinating polyneuropathy in children. *Neurology*, 2005; 64:1786-1788.
[16] Rossignol E., D'Anjou G., Lapointe N., Haddad E., Vanasse M. Evolution and treatment of childhood chronic inflammatory polyneuropathy. *Pediatr. Neurol.*, 2007; 36:88-94.
[17] Uncini A., Parano E., Lange D. J., De Vivo D. C., Lovelace R. E. Chronic inflammatory demyelinating polyneuropathy in childhood: clinical and electrophysiological features. *Childs Nerv. Syst.,* 1991; 7:191-196.
[18] Colan RV, Snead OC, 3rd, Oh SJ, Benton JW, Jr. Steroid-responsive polyneuropathy with subacute onset in childhood. J Pediatr 1980; 97:374-377.
[19] Vedanarayanan V. V., Kandt R. S., Lewis D. V., Jr., DeLong G. R. Chronic inflammatory demyelinating polyradiculoneuropathy of childhood: treatment with high-dose intravenous immunoglobulin. *Neurology,* 1991; 41:828-830.
[20] Korinthenberg R. Chronic inflammatory demyelinating polyradiculoneuropathy in children and their response to treatment. *Neuropediatrics*, 1999; 30:190-196.
[21] Jo H. Y., Park M. G., Kim D. S., Nam S. O., Park K. H. Chronic inflammatory demyelinating polyradiculoneuropathy in children: characterized by subacute,

predominantly motor dominant polyeuropathy with a favorable response to the treatment. *Acta. Neurol. Scand.*, 2010; 121:342-347.

[22] Luan X., Zheng R., Chen B., Yuan Y. Childhood chronic inflammatory demyelinating polyneuropathy with nonuniform pathologic features. *Pediatr. Neurol.*, 2010; 43:103-109.

[23] Simmons Z., Wald J. J., Albers J. W. Chronic inflammatory demyelinating polyradiculoneuropathy in children: II. Long-term follow-up, with comparison to adults. *Muscle Nerve*, 1997; 20:1569-1575.

[24] Hattori N., Misu K., Koike H., et al. Age of onset influences clinical features of chronic inflammatory demyelinating polyneuropathy. *J. Neurol. Sci.*, 2001; 184:57-63.

[25] Hughes R., Sanders E., Hall S., Atkinson P., Colchester A., Payan P. Subacute idiopathic demyelinating polyradiculoneuropathy. *Arch. Neurol.*, 1992; 49:612-616.

[26] Polat M., Tosun A., Serdaroglu G., et al. Chronic inflammatory demyelinating polyradiculopathy: an atypical pediatric case complicated with phrenic nerve palsy. *Turk. J. Pediatr.*, 2007; 49:210-214.

[27] Rotta F. T., Sussman A. T., Bradley W. G., Ram Ayyar D., Sharma K. R., Shebert R. T. The spectrum of chronic inflammatory demyelinating polyneuropathy. *J. Neurol. Sci.*, 2000; 173:129-139.

[28] Nevo Y., Topaloglu H. 88th ENMC international workshop: childhood chronic inflammatory demyelinating polyneuropathy (including revised diagnostic criteria), Naarden, The Netherlands, December 8-10, 2000. *Neuromuscular Disord.*, 2002; 12:195-200.

[29] McDonald D. G., Farrell M. A., McMenamin J. B. Focal upper limb neuropathy in a child. *Eur. J. Paediatr. Neurol.*, 2000; 4:283-287.

[30] Gutierrez A., England J. D., Sumner A. J., et al. Unusual electrophysiological findings in X-linked dominant Charcot-Marie-Tooth disease. *Muscle Nerve*, 2000; 23:182-188.

[31] Sakaguchi H., Yamashita S., Miura A., et al. A novel GJB1 frameshift mutation produces a transient CNS symptom of X-linked Charcot-Marie-Tooth disease. *J. Neurol.*, 2011; 258:284-290.

[32] Chaudhry V., Moser H. W., Cornblath D. R. Nerve conduction studies in adrenomyeloneuropathy. *J. Neurol. Neurosurg. Psychiatry*, 1996; 61:181-185.

[33] Cameron C. L., Kang P. B., Burns T. M., Darras B. T., Jones H. R., Jr. Multifocal slowing of nerve conduction in metachromatic leukodystrophy. *Muscle Nerve*, 2004; 29:531-536.

[34] Wanders R. J., Jansen G. A., Skjeldal O. H. Refsum disease, peroxisomes and phytanic acid oxidation: a review. *J. Neuropathol. Exp. Neurol.*, 2001; 60:1021-1031.

[35] Kuwabara S., Kai M. R., Nagase H., Hattori T. n-Hexane neuropathy caused by addictive inhalation: clinical and electrophysiological features. *Eur. Neurol.*, 1999; 41:163-167.

[36] Hagberg B., Lyon G. Pooled European series of hereditary peripheral neuropathies in infancy and childhood. A "correspondence work shop" report of the European Federation of Child Neurology Societies (EFCNS). *Neuropediatrics,* 1981; 12:9-17.

[37] Midroni G., de Tilly L. N., Gray B., Vajsar J. MRI of the cauda equina in CIDP: clinical correlations. *J. Neurol. Sci.*, 1999; 170:36-44.

[38] Likasitwattanakul S., Visrutaratna P. Chronic inflammatory demyelinating polyneuropathy in a child: clinical-spinal MR imaging correlation. *Singapore Med. J.*, 2004; 45:536-537.
[39] Liao J. P., Waclawik A. J. Nerve root hypertrophy in CMT type 1A. *Neurology,* 2004; 62:783.
[40] Ishigami N., Kondo M., Nakagawa M. [Case of Charcot-Marie-Tooth disease type 1A with increased cerebrospinal fluid proteins and nerve root hypertrophy]. *Rinsho Shinkeigaku* 2008; 48:419-421.
[41] Mulkey S. B., Glasier C. M., El-Nabbout B., et al. Nerve root enhancement on spinal MRI in pediatric Guillain-Barre syndrome. *Pediatr. Neurol.*, 2010; 43:263-269.
[42] Mohamed A. R., Rodriguez-Casero M. V., Ryan M. M. Atypical childhood chronic inflammatory demyelinating polyneuropathy. *Muscle Nerve*, 2010; 42:293-295.
[43] Koller H., Kieseier B. C., Jander S., Hartung H. P. Chronic inflammatory demyelinating polyneuropathy. *N. Engl. J. Med.,* 2005; 352:1343-1356.
[44] Dalakas M. C., Medscape. Advances in the diagnosis, pathogenesis and treatment of CIDP. *Nat. Rev. Neurol.*, 2011; 7:507-517.
[45] Dalakas M. C., Engel W. K. Immunoglobulin and complement deposits in nerves of patients with chronic relapsing polyneuropathy. *Arch. Neurol.*, 1980; 37:637-640.
[46] Yan W. X., Taylor J., Andrias-Kauba S., Pollard J. D. Passive transfer of demyelination by serum or IgG from chronic inflammatory demyelinating polyneuropathy patients. *Ann. Neurol.*, 2000; 47:765-775.
[47] Yan W. X., Archelos J. J., Hartung H. P., Pollard J. D. P0 protein is a target antigen in chronic inflammatory demyelinating polyradiculoneuropathy. *Ann. Neurol.,* 2001; 50:286-292.
[48] Melendez-Vasquez C., Redford J., Choudhary P. P., et al. Immunological investigation of chronic inflammatory demyelinating polyradiculoneuropathy. *J. Neuroimmunol.,* 1997; 73:124-134.
[49] Kuwahara M., Suzuki S., Takada K., Kusunoki S. Antibodies to LM1 and LM1-containing ganglioside complexes in Guillain-Barre syndrome and chronic inflammatory demyelinating polyneuropathy. *J. Neuroimmunol.*, 2011; 239:87-90.
[50] Kwa M. S., van Schaik I. N., De Jonge R. R., et al. Autoimmunoreactivity to Schwann cells in patients with inflammatory neuropathies. *Brain*, 2003; 126:361-375.
[51] Weiss M. D., Luciano C. A., Semino-Mora C., Dalakas M. C., Quarles R. H. Molecular mimicry in chronic inflammatory demyelinating polyneuropathy and melanoma. *Neurology*, 1998; 51:1738-1741.
[52] Thompson N., Choudhary P., Hughes R. A., Quinlivan R. M. A novel trial design to study the effect of intravenous immunoglobulin in chronic inflammatory demyelinating polyradiculoneuropathy. *J. Neurol.*, 1996; 243:280-285.
[53] Hahn A. F., Bolton C. F., Zochodne D., Feasby T. E. Intravenous immunoglobulin treatment in chronic inflammatory demyelinating polyneuropathy. A double-blind, placebo-controlled, cross-over study. *Brain*, 1996; 119:1067-1077.
[54] Mendell J. R., Barohn R. J., Freimer M. L., et al. Randomized controlled trial of IVIg in untreated chronic inflammatory demyelinating polyradiculoneuropathy. *Neurology,* 2001; 56:445-449.
[55] Hughes R. A., Donofrio P., Bril V., et al. Intravenous immune globulin (10% caprylate-chromatography purified) for the treatment of chronic inflammatory demyelinating

polyradiculoneuropathy (ICE study): a randomised placebo-controlled trial. *Lancet Neurol.*, 2008; 7:136-144.
[56] Hughes R., Bensa S., Willison H., et al. Randomized controlled trial of intravenous immunoglobulin versus oral prednisolone in chronic inflammatory demyelinating polyradiculoneuropathy. *Ann. Neurol.*, 2001; 50:195-201.
[57] Dyck P. J., Litchy W. J., Kratz K. M., et al. A plasma exchange versus immune globulin infusion trial in chronic inflammatory demyelinating polyradiculoneuropathy. *Ann. Neurol.,* 1994; 36:838-845.
[58] Jolles S., Sewell W. A., Misbah S. A. Clinical uses of intravenous immunoglobulin. *Clin. Exp. Immunol.*, 2005; 142:1-11.
[59] Cocito D., Serra G., Falcone Y., Paolasso I. The efficacy of subcutaneous immunoglobulin administration in chronic inflammatory demyelinating polyneuropathy responders to intravenous immunoglobulin. *J. Peripher. Nerv. Syst.,* 2011; 16:150-152.
[60] Borte M., Pac M., Serban M., et al. Efficacy and safety of hizentra(R), a new 20% immunoglobulin preparation for subcutaneous administration, in pediatric patients with primary immunodeficiency. *J. Clin. Immunol.,* 2011; 31:752-761.
[61] Gallagher J. L., Patel N. C. Subcutaneous immunoglobulin replacement therapy with Hizentra(R) is safe and effective in two infants. *J. Clin. Immunol.*, 2012; 32:474-476.
[62] Sladky J. T. What is the best initial treatment for childhood chronic inflammatory demyelinating polyneuropathy: corticosteroids or intravenous immunoglobulin? *Muscle Nerve,* 2008; 38:1638-1643.
[63] Teasley J. E. Initial treatment of childhood chronic inflammatory demyelinating polyradiculoneuropathy. *Muscle Nerve*, 2008; 38:1640-1643.
[64] Dyck P. J., Daube J., O'Brien P., et al. Plasma exchange in chronic inflammatory demyelinating polyradiculoneuropathy. *N. Eng. J. Med.,* 1986; 314:461-465.
[65] Hahn A. F., Bolton C. F., Pillay N., et al. Plasma-exchange therapy in chronic inflammatory demyelinating polyneuropathy. A double-blind, sham-controlled, cross-over study. *Brain,* 1996 119:1055-1066.
[66] Gorson K. C., Allam G., Ropper A. H. Chronic inflammatory demyelinating polyneuropathy: clinical features and response to treatment in 67 consecutive patients with and without a monoclonal gammopathy. *Neurology*, 1997; 48:321-328.
[67] Dalakas M. C., Engel W. K. Chronic relapsing (dysimmune) polyneuropathy: pathogenesis and treatment. *Ann. Neurol.,* 1981; 9:134-145.
[68] McCombe P. A., Pollard J. D., McLeod J. G. Chronic inflammatory demyelinating polyradiculoneuropathy. A clinical and electrophysiological study of 92 cases. *Brain,* 1987; 110:1617-1630.
[69] Dyck P. J., O'Brien P., Swanson C., Low P., Daube J. Combined azathioprine and prednisone in chronic inflammatory-demyelinating polyneuropathy. *Neurology,* 1985; 35:1173-1176.
[70] Fialho D., Chan Y. C., Allen D. C., Reilly M. M., Hughes R. A. Treatment of chronic inflammatory demyelinating polyradiculoneuropathy with methotrexate. *J. Neurol. Neurosurg. Psychiatry,* 2006; 77:544-547.
[71] Tzaribachev N., Koetter I., Kuemmerle-Deschner J. B., Schedel J. Rituximab for the treatment of refractory pediatric autoimmune diseases: a case series. *Cases J.* 2009; 2:6609.

[72] D'Amico A., Catteruccia M., De Benedetti F., et al. *Rituximab in a childhood-onset idiopathic refractory chronic inflammatory demyelinating polyneuropathy.* 2012; 16:301-303.

[73] Gorson K. C., Amato A. A., Ropper A. H. Efficacy of mycophenolate mofetil in patients with chronic immune demyelinating polyneuropathy. *Neurology,* 2004; 63:715-717.

[74] Benedetti L., Grandis M., Nobbio L., et al. Mycophenolate mofetil in dysimmune neuropathies: a preliminary study. *Muscle Nerve*, 2004; 29:748-749.

[75] Kazmi M. A., Mahdi-Rogers M., Sanvito L. Chronic inflammatory demyelinating polyradiculoneuropathy: a role for haematopoietic stem cell transplantation? *Autoimmunity*, 2008; 41:611-615.

[76] Riekhoff A. G., Jadoul C., Mercelis R., Cras P., Ceulemans B. P. Childhood chronic inflammatory demyelinating polyneuroradiculopathy--three cases and a review of the literature. *Eur. J. Paediatr. Neurol.*, 2012; 16:315-331.

In: Contemporary Issues in Peripheral Neuropathy
Editor: Daniel L. Menkes
ISBN: 978-1-62948-681-9

Chapter VII

Monoclonal Gammopathy of Undetermined Significance and Polyneuropathy

Kam Newman[1,#], ***Ihab El-Hemaidi***[2,†], ***Jagar A. Jasem***[3,‡] ***and Mojtaba Akhtari***[4,*]

[1]Section of Transfusion Medicine, Cleveland Clinic Foundation, Cleveland, OH, US
[2]Adult Hematology/BMT, Princess Noorah Oncology Center MBC-6447, King Abdulaziz Medical City-Western Region, National Guard Health Affairs, Kingdom of Saudi Arabia
[3]Department of Neurology, Ohio State University, Columbus, Ohio, US
[4]Division of Hematology and Oncology, Department of Internal Medicine, University of Nebraska Medical Center, Omaha, NE, US

Abstract

Monoclonal gammopathies are heterogeneous group of disorders characterized by unregulated production and deposition of monoclonal (M) protein or paraproteins by proliferation of a clone of plasma cells or B lymphocytes. Paraproteins are consist of two same class and subclass heavy polypeptide chains (G, M, or A) and two same type light polypeptide chains (kappa or lambda). IgG is the most common paraproteins, and less than 15% is IgM. Monoclonal gammopathy without any association with plasma cell dyscrasia occurs in 1% of general population and increases to 10% in older than 80 years. Monoclonal gammopathy with undetermined significance (MGUS) is the most common type of gammopathies which occurs in the absence of malignancy but multiple myeloma

[#] E-mail: Newmank3@ccf.org.
[†] Email: HemaidiIH@NGHA.MED.SA.
[‡] E-mail: jagar.abdullah@yahoo.com.
[*] Tel: 402-559-3834; Fax: 402-559-6520; E-mail: mojtaba.akhtari@unmc.edu.

and Waldenstrom's macroglobulinemia occur in the context of systemic malignant disorder.

Neuropathies are defined as damage to or degeneration of sensory, motor, or autonomic nerves, and association of monoclonal gammopathy and neuropathy is commonly seen in clinical practice. Neuropathy is highly prevalent in MGUS, and estimated 30-50% in IgM, 10-15% in IgA, and 5% in IgG paraproteins. Symmetrical paresthesia, tingling and numbness of the hands and feet in a socks and gloves pattern are the common presentation features. There is large body of evidences that IgM paraproteins induced neuropathy is an immune-mediated neuropathy, and IgM antibodies may bind directly to myelin-associated glycoprotein (MAG) and disrupt interactions between Schwann cells and axons. Peripheral neuropathy is highly variable in IgM MGUS neuropathy, but a phenotypically characteristic IgM MGUS neuropathy progresses slowly and first involves longest nerves symmetrically, and then may progress to proximal nerves.

This is the classic description of distal acquired demyelinating symmetric (DADS) sensory and motor neuropathy. In about half of IgM MGUS patients, the IgM M protein binds to carbohydrate moiety of MAG and results in widening of myelin lamella. Anti-MAG antibody induced neuropathy is less common in other monoclonal gammopathies. Motor neuropathies present with muscle cramps, tremors or weakness, and are less frequent than sensory neuropathies. Diabetes mellitus, alcohol abuse, vitamin deficiencies, and viral infections are predisposing factors which may aggravate IgM MGUS neuropathies. A history of already existing neuropathy is a strong risk factor for IgM MGUS neuropathy. Identification of IgM paraproteins by serum protein electrophoresis and presence of high titer (more than 1:6400) anti-MAG antibody are diagnostic of IgM MGUS neuropathy.

Sensory action potentials are severely attenuated in electrophysiological studies. Motor nerve conduction velocity is significantly decreased and can be quantified by the terminal latency index which is highly specific for anti-MAG neuropathies. In about 80% of patients CSF protein is increased with normal cellularity. In electron microscopy, there is deposition of IgM on nerve myelin, and myelin lamella is widely open. Serum level of IgM shows correlation with anti-MAG antibodies, and appearance of axonal degeneration in skin nerve biopsies. Patients with IgG/IgA neuropathies have more motor weakness, and less balance problem.

The presence of demyelination in nerve conduction studies, the absence of anti-MAG antibodies, and higher age at the onset of disease are three different prognostic factors which can help to classify patients. Patients with demyelinating IgM MGUS neuropathy have more severe nervous symptoms than MAG-positive patients. It has been shown that the disease progress reach at a plateau phase after 10-15 years, and treatment modalities should start at the first 10 years of disease duration.

Treatment should target lowering IgM paraproteins levels. It is appropriate to start treatment in younger patients, but timing of treatment is not clear in older patients. Plasma exchange, cytotoxic alkylating drugs, nucleoside analogs, IVIg, and rituximab are tested modalities but no randomized clinical trial supports any of them. IVIg has only short-term benefits, but studies showed that targeting the B-cell surface antigen CD20 by rituximab is promising. Rituximab may improve or stabilize the anti-MAG antibody neuropathy, and has direct correlation with its serum levels. However, rituximab increase progressive multifocal leukoencephalopathy, and it is prudent to check serum antibodies to JC virus before starting treatment.

Introduction

Peripheral neuropathy (PN) refers to disorders that result from pathology that affects sensory, motor, or autonomic nerve fibers. PN is a common condition with a prevalence of 8% in persons over 60 years of age [1]. One significant cause of PN is its association with monoclonal gammopathies (MG). The proper diagnosis and treatment of MG requires close collaboration between hematologist/oncologists and neurologists. The American Academy of Neurology Practice Guidelines recommends that all patients with PN undergo an evaluation for MG with a serum protein immunofixation electrophoresis [IFE] [2].

MG are a heterogeneous group of single clone proliferation of plasma cells or B lymphocytes characterized by production and deposition of aberrant proteins known as monoclonal (M) proteins or paraproteins. MG may occur either in a premalignant, subclinical condition known as monoclonal gammopathy of undetermined significance (MGUS) or in association with systemic disorders. These systemic disorders include multiple myeloma, Waldenstrom's macroglobulinemia, POEMS syndrome (polyneuropathy, organomegaly, endocrinopathy, M-spike, and skin changes), AL amyloidosis, and cryoglobulinemia [3, 4].

MGUS is the most common plasma cell dyscrasia. It is characterized by a serum M component concentration of 3 g/dl or less, fewer than 10% plasma cells in the bone marrow, absence of another B cell proliferative disorder, absent or low levels of Bence Jones protein in the urine, and absence of end organ damage. The diagnosis of MGUS also requires the absence of hypercalcemia, anemia, lytic bone lesions, and stability of the monoclonal protein.

Osteoporosis, osteopenia, increased risk of fractures, thromboembolic events, and PN are more common in MGUS patients [5]. Nonetheless, PN is the sole clinical manifestation of MGUS in most patients. The annual risk of MGUS malignant transformation to multiple myeloma or related malignancies is approximately 1% a year [5-6]. Thus, these patients need indefinite hematological monitoring. This risk is independent of age or disease duration. The M component or M spike is produced by a single clone of plasma cells comprised of two same class and subclass heavy chains (IgM, IgG, IgA, or IgD) and two same type light chains (κ or λ). Kappa light chain is the most common paraprotein [4-7].

Given their different pathological and therapeutic implications, MGUS-associated neuropathy may be subdivided into IgM and non-IgM associated types. IgG isotype, found in more than two-thirds of cases, is the most common-immunoglobulin in MGUS. In contrast, only 17% of patients have an IgM isotype [9]. Nonetheless, the IgM isotype is more likely to result in a PN than IgG or IgA MGUS. IFE is the most sensitive diagnostic measure. IFE may demonstrate single heavy and light chains and should be performed in all patients with polyneuropathy [2, 10, 11].

Epidemiology

The precise prevalence of MGUS-associated PN is not known as it may be influenced by patient selection and the criteria by which PN is diagnosed. Notwithstanding, idiopathic PN is associated with paraproteinemia in about 10% of patients with MG. Notably, MG is ten times more common in patients with idiopathic PN than with a PN of another known cause. It is also 6-10 times more common in patients with PN as compared to general population [12,

13]. The presence of IgM paraproteinemia in PN is more than coincidental as the prevalence of a PN associated with an IgM paraprotein MG is about 50-80%. In contrast, IgG paraproteins have been found in 20-30% and IgA in only 10% of patients with PN. Conversely, PN has been diagnosed in 15.4% of patients with an IgM paraprotein, 7.1% of patients with IgA paraproteins, and 3% of IgG MGUS [14-16]. The risk of progression to malignancy is higher in patients with MGUS-associated PN in that the annual risk is about 2.7% versus 1% in the general population. IgM and IgA isotype MGUS, serum M protein more than 1.5 g/dl, and an elevated free κ to λ ratio in serum are other risk factors that predict progression to malignancy [17].

Pathogenesis

There is a large body of literature that IgM paraproteins have autoimmune activity and cross-react with different neural antigens of the myelin sheath. Identification and characterization of these antigens may shed some light on the pathogenic mechanisms involved in IgM paraproteinemic neuropathies. It has been shown that deposition of IgM antibodies in the myelin sheath damages myelin-axon interactions with a resultant neuropathy [13, 16, 18-22]. There is no immune cell infiltration observed on nerve biopsy specimens [19, 21]. In 50-75% of patients, complement fixing IgM isotype paraproteins react with oligosaccharide determinants of a 100 kDa transmembrane immunoglobulin superfamily known as myelin associated glycoprotein (MAG). MAG is a constituent of the myelin sheaths formed by Schwann cells in peripheral nerves [18, 19].

Due to its location on the membrane surface, MAG is an exposed and accessible antigen. MAG, which comprises about 1% of peripheral myelin, was the first discovered antigen that has reactivity with IgM paraproteins. IgM antibodies react with carbohydrate moiety of MAG that constitutes 30% of its structure. MAG is a major component of non-compact myelin in the paranodal loops of the nodes of Ranvier, Schmidt-Lanterman incisures, internal and external mesaxons, and periaxonal Schwann cell membrane. Thus, anti-MAG antibodies attach to Schwann cell membranes in those areas. Anti-MAG antibody presents in about 56% of patients and is the most frequent antibody reactive to myelin components in IgM MGUS associated neuropathy [20]. Western blot (WB) is the gold standard technique used in identifying anti-MAG antibodies. However, ELISA is a more sensitive assay used to detect anti-MAG antibody than WB in IgM MGUS associated demyelinating neuropathy; (more than 70% for ELISA versus 44-54% for WB) [21].

Systemic transfusion of circulating monoclonal IgM antibodies of some PN patients may strongly react with human MAG [18]. Animal studies on chickens have demonstrated myelin reactivity similar to that found in humans. Tatum et al. reported that intraperitoneal injection of human IgM anti-MAG antibody into two-day-old roosters induced segmental demyelination and clinical neuropathy associated with a 50% compound muscle action potential amplitude reduction on motor nerve conduction studies [22]. Nerve biopsies demonstrated demyelination and remyelination, large intramyelin vacuoles, and myelin edema [22]. Sulfated glucuronic glycolipids (SGGLs), peripheral myelin protein-22 (PMP-22), and myelin protein zero (MPZ) are other nerve glycoconjugates that share the same sulfated trisaccharide epitope termed HNK-1 with MAG. Therefore, they are targets for anti-

MAG antibodies in myelinated peripheral nerves. Active immunization of cats with sulfated glucuronyl paragloboside (SGPG) can induce anti-SGPG antibodies that result in clinical signs of a large fiber sensory neuropathy and ataxia. SGPG-immunized cats developed sensory ganglionitis with inflammatory infiltrates noted on pathological examination of dorsal root ganglia [23]. These experiments provide compelling evidence for a cause and effect relationship between anti-MAG/SGPG IgM antibodies and peripheral neuropathy. MPZ is a 28 kDa glycoprotein with adhesion molecule function. It represents approximately 50% of peripheral nerve myelin protein and is responsible for maintaining the integrity of peripheral nerves. MPZ is the key $CD4^+$ T-cell antigen. B cells of MGUS patients with PN bind to the oligosaccharide epitope of MPZ and trigger myelin-specific autologous T cells to produce IL2 and IFNγ cytokines. These anti-MPZ autoreactive B cells subsequently present myelin peptide antigens to autologous T cells, thereby inducing activation of both $CD4^+$ and $CD8^+$ autologous T cells to produce the Th1 cytokine IFNγ [24].

It has been reported that IL-10 levels are elevated in IgM anti-MAG antibody neuropathy [25]. IL-10 is a potent anti-inflammatory cytokine that stimulates antibody production by B cells, which is secreted by T cells and macrophages. This observation suggests that IL-10 promotes B cell secretion of anti-MAG antibodies. This finding may explain the paucity of immune infiltration observed in IgM anti-MAG antibody polyneuropathy [25].

Although MAG is the most common target in IgM MGUS-associated PN, some patients' IgM does not react with MAG but with some entity. Gangliosides or other acidic glycolipid antigens are another common target for antibody deposition on the myelin sheaths in this group of patients [26]. The antigenic lipids that react with the human antibodies are gangliosides G_{M2}, $IV^4GalNA_cG_{M1b}$, and $IV^4GalNA_CG_{D1a}$. These three minor gangliosides have a common terminal moiety which appears to be antigenic for IgM paraproteins [27]. GD2, GD3, GT1a, GT1b, and GQ1b are some other members of cell surface glycosphingolipids that contain sialic acid epitopes, which may also react with IgM antiganglioside antibodies. Intraperitoneal injection of human IgM antiganglioside antibody in a mouse model impaired phrenic nerve excitability and release of neurotransmitters, suggesting a role for antiganglioside antibodies in IgM MGUS mediated neuropathy [28, 29].

The presence of IgM anti-MAG and other anti-neural antigen antibodies has been associated with a heterogeneous group of neuropathies, which may have a direct pathogenic action on the myelin sheath. However, the presence of these antibodies is not diagnostic of a PN such that their pathogenic relevance is still debated. Approximately 90% of patients with anti-MAG antibody have a clinically detectable polyneuropathy. However, the presence of anti-MAG antibody in the serum does not provide any additional clinical or prognostic information. Paraprotein deposition on peripheral nerves may only be confirmed by nerve biopsy. Widening of myelin lamella (WML), axonal atrophy, demyelination, tomaculous changes, and granular deposits in Schwann cell cytoplasm are the characteristic histopathologic changes of IgM MGUS neuropathy. Ultrastructural analysis, which requires confirmation with electron microscopy (EM), demonstrates severe abnormalities of myelin compaction. The detection of IgM paraprotein at the sites of WML by immunoelectron microscopy may be associated with direct IgM infiltration into the myelin sheath and abnormal myelin spacing. However, WML has been observed in only 36% of IgM anti-MAG PN patients. It has been suggested that WML is one of the earliest changes at paranodal regions which disrupts axon-Schwann cell signaling, myelin terminal and paranodal axolemma attachment, and induces widening and demyelination at the nodes of Ranvier [30-32]. Widening of the outer lamella is greater than that observed with the inner lamella such that the separation of two leaflets is about 22-23 nm [33].

Although IgM deposition on myelinated nerve fascicles has a linear relation with the serum IgM level, the severity of nerve injury is not related to serum IgM level, clinical severity, or disease duration. Both small and large diameter nerves are affected in IgM anti-MAG PN. Sural nerve biopsy provides a useful tool in diagnosing IgM paraprotein PN. Owing to microheterogeneity of IgM anti-MAG PN, individual sural nerve fascicles may manifest different pathologic findings even in the same patient. Repeated nerve biopsy may predict response to therapy [34]. However, this often results in a significant sensory deficit. Therefore, other authors recommend repeated skin biopsy as an alternative [34, 35].

As previously mentioned, non-IgM paraprotein-associated PN is less frequent and its pathology is not as well understood. IgG and IgA demyelinating and axonal neuropathy patterns are more heterogeneous than IgM paraprotein PN [36]. Moreover, their primary antigenic targets have not been as well characterized. One hypothesis is that LM1 ganglioside is immunoreactive with IgA paraprotein such that it may be pathogenic [36]. While there are some reported cases in which there is infiltration and annular binding of monoclonal IgA to myelinated fibers, IgA binding to the myelin sheath is relatively uncommon [36, 37]. There are very few reports with respect to the neural antigens binding with IgG paraproteins. In general, nerve biopsies do not demonstrate endoneurial monoclonal IgG deposition and WML has not been reported in IgG and IgA paraprotein associated PN [38, 39]. Direct immunofluorescence examination of nerve biopsies in IgA paraprotein associated PN demonstrates decreased number of myelinated fibers and axonal degeneration but electron microscopy has not revealed IgA deposition [40]. There is one report of the presence of numerous crystalline inclusions in endoneurial macrophage cytoplasm but its role in IgA paraprotein PN has yet to be determined [41].

Clinical Syndromes

Paraproteinemic polyneuropathies are separate clinical syndromes that may be divided to IgM and non-IgM related PN. Different clinical patterns such as sensory, motor, monofocal or multifocal, and axonal or demyelinating types may be observed (table 1).

IgM anti-MAG neuropathy is the most common IgM MGUS neuropathy, which has a homogenous presentation. Patients are typically older men (2:1 male to female ratio) in their sixth to ninth decade who present with slowly progressive, distal, predominantly large fiber sensory signs and symptoms such as paresthesias and ataxia. Neurological examination may confirm vibratory impairment in the distal portions of the lower extremity. Limb weakness, if present, tends to be mild and appears later in the course of disease. The acronym DADS (distal, acquired, demyelinating sensory neuropathy) summarizes the characteristic presentation of anti-MAG neuropathy. DADS is a slowly progressive sensory neuropathy with frequent sensory ataxia associated with both intention and postural tremors in the upper extremities. Intention tremors can also present early in the course of the disease. A Romberg sign may be present whereas cranial nerve and autonomic nerve symptoms are rare.

Table 1. Summary of the clinical features, pathogenesis, electrophysiological findings and treatment of paraproteinemic polyneuropathies

Paraproteinemic polyneuropathies	Clinical features	Pathogenesis	Electrophysiology	Treatment
IgM- paraproteinemic polyneuropathies				
IgM anti-MAG antibody polyneuropathy	- Slowly progressive, distal, sensory dysfunction (paresthesia, numbness, and loss of vibration, light touch, and proprioception more than pain and temperature) -Weakness, if occurs, is a late manifestation	IgM antibodies against MAG	Predominantly demyelinating: Prolonged DML, slowed MCNV, delayed or absent F waves, and partial conduction block	Rituximab, IVIG interferon alpha, plasmapheresis, cyclophosphamide, fludarabine, prednisone, chlorambucil, and neurosurgical interventions have been used with mixed success
IgM anti-GM1 antibody polyneuropathy	- Weakness is asymmetric, and more in distal upper than lower extremities - Weakness without muscle atrophy is a common finding	IgM anti-GM1 antibodies react with Gal(β1-3) GalNAc epitopes	Slow NCV	Very poor response to treatment. NOTE: Treatment may even aggravate the condition
IgM anti-ganglioside GD1b/GQ1b antibody polyneuropathy	Chronic ataxia, ophthalmoplegia, M-protein, anemia due to cold agglutinin antibodies	IgM anti-ganglioside Ab react with gangliosides containing NeuNAc(α2-8-NeuNAc(α2-3) Gal epitope	Slow NCV	IVIG
Non-IgM- paraproteinemic polyneuropathies				
IgG monoclonal gammopathy associated polyneuropathy	Heterogeneous, of 2 main clinical presentations: 1- Moderate-severe chronic progressive or relapsing demyelinating polyneuropathy, which is predominantly motor and more common in middle age 2- Mild, chronic progressive, distal sensory axonopathy, more common in older age groups	Not well understood	-Heterogeneous -Demyelinating pattern with conduction block in distal, proximal or intermediate motor nerves (less severe than IgM PN)	Plasmapheresis
IgA monoclonal gammopathy associated polyneuropathy	IgA antibody PN can be insidious or rapidly progressive, and mean age of onset is about 55. Male to female ratio is 4 to 1	Not well understood	Similar to that of IgG monoclonal gammopathy associated polyneuropathy	Plasmapheresis

Abbreviations: Ab=Antibody, DML= distal motor latency, IVIG=Intravenous immunoglobulin, MAG= myelin-associated glycoprotein, MCNV= motor conduction nerve velocity, NCV= nerve conduction velocity.

Deep tendon reflexes tend to be absent in the lower extremities and decreased in the upper extremities. DADS associated with IgM-kappa MGUS (DADS-M) is twice as common as idiopathic DADS, such that it may be is a different entity. Anti-MAG antibody positive PN patients are less responsive to therapy [42, 43]. There are a few exceptional cases of IgM anti-MAG neuropathy with predominantly motor symptoms manifesting with extensive lower extremity muscular atrophy [44].

Electrophysiological studies of IgG/IgA MGUS PN are heterogeneous and are rarely similar to anti-MAG/SGPG PN. IgG/IgA MGUS PN tends to present as a demyelinating neuropathy with conduction block in distal, proximal or intermediate motor nerves. However, demyelination is more severe in anti-MAG/SGPG PN than in IgG/IgA MGUS PN [54, 59].

Treatment

Given the evidence that anti-MAG antibodies are pathogenic to the myelin sheath, current therapeutic modalities focus on reducing the number of circulating antibodies (table 2). Nonetheless, there is no consensus regarding when to initiate treatment or which medication will produce the optimal effect with the best long term outcome. Clinicians should consider a variety of factors in developing their treatment strategy. This would include patient age, the patient's ability to tolerate the therapy, the degree of functional impairment and life expectancy. More emphasis should be given to the clinical presentation, subtypes of polyneuropathy, and degree of disability.

Rituximab, intravenous immunoglobulin (IVIg), interferon alpha, plasmapheresis, cyclophosphamide, fludarabine, prednisone, chlorambucil, and neurosurgical interventions have all been used in many non-randomized or small clinical studies for IgM MGUS associated neuropathy. Nonetheless, there is insufficient evidence based medicine to support one treatment over another and the order of such treatments [60].

Rituximab is a humanized chimeric monoclonal antibody against CD20 antigen on the surface of pre-B and mature B cells. Rituximab induces apoptosis of $CD20^+$ cells through antibody-dependent cell- and complement-mediated cytotoxicity. Rituximab does not reduce IgG level, and is associated with a low risk of infection. It has been reported that rituximab reduces anti-MAG antibody and helps improving signs and symptoms of anti-MAG polyneuropathies. However, most of these reports are open label trials, case reports, and small size randomized controlled clinical trials.

In a randomized placebo-controlled trial of 26 patients, 13 patients received weekly infusions of 375 mg/m^2 of Rituximab and 13 patients received placebo; seven patients in the rituximab group clinically improved and were able to walk. Rituximab was well-tolerated and had no significant side effects as compared to placebo. Although anti-MAG antibody titers were reduced by 50%, no significant changes in the nerve conduction velocities were noted eight months later. There was no detectable $CD20^+$ B cell by the end of the second month and this state of B cell depletion lasted for 6-8 months [61]. In a prospective study of 10 patients with anti-MAG polyneuropathy responding to rituximab for 36 months, all patients had a reduction in sensory ataxia after the first year of treatment. A sustained clinical response lasting 24 months was observed in 80% of patients. This study speculated that patients with a higher baseline anti-MAG antibody titer may require additional rituximab courses [62].

In an uncontrolled open-label trial on 13 patients with anti-MAG polyneuropathy conducted by members of the Italian Peripheral Nerve Study Group, Rituximab was administered at a dosage of 375 mg/m^2 intravenous weekly infusion for four weeks. Improvement of both sensory and motor impairment was observed in eight patients (62%) along with an 87% decrease in the anti-MAG antibody titer after 12 months.

Table 2. Reports that demonstrate the effectiveness of various therapeutic modalities in treating patients with MGUS-associated PN

Study	Type of study	Study design	Conclusions
Dalakas et al. [61]	Randomized clinical trial	13 patients received weekly infusions of 375 mg/m^2 of Rituximab and 13 patients received placebo	7 patients in the Rituximab group clinically improved and were able to walk Rituximab was well-tolerated and had no significant side effects as compared to placebo. Although anti-MAG antibody titers were reduced by 50%, no significant changes in the nerve conduction velocities were noted eight months later
Benedetti et al. [62]	Prospective study	10 patients with anti-MAG polyneuropathy were given rituximab for 36 months	Sensory ataxia of all patients was reduced by 12 months. Sustained clinical response was noted in 80% of patients, lasting 24 months. Patients with a higher baseline anti-MAG antibody may need additional Rituximab courses
Benedetti et al. [63]	Uncontrolled open-label trial	Weekly I.V. infusion of Rituximab (375 mg/m^2) was administered for 13 patients with anti-MAG polyneuropathy for four weeks	Improvement of both sensory and motor impairment was observed in eight patients (62%) along with an 87% decrease in the anti-MAG antibody titer after 12 months. Reducing the antibody titers below a certain level may be necessary in order to achieve the therapeutic response
Renaud et al. [64]	Prospective study	High dose Rituximab (750 mg/m^2) was administered to eight patients with anti-MAG polyneuropathy, who had already received 375 mg/m^2 before enrollment	Patients demonstrated a 23%, improvement in muscle strength and the anti-MAG antibody titer was reduced to 43% of its original value after two years
Renaud et al. [65]	Prospective, open-label study	Rituximab was administered to nine patients with anti-MAG polyneuropathy with various underlying disorders	Clinical improvement was reported in 4 patients and improvement on nerve conduction velocity in 7 patients. Patients with the longest duration of polyneuropathy had a better therapeutic response
Pestronk et al. [66]	Prospective study	21 patients with IgM MGUS PN on Rituximab were compared with 13 untreated controls over a period of 24 months	Muscle strength improved by at least 12% in 81% of treatment group at two years compared with 0% in the control group, and activities of daily living were improved in most treated patients
Levine et al. [67]	Open-label prospective study	5 patients with anti-MAG antibody or IgM anti GM1 ganglioside-related polyneuropathy received rituximab	All five patients showed more than 12% improvement in distal muscle strength after 3 months of treatment accompanied by functional improvement in daily activities
Kelly et al. [68]	Case report	A 73-year-old man with severe numbness of feet and ataxic gait secondary to anti-MAG/SGPG polyneuropathy for 3 years	Muscle strength significantly improved with Rituximab 4 months after treatment
Rojas-Garcia et al. [69]	Case report	2 patients with multifocal motor neuropathy and positive IgM anti-ganglioside antibody (AGA)	Peripheral B cells depleted effectively with rituximab without any clinical benefit. Serum level of IgM AGA did not decrease, and even increased after three months of Rituximab treatment

Table 2. (Continued)

Study	Type of study	Study design	Conclusions
Broglio et al. [70]	Case report	A 75-year-old female with anti-MAG polyneuropathy resistant to steroids, IVIg, and cyclophosphamide, then treated with Rituximab	Rituximab did not reduce anti-MAG antibody titer while both $CD20^{+}$ B cell count and IgM titer decreased while the patient continued to lose distal muscle strength
Delmont et al. [71]	Case report	Rituximab	Rituximab reduced the degree of disability
Comi et al. [72]	Randomized clinical trials	22 patients with IgM anti-MAG were evenly randomized to receive either placebo or IVIg (11 patients each)	Patients who received IvIg had significantly less disability and improved median and ulnar nerve function as demonstrated by an increase in the compound muscle action potential amplitude
Dalakas et al. [73]	Randomized controlled trial	11 patients with IgM demyelinating PN were randomized to two groups; placebo infusion (4 patients) and IVIg (7 patients). Infusions of IVIg was administered at 1 g/kg/day for 2 consecutive days on a monthly basis for three consecutive months	IVIg improved activities of daily living in two patients while nerve conduction studies remained unchanged
Attarian et al. [74]	Uncontrolled retrospective study	13 patients with chronic sensory ataxic neuropathy with high anti-GD1b IgM (CANOMAD) were treated with 2 g/kg of IVIg for 3-5 days every six weeks, then followed for 12 months. On average, each patient received 24 doses of 2 g/kg of IVIg.	9 of 13 patients (68%) demonstrated an improvement in their disability score and six patients had sustained improvement
Oksenhendler et al. [75]	Prospective open trial	44 patients were randomly assigned to two groups of chlorambucil alone and chlorambucil associated with plasma exchange	The difference of MNCV and DML in these two groups was not significant by month 12 such that adding plasma exchange to chlorambucil had no effect on the outcome
Dyck et al. [76]	Randomized clinical trial	39 patients with MGUS of IgM, IgG, and IgA were randomly assigned to receive sham exchange or plasma exchange 6 times in three weeks	The difference between plasma exchange and sham exchange in IgM antibody PN group was not statistically significant
Niermeijer et al. [77]	Prospective study	16 patients with IgM MGUS PN treated with fludarabine	5 patients (31%) showed clinical improvement with their PN being stabilized and without significant side effects after one year of follow up
Wilson et al. [78]	Case report	two patients with IgM anti-MAG PN were treated with fludarabine	Clinical and electrodiagnostic improvement reported
Niermeijer et al. [79]	Randomized clinical trial	35 patients with IgM PN were randomly assigned into the treatment group of cyclophosphamide and prednisone (16), and placebo (19) arms with follow ups at 3, 6, 12, and 24	RMI did not demonstrate any difference between the two groups

Study	Type of study	Study design	Conclusions
		months intervals. The revised Rivermead mobility index (RMI) was used as the primary outcome measure to compare CP from placebo group	
Notermans et al. [80]	Open, prospective study	Combination of cyclophosphamide and prednisone (CP) was administered to 16 patients with IgM (11) and IgG (5) associated PN and patients were followed for three years. Quantitative neurologic exam, the Rankin disability scale and nerve conduction studies were used for assessment.	After six months of therapy, neuropathy progression improved in 50% of patients whereas progression was halted in 38%. There was no difference in the degree of improvement between IgM and IgG MGUS PN patients
Mc Master et al. [81]	Case report	A patient with anti-MAG PN refractory to corticosteroids, IVIg, and plasma exchange in treated with unilateral thalamic deep brain stimulation	Unilateral thalamic deep brain stimulation significantly improved patient's tremor and quality of life after six months
Cortese et al. [82]	Randomized clinical trial	39 patients were randomized to two groups of sham exchange (10 IgM and 10 IgG/IgA associated PN) and plasma exchange (11 with IgM and 8 with IgG/IgA associated PN)	Weakness and neuropathy disability scores were significantly improved in IgG/IgA PN with plasma exchange group
Notermans et al. [83]	Case report	Pulsed high dose dexamethasone therapy was used to treat IgG associated MGUS polyneuropathy	Paresthesias and motor strength improved before the treatment had to be stopped due to proximal lower limb weakness

DML: distal motor latency, IVIg: intravenous immunoglobulin, MAG: myelin-associated glycoprotein, MGUS: monoclonal gammopathy with uncertain significance, MNCV: motor nerve conduction velocity, PN: polyneuropathy, SGPG: sulfated glucuronic acid paragloboside.

These authors speculated that reducing the antibody titers below a certain level may be necessary in order to achieve a therapeutic response [63].

High dose Rituximab (750 mg/m^2) was administered in four weekly infusions to8 patients with anti-MAG polyneuropathy, who had already received 375 mg/m^2 before enrollment. These patients were diagnosed as anti-MAG polyneuropathy secondary to either MGUS or an indolent non-Hodgkin B cell lymphoma, [64]. After retreatment, these patients demonstrated a 23% improvement in muscle strength while the anti-MAG antibody titer was reduced to 43% of its original value after two years. In a prospective, open label study, Rituximab was administered to nine patients with anti-MAG polyneuropathy with various underlying disorders. This study reported clinical improvement in four patients and improvement on nerve conduction velocity in seven patients. Patients with the longest duration of polyneuropathy had a better therapeutic response [65].

In a prospective study, 21 patients with IgM MGUS PN on Rituximab were compared with 13 untreated controls over a period of 24 months. Rituximab was administered weekly for four weeks, resulting in elimination of B cells from circulation following the first dose, which remained below normal levels for one year following the treatment. Muscle strength improved by at least 12% in 81% of treatment group at two years compared with 0% in the control group along with an improvement in the treated patients' activities of daily living

[ADL] [66]. In another study, five patients with anti-MAG antibody or IgM anti GM1 ganglioside-related polyneuropathy received Rituximab. All five patients manifested more than 12% improvement in distal muscle strength after 3 months of treatment accompanied by functional improvement in their ADL [67]. In a case report of 73 year old man with severe numbness of feet and ataxic gait secondary to anti-MAG/SGPG polyneuropathy of three years' duration, his muscle strength significantly improved with Rituximab four months after treatment [68].

There are some reports that Rituximab does not improve the IgM anti-ganglioside PN, or may even make it worse. In two patients with multifocal motor neuropathy and positive IgM anti-ganglioside antibody (AGA), peripheral B cells were effectively depleted by Rituximab without any clinical benefit. Furthermore, the serum level of IgM AGA actually increased after three months of Rituximab treatment [69]. In a 75 year old female with anti-MAG polyneuropathy resistant to steroids, IVIg, cyclophosphamide, and Rituximab did not reduce anti-MAG antibody titers while both $CD20^+$ B cell count and IgM titers decreased and patient continued to lose distal muscle strength [70]. There is another case report that Rituximab improved disabling neuropathy in a patient with CANOMAD [71]. In summary, there is insufficient evidence to recommend Rituximab as a treatment for any type of MGUS syndrome.

The immunomodulating effect of IVIg on IgM associated PN has yet to be determined. It has been reported in two different randomized clinical trials that IVIg improves nerve function for a short period of time in IgM anti-MAG polyneuropathy. In one trial, 22 patients with IgM anti-MAG were evenly randomized to receive either placebo or IVIg. The IvIg treatment group had significantly less disability and improved median and ulnar nerve function as demonstrated by an increase in the compound muscle action potential amplitude [72]. In another randomized placebo-controlled trial, 11 patients with IgM demyelinating PN were randomized to two groups; placebo infusion (4 patients) and IVIg (7 patients). Infusions of IVIg were administered at 1 g/kg/day for 2 consecutive days on a monthly basis for three consecutive months. IVIg improved activities the ADL in two patients although their nerve conduction studies remained unchanged [73].

In an uncontrolled retrospective study, 13 patients with chronic sensory ataxic neuropathy with high anti-GD1b IgM (CANOMAD) were treated with 2 g/kg of IVIg for 3-5 days every six weeks, then followed for 12 months. On average, each patient received 24 doses of 2 g/kg of IVIg. Nine of 13 patients (68%) demonstrated an improvement in their disability score and six patients had sustained improvement [74].

No study has conclusively demonstrated any significant benefit of plasma exchange in IgM antibody mediated PN. In a prospective open trial, 44 patients were randomly assigned to two groups of chlorambucil alone and chlorambucil associated with plasma exchange. The difference of MNCV and DML in these two groups was not significant after one year such that adding plasma exchange to chlorambucil did not change the outcome [75]. In a double blind trial of polyneuropathy and MGUS of IgM, IgG, and IgA, 39 patients were randomly assigned to receive sham exchange or plasma exchange six times in three weeks. The difference between plasma exchange and sham exchange in IgM antibody PN group was not statistically significant [76].

A fluorinated purine analogue, fludarabine, has been used in IgM antibody PN in some uncontrolled trials and case reports. In a prospective study of 16 patients with IgM MGUS PN, five patients (31%) showed clinical improvement with their PN being stabilized and without significant side effects after one year of follow up [77]. In a case report of two patients with IgM anti-MAG PN, fludarabine has demonstrated clinical and electrodiagnostic improvement. Nonetheless, myelosuppression as well as atypical and opportunistic infections are well-known side effects of fludarabine that limit its use [78].

There is only one randomized, double blinded, placebo-controlled study using the combination of cyclophosphamide and prednisone (CP) in treating IgM antibody associated PN. In this study, 35 patients were randomly assigned into treatment (16) and placebo (19) arms with reevaluation at 3, 6, 12, and 24 months intervals. The revised Rivermead mobility index (RMI) was used as the primary outcome measure to compare CP to the placebo group. RMI did not demonstrate any difference between the two groups [79]. In an open progressive study, this combination of cyclophosphamide and prednisone (CP) was administered to 16 patients with IgM (11) and IgG (5) associated PN and these patients were followed for three years. Quantitative neurologic exam, the Rankin disability scale and nerve conduction studies were used for assessment. After six months of therapy, neuropathy progression stopped in 38% of patients or improved in 50% of them. There was no difference in the degree of improvement between IgM and IgG MGUS PN patients [80].

There is a single case report in a patient with anti-MAG PN refractory to corticosteroids, IVIg, and plasma exchange in whom unilateral thalamic deep brain stimulation significantly improved the patient's tremor and quality of life after six months [81].

There is a general agreement that plasmapheresis has a possible role in IgG/IgA associated polyneuropathy. In a double-blinded trial, 39 patients were randomized to two groups of sham exchange (10 IgM and 10 IgG/IgA associated PN) and plasma exchange (11 with IgM and 8 with IgG/IgA associated PN). Weakness and neuropathy disability scores were significantly improved in IgG/IgA PN with plasma exchange group [75, 82]. In a separate case report, pulsed high dose dexamethasone therapy was used to treat IgG associated MGUS polyneuropathy. These authors reported that paresthesias and motor strength improved before the treatment had to be stopped due to proximal lower limb weakness [83].

Five patients with IgG-associated sensorimotor polyneuropathy received cyclophosphamide and prednisone (CP) for six months in an open prospective study with a subsequent three year follow-up. One patient was removed from the trial for severe leukopenia. These authors reported significant improvement after three months of therapy [79].

Prognosis and Monitoring

The long-term prognosis of MGUS-associated polyneuropathy depends on different factors including the clinical subtype, pathologic findings, time course of treatment, and the type of therapy. The incidence of malignant transformation of IgG MGUS is 1% per year whereas the value for IgM MGUS is 1.5% per year [84]. In one study, the malignant transformation rate of MGUS with PN was 22% in a median of six years of follow up suggesting that malignant transformation rate is higher in MGUS PN than MGUS without polyneuropathy.

In a prospective study of 176 patients with MGUS PN, there was 2.7/100 patient-years incidence of MGUS PN malignant transformation. This study reported that weight loss, nocturnal fevers or sweating, progression of polyneuropathy, and M protein level are other independent predictors of MGUS malignant transformation. Of these factors, M protein level is the most important prognostic factor in malignant transformation [84].

It has been reported that anti-MAG antibody titers are not related to the severity of the neuropathy as it is the duration of exposure to the anti-MAG antibody that may be responsible for the neuropathy's severity. One study reported a mortality of 32% and a disability rate of 42% in patients with a mean anti-MAG antibody PN duration of 11.8 years. However, these deaths were either due to a hematological disorder or other comorbidities such that a direct correlation between death and neuropathy has not been confirmed [19, 85]. A prospective cohort study of 140 patients suggests three different risk factors for MGUS PN: higher age at presentation, demyelination in electrodiagnostic studies, and presence of anti-MAG antibody. This study categorized MGUS PN patients into three groups: anti-MAG positive demyelinating PN, anti-MAG negative demyelinating PN, and axonal type PN. Sensorimotor symptoms were more severe in demyelinating IgM MGUS than the axonal type at presentation.

It has been reported that MGUS PN may reach a plateau phase after 10 years, indicating that the progression of the polyneuropathy is faster in the first few years [86]. Diagnosis, proper classification, and prompt treatment of MGUS PN may help to lessen the morbidity and mortality associated with this disorder.

Conclusion

Monoclonal gammopathies are heterogeneous group of disorders characterized by unregulated production and deposition of monoclonal (M) protein or paraproteins by proliferation of a clone of plasma cells or B lymphocytes. Paraproteins are consist of two same class and subclass heavy polypeptide chains (G, M, or A) and two same type light polypeptide chains (kappa or lambda). IgG is the most common paraproteins, and less than 15% is IgM. Monoclonal gammopathy without any association with plasma cell dyscrasia occurs in 1% of general population and increases to 10% in older than 80 years. Monoclonal gammopathy of undetermined significance (MGUS) is the most common type of gammopathies which occurs in the absence of malignancy whereas multiple myeloma and Waldenstrom's macroglobulinemia occur in the context of systemic malignant disorder.

Polyneuropathy [PN] is defined as dysfunction of the peripheral nervous system that may affect sensory, motor, and autonomic nerves. It commonly occurs in association with a monoclonal gammopathy. PN is highly prevalent in MGUS, estimated at 30-50% in IgM, 10-15% in IgA, and 5% in IgG associated paraproteins. Symmetrical paresthesia, numbness and tingling, in the hands and feet in a "stocking and glove" pattern is a common presenting feature. There is a significant body of evidence that IgM paraproteins induced an immune-mediated neuropathy. IgM antibodies may bind directly to myelin-associated glycoprotein (MAG) and disrupt interactions between Schwann cells and axons. Although the IgM associated PN is highly variable, one phenotypically characteristic IgM MGUS neuropathy presents as a distal, symmetric slowly progressive neuropathy with demyelinating features known as "distal acquired demyelinating sensory neuropathy."

However, it should be recalled that the large myelinated motor fibers are affected as well. In 50% of IgM MGUS patients, the IgM protein binds to carbohydrate moiety of MAG and results in widening of the myelin lamellae. Anti-MAG antibody induced neuropathy is less common in other monoclonal gammopathies. Motor neuropathies may present with muscle cramps, tremors or weakness, and are less frequent than sensory neuropathies. Patients with pre-existing comorbid conditions such as an inherited PN, diabetes mellitus, alcohol abuse, and vitamin deficiencies, may present with a more rapidly progressive course and a greater degree of disability with superimposed IgM MGUS neuropathies. Identification of IgM paraproteins by serum protein electrophoresis and the presence of a high titer of anti-MAG antibody (> 1:6400) are diagnostic of IgM MGUS neuropathy. Sensory nerve action potentials are reduced or absent in electrophysiological studies.

The motor nerve conduction velocities are progressively slowed in more distal segments that may be quantified by the terminal latency index [TLI], which is highly specific for anti-MAG neuropathies.

In about 80% of patients, the CSF protein is increased with normal cellularity characterized as albuminocytological dissociation. Electron microscopy reveals deposition of IgM on nerve myelin with widely spaced myelin lamellae. The serum level of IgM correlates with the presence of anti-MAG antibodies, and the appearance of axonal degeneration in the nerve fibers as observed in intraepidermal skin biopsies. In contrast, patients with IgG/IgA MGUS neuropathies tend to have motor greater than large fiber sensory dysfunction than patients with IgM MGUS.

The presence of demyelinating features on nerve conduction studies, the absence of anti-MAG antibodies, and greater age at disease onset are three important prognostic factors such that the patients may be stratified.

Patients with a demyelinating IgM MGUS associated neuropathy have more profound PN symptoms than MAG-positive patients. MAG-negative IgM MGUS patients tend to have more profound motor weakness, paresthesia and ataxia. The medical literature indicates that MGUS neuropathies tend to be relentlessly progressive at first but reach a plateau phase after 10-15 years. Therefore, most authorities recommend that treatments should be initiated within the first 10 years after diagnosis.

In theory, effective treatment should target lowering the IgM paraprotein levels. While it is appropriate to initiate treatment in younger patients, the optimal timing of treatment is older patients has yet to be established.

Various clinical trials have utilized plasma exchange, cytotoxic alkylating drugs, nucleoside analogs, IVIg, and Rituximab are tested modalities but there are no Class I or Class II trials that have conclusively demonstrated that any of these agents by themselves or in combination result in an improvement in patient outcomes. While IVIg has only short-term benefits, there is accruing evidence that targeting the B-cell surface antigen CD20 by Rituximab is promising.

Rituximab may improve or stabilize the PN associated with anti-MAG antibody neuropathy, whose reduction in titer correlates with clinical improvement. However, Rituximab increase the risk for the development of progressive multifocal leukoencephalopathy. Therefore, it is prudent to assess for serum antibodies to the JC virus before starting treatment.

Although neither Class I nor Class II studies have confirmed this, there is a general agreement that plasmapheresis may be effective in IgG/IgA associated polyneuropathy. Therefore, this would be a reasonable course of action in a patient with an IgG or IgA associated MGUS neuropathy within the first ten years of the associated neuropathy's onset.

References

[1] Rajabally Y. A. Neuropathy and paraproteins: review of a complex association. *Eur. J. Neurol.,* 2011; 18 (11): 1291-8.

[2] England J. D., Gronseth G. S., Franklin G., Carter G. T., Kinsella L. J., Cohen J. A., Asbury A. K., Szigeti K., Lupski J. R., Latov N., Lewis R. A., Low P. A., Fisher M. A., Herrmann D. N., Howard J. F. Jr, Lauria G., Miller R. G., Polydefkis M., Sumner A. J.; American Academy of Neurology. Practice parameter: evaluation of distal symmetric polyneuropathy: role of laboratory and genetic testing (as evidence-based review). Report of the American Academy of Neurology, American Association of Neuromuscular and Electrodiagnostic Medicine, and American Academy of Physical Medicine and Rehabilitation. *Neurology,* 2009 Jan 13;72(2):185-92.

[3] Ramchandren S., Lewis R. A. Monoclonal gammopathy and neuropathy. *Curr. Opin. Neurol.,* 2009; 22: 480-485.

[4] Sonneveld P., Jongen J. L. M. Dealing with neuropathy in plasma-cell dyscrasia. *Hematology*, 2010; 2010: 423-30.

[5] Berenson J. R., Anderson K. C., Audell R. A., Boccia R. V., Coleman M., Dimopoulos M. A., Drake M. T., Fonseca R., Harousseau J. L., Joshua D., Lonial S., Niesvizky R., Palumbo A., Roodman G. D., San-Miguel J. F., Singhal S., Weber D. M., Zangari M., Wirstchafter E., Yellin O., Kyle R. A. Monoclonal gammopathy of undetermined significance: a consensus statement. *Br. J. Haematol.,* 2010; 150 (1): 28-38.

[6] Silberman J., Lonial S. Review of peripheral neuropathy in plasma cell disorders. *Hematol. Oncol.,* 2008; 26: 55-65.

[7] Nobile-Orazio E. Paraproteinemia related neuropathies. *Haematologica,* 2007; 92 (S2): 62-64.

[8] Ramchandren S., Lewis R. A. An update on monoclonal gammopathy and neuropathy. *Curr. Neurol. Neurosci. Rep.,* 2012; 12: 102-110.

[9] Kyle R. A., Therneau T. M., Rajkumar S. V., Larson D. R., Plevak M. F., Offord J. R., Dispenzieri A., Katzmann J. A., Melton III J. Prevalence of monoclonal gammopathy of undetermined significance. *N. Engl. J. Med.*, 2006; 354: 1362-9.

[10] Kelly J. J. Peripheral neuropathies associated with monoclonal gammopathies of undetermined significance. *Rev. Neurol. Dis.,* 2008; 5 (1): 14-22.

[11] Gorson K. C. Clinical features, evaluation, and treatment of patients with polyneuropathy associated with monoclonal gammopathy of undetermined significance (MGUS). *J. Clin. Apher.,* 1999; 14 (3): 149-53.

[12] Kelly J. J., Kyle R. A., O'Brien P. C., Dyck P. J. Prevalence of monoclonal protein in peripheral neuropathy. *Neurology (NY),* 1981; 31: 1480-3.

[13] Dalakas M. C. Pathogenesis and treatment of anti-MAG neuropathy. *Curr. Treat. Options Neurol.,* 2010; 12: 71-83.

[14] Nobile-Orazio E., Barbieri S., Baldini L., Marmiroli P., Carpo M., Premoselli S., Manfredini E., Scarlato G. Peripheral neuropathy in monoclonal gammopathy of undetermined significance: prevalence and immunopathogenetic studies. *Acta. Neurol. Scand.,* 1992; 85: 383-390.

[15] Nobile-Orazio E., Marmiroli P., Baldini L., Spagnol G., Barbieri S., Moggio M., Polli N., Polli E., Scarlato G. Peripheral neuropathy in macroglobulinemia: incidence and antigen-specificity of M proteins. *Neurology,* 1987; 37: 1506-1514.

[16] Vrethem M., Cruz M., Wen-Xin H., Malm C., Holmgren H., Ernerudh J. Clinical, neurophysiological and immunological evidence of polyneuropathy in patients with monoclonal gammopathies. *J. Neurol. Sci*., 1993; 114: 193-199.

[17] Lozeron P., Adams D. Monoclonal gammopathy and neuropathy. *Curr. Opin. Neurol.,* 2007; 20: 536-541.

[18] Latov N., Braun P. E., Gross R. B., Sherman W. H., Penn A. S., Chess L. Plasma cell dyscrasia and peripheral neuropathy: identification of the myelin antigen that react with human proteins. *Proc. Natl. Acad. Sci. USA,* 1981; 78 (11): 7139-7142.

[19] Ellie E., Vital A., Steck A., Boiron J-M., Vital C., Julien J. Neuropathy associated with "benign" anti-myelin-associated glycoprotein IgM gammopathy: clinical, immunological, neurophysiological pathological findings and response to treatment in 33 cases. *J. Neurol.,* 1996; 243: 34-43.

[20] Nobile-Orazio E., Manfredini E., Carpo M., Meucci N., Monaco S., Ferrari S., Allaria S., Sgarzi M., Scarlato G. Frequency and clinical correlates of anti-neural IgM antibodies in neuropathy associated with IgM monoclonal gammopathy. *Ann. Neurol.,* 1994; 36: 416-424.

[21] Kuijf M. L., Eurelings M., Tio-Gillen A. P., van Doorn P. A., van den Berg L. H., Hooijkaas H., Stork J., Notermans N. C., Jacobs B. C.. Detection of anti-MAG antibodies in polyneuropathy associated with IgM monoclonal neuropathy. *Neurology,* 2009; 73: 688-695.

[22] Tatum A. H. Experimental paraproteins neuropathy, demyelination by passive transfer of human IgM anti-myelin-associated glycoprotein. *Ann. Neurol*., 1993; 33: 502-506.

[23] Ilyas A. A., Gu Y., Dalakas M. C., Quarles R. H., Bhatt S. Induction of experimental ataxic sensory neuropathy in cats by immunization with purified SGPG. *J. Neuroimmunol.,* 2008; 193: 87-93.

[24] Hellqvist E., Kvarnstrom M., Soderberg A., Vrethem M., Ernerudh J., Rosen A. Myelin protein zero is naturally processed in the B cells of monoclonal gammopathy of undetermined significance of immunoglobulin M isotype: aberrant triggering of a patient's T cells. *Haematologica*, 2010; 95: 627-636.

[25] Gironi M., Saresella M., Marventano I., Guerini F. R., Gatti A., Antonini G., Ceresa L., Morino S., Beghi E., Angelici A., Mariani E., Nemni R., Clerici M. Distinct cytokine patterns associated with different forms of chronic dysimmune neuropathy. *Muscle Nerve,* 2010; 42: 864-870.

[26] Ilyas A. A., Quarles R. H., Dalakas M. C., Brady R. O. Polyneuropathy with monoclonal gammopathy: glycolipids are frequently antigens for IgM paraproteins. *Proc. Natl. Acad. Sci. USA,* 1985; 82: 6697-6700.

[27] Ilyas A. A., Li S. C., Chou D. K., Li Y. T., Jungalwala F. B., Dalakas M. C., Quarles R. H. Gangliosides G_{M2}, $IV^4GalNA_CG_{Mab}$, and $IV^4GalNA_CG_{D1a}$ as antigens for monoclonal

immunoglobulin M in neuropathy associated with gammopathy. *J. Biol. Chem.,* 1988; 263 (9): 4369-4373.

[28] Williamson H. J., O'Hanlon G. M., Paterson G., Veitch J., Wilson G., Roberts M., Tang T., Vincent A. A somatically mutated human antiganglioside IgM antibody that induces experimental neuropathy in mice is encoded by variable region heavy chain gene, V1-18. *J. Clin. Invest.,* 1996; 97: 1155-1164.

[29] Quarles R. H., Dalakas M. C. Do anti-ganglioside antibodies cause human cause human peripheral neuropathies? *J. Clin. Invest.,* 1996; 97 (5): 1136-1137.

[30] Nobile-Orazio E., Gallia F., Terenghi F., Allaria S., Giannotta C., Carpo M. How useful are anti-neural IgM antibodies in the diagnosis of chronic immune-mediated neuropathies? *J. Neurol. Sci.*, 2008; 266: 156-163.

[31] Vallat J. M., Magy L., Richard L., Sturtz F., Couratier P. Contribution of electron microscopy to the study of neuropathies associated with an IgG monoclonal paraproteinemia. *Micron.*, 2008; 39: 61-70.

[32] Kawagashira Y., koike H., Tomita M., Morozumi S., Iijima M., Nakamura T., Katsuno M., Tanaka F., Sobue G. Morphological progression of myelin abnormalities in IgM-monoclonal gammopathy of undetermined significance anti-myelin-associated glycoprotein neuropathy. *J. Neuropathol. Exp. Neurol.*, 2010; 69 (11): 1143-1157.

[33] Vital A. Paraproteinemic neuropathies. Brain Pathol. 2001; 11: 399-407.

[34] Lombardi R., Erne B., Lauria G., Pareyson D., Borgna M., Morbin M., Arnold A., Czaplinski A., Fuhr P., Schaeren-Wiemers N., Steck A. J. IgM deposits on skin nerves in anti-MAG-associated glycoprotein neuropathy. *Ann. Neurol.,* 2005; 57: 180-187.

[35] Stalder A. K., Erne B., Reimann R., Renaud S., Fuhr P., thomann S., Arnold A., Probst A., Schaeren-Wiemers N., Steck A. J. Immunoglobulin M deposition in cutaneous nerves of anti-myelin-associated glycoprotein polyneuropathy patients correlates with axonal degeneration. *J. Neuropathol. Exp. Neurol.,* 2009; 68 (2): 148-158.

[36] Farrer R. G., Dalakas M. C., Quarles R. H. Multiple antibodies to nerve glycoconjugates in a patient with neuropathy and monoclonal IgA gammopathy. *J. Neuroimmunol.*, 1996; 66: 71-76.

[37] Vallat J. M., Tabaraud F., Sindou F., Preux P. M., Vandenberghe A., Steck A. Myelin widenings and MGUS-IgA: an immunoelectron microscopic study. *Ann. Neurol.*, 2000; 47: 808-811.

[38] Yeung K. B., Thomas P. K., King R. H. M., Waddy H., Will R. G., Hughes R. G., Gregson N. A., Leibowitz S. The clinical spectrum of peripheral neuropathies associated with benign monoclonal IgM, IgG and IgA paraproteinemia. Comparative clinical, immunological and nerve biopsy findings. *J. Neurol.,* 1991; 238: 383-391.

[39] Di Troia A., Carpo M., Meucci N., Pellegrino C., Allaria S., Gemignani F., Marbini A., Mantegazza R., Sciolla R., Manfredini E., Scarlato G., Nobile-Orazio E. Clinical features and anti-neural reactivity in neuropathy associated with IgG monoclonal gammopathy of undetermined significance. *J. Neurol. Sci.,* 1999; 164: 64-71.

[40] Nemni R., Mamoli A., Fazio R., Camerlingo M., Quattrini A., Lorenzetti I., Comola M., Galardi G., Canal N. Polyneuropathy associated with IgA monoclonal gammopathy: a hypothesis of its pathogenesis. *Acta. Neuropathol.,* 1991; 81: 371-376.

[41] Vital A., Nedelec-Ciceri C., Vital C. Presence of crystalline inclusions in the peripheral nerve of a patient with IgA lambda monoclonal gammopathy of undetermined significance. *Neuropathology,* 2008; 28: 526-531.

[42] Chacko J. M., Spinner W. D. Paraproteinemic neuropathies. *J. Clin. Neuromuscul. Dis.*, 2006; 7 (4): 185-197.

[43] Rotta F. T., Sussman A. T., Bradley W. G., Ram Ayyar D., Sharma K. R., Shebert R. T. The spectrum of chronic inflammatory demyelinating polyneuropathy. *J. Neurol. Sci.*, 2000; 173: 129-139.

[44] Kawagashira Y., Kondo N., Atsuta N., Iijima M., Koike H., Katsuno M., Tanaka F., Kusunoki S., Sobue G. IgM MGUS anti-MAG neuropathy with predominant muscle weakness and extensive muscle atrophy. *Muscle Nerve,* 2010; 42: 433-435.

[45] Latov N. Pathogenesis and therapy of neuropathies associated with monoclonal gammopathies. *Ann. Neurol.,* 1995; 37 (S1): S32-S42.

[46] Saperstein D. S., Katz J. S., Amato A. A., Barohn R. J. Clinical spectrum of chronic acquired demyelinating polyneuropathies. *Muscle Nerve,* 2001; 24: 311-324.

[47] Nobile-Orazio E. Update on neuropathies associated with monoclonal gammopathy of undetermined significance (2008-2010). *J. Peripher. Nerv. Syst.,* 2010; 15: 302-306.

[48] Joint Task Force of the EFNS and the PNS. European Federation of Neurological Societies/Peripheral Nerve Society Guideline on management of paraproteinemic demyelinating neuropathies. Report of a Joint Task Force of the European Federation of Neurological Societies and the Peripheral Nerve Society-first revision. *J. Peripher. Nerv. Syst.*, 2010; 15: 185-195.

[49] Willison H. J., O'Leary C. P., Veitch J., Blumhardt L. D., Busby M., Donaghy M., Fuhr P., Ford H., Hahn A., Renaud S., Katifi H. A., Ponsford S., Reuber M., Steck A., Sutton I., Schady W., Thomas P. K., Thompson A. J., Vallat J. M., Winer J. The clinical and laboratory features of chronic sensory ataxic neuropathy with anti-disialosyl IgM antibodies. *Brain,* 2001; 124: 1968-1977.

[50] Larue S., Bombelli F., Viala K., Neil J., Maisonobe T., Bouche P., Musset L., Fournier E., Leger J. M. Non-anti-MAG DADS neuropathy as a variant of CIDP: clinical, electrophysiological, laboratory features and response to treatment in 10 cases. *Eur. J. Neurol.,* 2011; 18: 899-905.

[51] Vrethem M., Reiser N., Lauermann C., Svanborg E. Polyneuropathy associated with IgM vs IgG monoclonal gammopathy: comparison between clinical and electrophysiological findings. *Acta. Neurol. Scand.,* 2010; 122: 52-57.

[52] Magy L., Chassande B., Malsonobe T., Bouche P., Vallat J. M., Leger J. M. Polyneuropathy associated with IgG/IgA monoclonal gammopathy: a clinical and electrophysiological study of 15 cases. *Eur. J. Neurol.,* 2003; 10: 677-685.

[53] Mehndiratta M. M., Sen K., Tatke M., Bajaj B. K. IgA monoclonal gammopathy of undetermined significance with peripheral neuropathy. *J. Neurol. Sci., 2004;* 221: 99-104.

[54] Simmons Z., Bromberg M. B., Feldman E. L., Blaivas M. Polyneuropathy associated with IgA monoclonal gammopathy of undetermined significance. *Muscle Nerve*, 1993; 16: 77-83.

[55] Kaku D. A., England J. D., Sumner A. J. Distal accentuation of conduction slowing in polyneuropathy associated with antibodies to myelin-associated glycoprotein and sulphated glucuronyl paragloboside. *Brain,* 1994; 117: 941-947.

[56] Lupu V. D., Mora C. A., Dambrosia J., Meer J., Dalakas M., Floeter M. K. Terminal latency index in neuropathy with antibodies against myelin-associated glycoproteins. *Muscle Nerve*, 2007; 35: 196-202.

[57] Attarian S., Azulay J. P., Boucraut J., Escande N., Pouget J. Terminal latency index and modified F ratio in distinction of chronic demyelinating neuropathies. *Clin. Neurophysiol.*, 2001; 112: 457-463.

[58] Klein C. J., Moon J-S., Mauermann M. L. The neuropathies of Waldenstrom's macroglobulinemia (WM) and IgM-MGUS. *Can. J. Neurol. Sci.*, 2011; 38: 289-295.

[59] Simovic D., Gorson K. C., Ropper A. H. Comparison of IgM-MGUS and IgG-MGUS polyneuropathy. *Acta. Neurol. Scand.,* 1998; 97: 194-200.

[60] Lunn M. P. T., Nobile-Orazio E. Immunotherapy for IgM anti-myelin-associated glycoprotein paraprotein-associated peripheral neuropathies. *The Cochrane Data Base Syst. Rev.*, 2012. Issue 5: CD002827.

[61] Dalakas M. C., Rakocevic G., Salajegheh M., Dambrosia J. M., Hahn A. F., Raju R., McElroy B. Placebo-controlled trial of rituximab in IgM anti-myelin-associated glycoprotein antibody demyelinating neuropathy. *Ann. Neurol.,* 2009; 65: 286-293.

[62] Benedetti L., Briani C., Franciotta D., Carpo M., Padua L., Zara G., Zambello R., Sormani M. P., Mancardi G. L., Nobile-Orazio E., Schenone A. Long-term effect of rituximab in anti-MAG polyneuropathy. *Neurology*, 2008; 71: 1742-1744.

[63] Benedetti L., Briani C., Grandis M., Vigo T., Gobbi M., Ghiglione E., Carpo M., Cocito D., Caporale C. M., Sormani M. P., Mancardi G. L., Nobile-Orazio E., Schenone A. Predictors of response to rituximab in patients with neuropathy and anti-myelin associated glycoprotein immunoglobulin M. *J. Peripher. Nerv. Syst.,* 2007; 12: 102-107.

[64] Renaud S., Fuhr P., Gregor M., Schweikert K., Lorenz D., Daniels C., Deuschl G., Gratwohl A., Steck A. J. High-dose rituximab and anti-MAG-associated polyneuropathy. *Neurology*, 2006; 66: 742-744.

[65] Renaud S., Gregor M., Fuhr P., Lorenz D., Deuschl G., Gratwohl A., Steck A. J. Rituximab in the treatment of polyneuropathy associated with anti-MAG antibodies. *Muscle Nerve*, 2003; 27: 611-615.

[66] Pestronk A., Florence J., Miller T., Choksi R., Al-Lozi M. T., Levine T. D. Treatment of IgM antibody associated polyneuropathies using rituximab. *J. Neurol. Neurosurg. Psychiatry,* 2003; 74: 485-489.

[67] Levine T., Pestronk A. IgM antibody-related polyneuropathies: B-cell depletion chemotherapy using rituximab. *Neurology,* 1999; 52 (8): 1702-1705.

[68] Kelly J. J. Chronic peripheral neuropathy responsive to rituximab. *Rev. Neurol. Dis.,* 2006; 3 (2): 78-81.

[69] Rojas-Garcia R., Gallardo E., de Andres I., de Luna N., Juarez C., Sanchez P., Illa I. Chronic neuropathy with IgM anti-ganglioside antibodies: lack of long term response to rituximab. *Neurology,* 2003; 61: 1814-1816.

[70] Broglio L., Lauria G. Worsening after rituximab treatment in anti-MAG neuropathy. *Muscle Nerve*, 2005; 32 (3): 378-9.

[71] Delmont E., Jeandel P. Y., Hubert A. M., Marc L., Boucraut J., Desnuelle C. Successful treatment with rituximab of one patient with CANOMAD neuropathy. *J. Neurol.*, 2010; 257: 655-657.

[72] Comi G., Roveri L., Swan A., Willison H., Bojar M., Illa I., Karageorgiou C., Nobile-Orazio E., van den Bergh P., Swan T., Hughs R., Aubry J., Baumann N., Hadden R., Lunn M., Knapp M., Leger J. M., Bouche P., Mazanec R., Meucci N., van der Meche F., Toyka K.; Inflammatory Neuropathy Case and Treatment Group. A randomized

controlled trial of intravenous immunoglobulin in IgM paraprotein associated demyelinating neuropathy. *J. Neurol.,* 2002; 249: 1370-1377.

[73] Dalakas M. C., Quarles R. H., Farrer R. G., Dambrosia J., Soueidan S., Stein D. P., Cupler E., Sekul E. A., Otero C. A controlled study of intravenous immunoglobulin in demyelinating neuropathy with IgM gammopathy. *Ann. Neurol.,* 1996; 40: 792-795.

[74] Attarian S., Boucraut J., Hubert A. M., Uzenot D., Delmont E., Verschueren A., Franques J., Azulay J. P., Pouget J. Chronic ataxic neuropathies associated with anti-GD1b IgM antibodies: response to IVIg therapy. *J. Neurol. Neurosurg. Psychiatry,* 2010; 81: 61-64.

[75] Oksenhendler E., Chevret S., Leger J. M., Louboutin J. P., Bussel A., Brouet J. C. Plasma exchange and chlorambucil in polyneuropathy associated with monoclonal IgM gammopathy. *J. Neurol. Neurosurg. Psychiatry*, 1995; 59: 243-247.

[76] Dyck P. J., Low P. A., Windebank A. J., Jaradeh S. S., Gosselin S., Bourque P., Smith B. E., Kratz K. M., Karnes J. L., Evans B. A., Pineda A. A., O'Brien P. C. Plasma exchange in polyneuropathy associated with monoclonal gammopathy of undetermined significance. *N. Engl. J. Med.,* 1991; 325: 1482-6.

[77] Niermeijer J. M. F., Eurelings M., Lokhorst H., Franssen H., Fijnheer R., Wokke J. H. J., Notermans N. C. Neurologic and hematologic response to fludarabine treatment in IgM MGUS polyneuropathy. *Neurology*, 2006; 67: 2076-2079.

[78] Wilson H. C., Lunn M. P. T., Schey S., Hughs R. A. C. Successful treatment of IgM paraproteinemic neuropathy with fludarabine. *J. Neurol. Neurosurg. Psychiatry*, 1999; 66: 575-580.

[79] Niermeijer J. M. F., Eurelings M., Lokhorst H. M., Franssen H., Fischer K., Teunissen L. L., van den Berg L. H., Schobben F., Wokke J. H. J., Notermans N. C. Intermittent cyclophosphamide with prednisone versus placebo for polyneuropathy with IgM monoclonal gammopathy. *Neurology,* 2007; 69: 50-59.

[80] Notermans M. C., Lokhorst H. M., Franssen H., van der Graaf Y., Teunissen L. L., Jennekens F. G. I., van den Berg L. H., Wokke J. H. J. Intermittent cyclophosphamide and prednisone treatment of polyneuropathy associated with monoclonal gammopathy of undetermined significance. *Neurology*, 1996; 47: 1227-1233.

[81] Mc Master J., Gibson G., Castro-Prado F., Vitali A., Honey C. R. Neurosurgical treatment of tremor in anti-myelin-associated glycoprotein neuropathy. *Neurology,* 2009; 73: 1707-1708.

[82] Cortese I., Chaudhry V., So Y. T., Cantor F., Cornblath D. R., Rae-Grant A. Evidence-based guideline update: Plasmapheresis in neurologic disorders: report of the Therapeutics and Technology Assessment Subcommittee of the American Academy of Neurology. *Neurology*, 2011; 76: 294-300.

[83] Notermans N. C., Vermeulen M., Lokhorst H. M., Van Doorn P. A., Van Den Berg L. H., Teunissen L. L., Wokke J. H. J. Pulsed high-dose dexamethasone treatment of polyneuropathy associated with monoclonal gammopathy. *J. Neurol.,* 1997; 244 (7): 462-3.

[84] Eurelings M., Lokhorst H. M., Kalmijn S., Wokke J. H. J., Notermans N. C. Malignant transformation in polyneuropathy associated with monoclonal gammopathy. *Neurology,* 2005; 64: 2079-2084.

[85] Nobile-Orazio E., Meucci N, Baldini L., Di Troia A., Scarlato G. Long-term prognosis of neuropathy associated with anti-MAG IgM M-proteins and its relationship to immune therapies. *Brain,* 2000, 123: 710-717.

[86] Niermeijer J. M. F., Fischer K., Eurelings M., Franssen H., Wokke J. H. J., Notermans N. C. Prognosis of polyneuropathy due to IgM monoclonal gammopathy. *Neurology,* 2010; 74: 406-412.

In: Contemporary Issues in Peripheral Neuropathy
Editor: Daniel L. Menkes
ISBN: 978-1-62948-681-9

Chapter VIII

Peripheral Neuropathies in HIV Infection

Maurizio Osio [1]***, Caterina Nascimbene*** [2]***,***
Alessandra Vanotti [1] ***and Cristoforo Comi*** [2]
[1]Neurology Department. University of Milan, "L. Sacco" Hospital, Milan, Italy
[2]Department of Translational Medicine, Section of Neurology,
University of Eastern Piedmont "Amedeo Avogadro", Novara, Italy

Abstract

While the introduction of HAART [Highly active anti retoriviral therapy] has resulted in an overall decline in the incidence and prevalence of nervous system complications, peripheral neuropathy (PN) continues to be a common neurologic complication at every stage of HIV infection. The treating physician has to determine if the patient is experiencing a neuropathy due to the immune system's reaction to the virus, direct toxic effects of the virus or if the neuropathy may be attributed to the effects of the antiretroviral agents used to reduce the viral load. The spectrum of peripheral nervous system involvement in HIV infection includes distal symmetrical polyneuropathy (DSP), toxic neuropathy from antiretroviral drugs, diffuse infiltrative lymphocytosis syndrome (DILS), inflammatory demyelinating polyneuropathies (IDPs), multifocal mononeuropathies, and progressive polyradiculopathy. On general principles, immune mediated neuropathies tend to occur in the earlier stages of HIV infection when the patient is relatively immunocompetent whereas neuropathies that result from antiretroviral therapy and direct viral toxicity tend to occur later in the course of the infection. This chapter addresses these conditions as well as the treatmentrs available for these disorders and the neuropathic pain that often accompanies them.

The incidence of HIV infection is slowly decreasing worldwide. The number of new cases declined from approximately 3.1 million people in 2002 to 2.7 million people in 2010 [1]. Moreover, significant improvements in both the efficacy and the availability of antiretroviral treatments have led to increased survival and a resultant increase in disease prevalence such that the total number of HIV positive persons reached 34 million people in 2010 [1] (Figure 1). Antiretroviral treatments also resulted in an overall reduction in central nervous system complications. In contrast, peripheral neuropathy (PN) continues to be a common neurological disorder encountered at every stage of HIV infection [2-5]. Peripheral nervous system (PNS) involvement with concomitant HIV infection may result from either direct or indirect viral effects as well as from comorbid diseases or treatment side-effects. Notwithstanding, it was recently reported that PNS pathology has a stronger correlation with CD4+ lymphocyte counts than with disease duration [6].

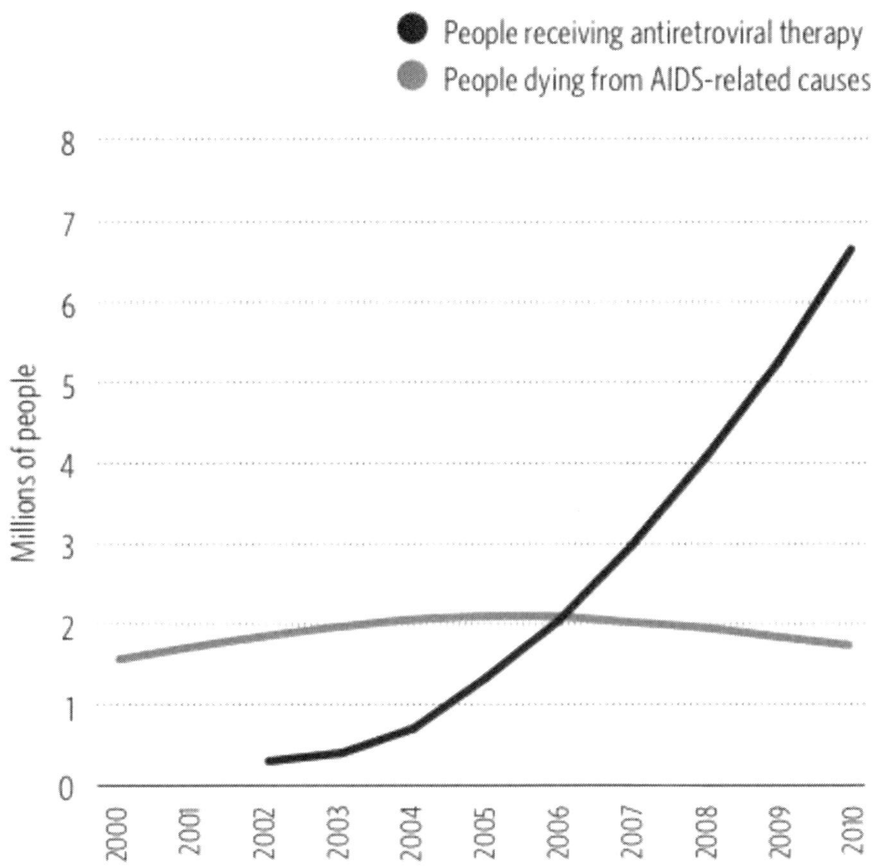

Figure 1. Number of people with access to antiretroviral therapy and the number of people dying from AIDS-related causes, low- and middle-income countries, 2000–2010 (After UNAIDS 2011 GLOBAL HIV/AIDS RESPONSE Epidemic update and health sector progress towards Universal Access Progress Report 2011).

The increased survival of HIV infected patients, as well as the increased frequency of new cases in the aging population, has resulted in a novel situation. As immune surveillance decreases with age, previously immunocompetent persons who are HIV positive may present with a PN [6]. PN tends to be more common in the elderly given this group's tendency to acquire comorbid disorders such that the added burden of HIV infection may increase the probability of developing a PN. Schifitto et al. systematically analyzed the risk factors of HIV related PN and reported that the main predictors are the presence of depressed mood and general signs of neurological dysfunction [7]. This implies that patients who display earlier nervous system involvement appear to have a higher risk of developing a PN.

The spectrum of PNS involvement in HIV infection includes distal symmetrical polyneuropathy (DSP), toxic neuropathy from antiretroviral drugs, diffuse infiltrative lymphocytosis syndrome (DILS), inflammatory demyelinating polyneuropathies (IDPs), multifocal mononeuropathies (MM), and progressive polyradiculopathies (PR). It should be recalled that HIV infection may involve different areas of the nervous system simultaneously (e.g. concurrent PN and myelopathy). As such, it may not be possible to localize the pathological site to just one specific location within in the nervous system. Moreover, the same patient may have more than one cause of their neurological dysfunction (e.g. HIV related PN appearing in a patient with a previous drug related neuropathy). Notwithstanding, the various types of PN encountered with HIV infection are summarized in the subsequent sections.

Distal Symmetrical Polyneuropathy

Distal symmetrical polyneuropathy (DSP) is the most frequent form of neuropathy encountered in HIV-1 infection. It typically presents as a length-dependent degeneration of both myelinated and unmyelinated nerve fibers in 30% of HIV infected patients [7, 8]. It is noteworthy that virtually every person diagnosed with acquired immunodeficiency syndrome (AIDS) has evidence of this disorder at autopsy [9]. DSP typically presents with the onset of painful lower extremity digital paresthesias that progress up the lower extremities over several weeks to months whereas the upper extremities are hardly ever involved [10, 11]. The sensory examination demonstrates loss of small fiber function (pain and temperature) out of proportion to large fiber dysfunction. More than two-thirds of patients display decreased or absent distal ankle reflexes whereas the others manifest either a superimposed myelopathy or a small fiber neuropathy [11, 12] (Figure 2). Electrodiagnostic evaluations should be performed in order to assess for the presence of large fiber dysfunction followed by a skin biopsy for an assessment of small fiber function in the event that the electrodiagnostic studies are normal (Table 1). In all HIV-positive patients, an increased thermal threshold on quantitative sensory testing (QST) may be detected, even when there are no clinical manifestations of a PN [11]. Notwithstanding, it has been reported that patients who display an early loss of thermal function do not have a higher incidence of symptomatic DSP such that an abnormal thermal threshold does not predict the subsequent development of a DSP [13]. Another study reported that the intraepidermal fiber density (IENF) is significantly decreased in patients with DSP as compared to controls and patients with abnormal thermal thresholds on QST [14]. Approximately 25% of patients with DSP patients report mild degrees of foot cramps, which tend to occur later in the course of the neuropathy [11, 12, 15]. DSP has the same frequency in children, (circa 34%), as in adults but the symptoms tend to be less severe [16].

The authors recommend that all HIV positive patients be evaluated for other potential causes of neuropathy (Table 2). The patient should be asked about a history of alcohol abuse [17], illicit drug use [18] or prior exposure to neurotoxic drugs, especially those containing dideoxynucleosides. In addition, the diagnostic work-up should include a fasting blood glucose, a hemoglobin A1c, serum vitamin B12 with or without a methylmalonic acid determination, folic acid, thyroid function studies, a serum immunoelectrophoresis [SIEP], a urine protein electrophoresis as well as HBV and HCV serology given the higher risk of viral coinfection [19]. DSP typically displays axonal features on nerve conduction studies [11]. Approximately 25% of asymptomatic patients demonstrate neurophysiological abnormalities whereas 20% of cases have symptoms of a DSP but a normal neurophysiological exam, which may indicate selective small fiber involvement [11].

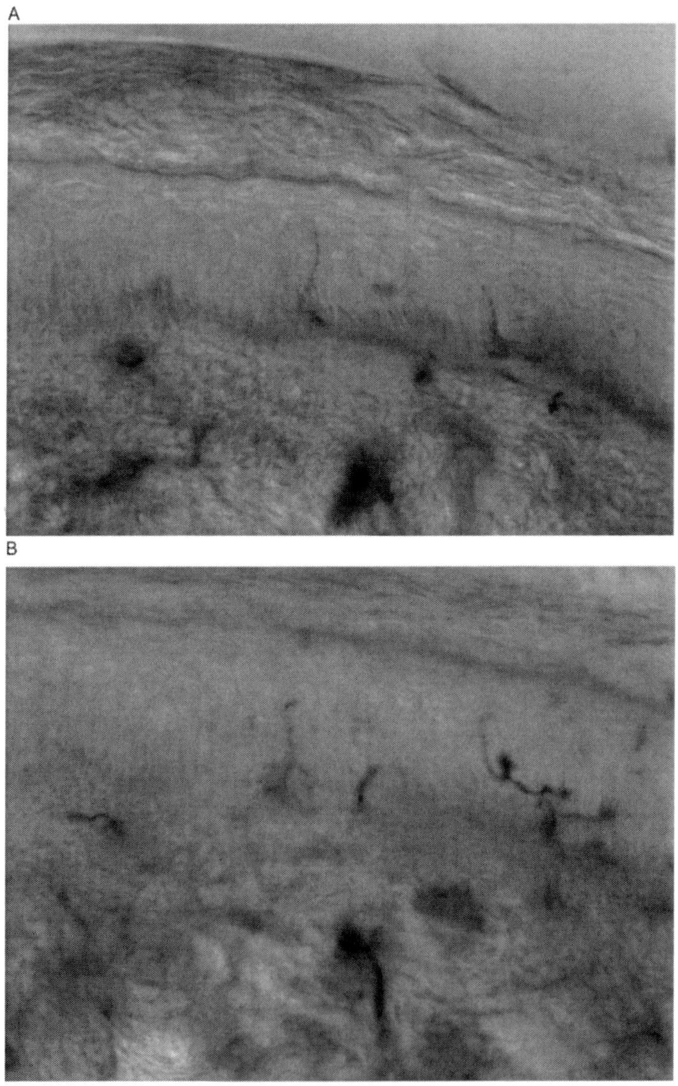

Figure 2. Skin biopsy performed on the ankle in two HIV subjects complaining of distal pain with a "stocking and glove" distribution associated with normal clinical neurophysiological findings. Patient A: normal intraepidermal nervous fibers density. Peripheral neuropathy was not demonstrated in this patient. Patient B: reduced number of intra-epidermal nerve fiber density consistent with the diagnosis of small fiber polyneuropathy.

Table 1. Diagnostic approach to HIV patients who complain of distal pain with glow-stocking distribution

	Nerve conduction data	Electromyography	Skin biopsy	Diagnosis
Distal pain	Normal motor conduction studies	Normal	Normal	No neuropathy
	Normal sensory conduction studies	Normal	Abnormal	Small fiber polyneuropathy
	Normal /Low amplitude CMAP	Normal	Not needed	Distal symmetric polyneuropathy
	Low amplitude/absent SNAP	Abnormal (Proximal/distal gradient)		
	Slow motor nerve conduction – Abnormal CMAP dispesion – Conduction block	Normal	Not needed	Demyelinating Polyradiculoneuropathy
	Prolonged SAP distal latencies – Low amplitude SNAP	Abnormal (No proximal/distal gradient)		

Legend: CMAP: Compound Muscle Action Potential; SNAP: Sensory Nerve Action Potential; Proximal/distal gradient: electromyographic signs of chronic involvement prominent in the distal muscles of limbs (usually lower limbs)

Table 2. Differential diagnosis of Distal Sensory Polyneuropathy (DSP)

	History	d-drugs	Blood lactate	Diagnosis	Therapy
Distal Sensory Polyneuropathy	CD4+ > 200 cells/mL*	No	Not needed	HIV-related DSP	Introduce ART therapy without d-drugs
	Consider**: Alimentary regimen Diabetes Alcohol abuse Drug abuse Chemiotherapy Other Neurotoxic therapies				Treat pain
		Yes	Normal		
			High	ART-related DSP	Interrupt d-drugs (possible "coasting") Change ART regiment

Legend: * DSP is possible even in patients with CD4+> 200 cells/mL; ** factors that may be cause of DSP but do not rule out HIV-related or ART-related polyneuropathy; d-drugs: zalcitabine (ddC), didanosine (ddI), stavudine (d4T) ; ART: Antiretroviral Therapy;

Pathophysiology of DSP

HIV related DSP is characterized by distal axonal degeneration [20-22], neuronal loss in the dorsal root ganglia (DRG) [23], and Wallerian degeneration or "dying-back" of peripheral and central terminals of peripheral nerve fibers [23-25]. Post-mortem neuro-anatomical studies have demonstrated immune cell infiltration and inflammatory mediator release in peripheral nerve trunks and the DRG of patients with advanced disease [20, 22, 26-29].

Because neurons do not express CD4 receptors, it is unlikely that neuronal damage in HIV-infected subjects occurs by direct infection. Otherwise peripheral nerve damage may occur indirectly through inappropriate activation of immunocompetent cells by the virus or viral proteins [8, 30]. Alternatively, this may result from direct viral-mediated neurotoxicity [31, 32].

The most important viral protein used, in vivo and in vitro, to investigate the pathogenesis of HIV-mediated neurotoxicity is gp120. This is a viral coat protein that mediates the binding to and the transmission of HIV into cells through interactions with the CD4 protein and the chemokine co-receptors CCR5 and CXCR4. Even in its soluble form, gp120 is able to activate antigen presenting cells [33]. In addition, HIV-1 viral protein R (Vpr) has been used experimentally to assess the neurotoxicity of viral proteins in vitro [32, 34]. It is an accessory protein that regulates HIV-1 infectivity that has been identified in macrophage-like cells in the DRGs of HIV-infected individuals.

Acute perineural application of gp120 to rat sciatic nerves resulted in acute axonal swelling and increased tumor necrosis factor (TNF)-α expression in the nerve trunks, DRG [35] and the dorsal horn of the spinal cord [36]. Macrophage accumulation in the nerve trunk was maximal approximately two weeks after gp120 application and was associated with dying-back of distal nerve fiber endings in the epidermis, macrophage infiltration, and inflammatory mediator production in the DRG [37, 38]. These changes were preceded by expression of ATF3; a marker of cellular stress and neuronal injury in DRG neurons.

Studies using cultured primary rat and human DRG neurons have demonstrated that the neurotoxic effects of gp120 may be directly mediated by activation of chemokine receptors on the surface of neurons, or indirectly through the activation of Schwann cells and macrophages [39-41].

The toxicity of gp120 required the presence of Schwann cells, which likely mediated the binding of gp120 to CXCR4 receptors on Schwann cells that subsequently stimulated the release of the chemokine CCL5, which activated CCR5 receptors on DRG neuronal cells. This neuronal activation induced TNF-α release from the neuronal cells which, through an autocrine and/or paracrine mechanism, activated neuronally expressed TNFR1 receptors, leading to cell death [28, 36, 39, 42]. Activation of a non-specific immune response might also contribute to the indirect neurotoxicity of the virus.

Hahn and colleagues [43] reported that supernatant from cultured human monocytic cells infected with HIV inhibited neurite growth in cultured human fetal DRGs even when neuronally expressed CCR5 and CXCR4 receptors were neutralized. Inhibition of neurite growth was associated with depolarization of the mitochondrial membrane and generation of reactive oxygen species presumably related to release of inflammatory substances such as interleukin (IL)-1β and TNF-α. Although the mechanism by which infection-induced mitochondrial dysfunction is unknown, some data indicate that mitochondrial dysfunction may contribute to the virally induced neuropathy [43, 44].

In addition to indirect neurotoxicity, there is experimental evidence for direct viral effect on peripheral nerve fibers, especially along axons, which may also contribute to the neuronal degeneration and dying-back of epidermal nerve fibers observed in affected patients [42, 45].

DSP Treatment

Treatment of HIV-related sensory neuropathy is primarily symptomatic. Neuropathic pain is often present and manifests a complex array of symptoms and signs that actually fluctuate over time. The pathophysiology and biochemistry of neuropathic pain and epilepsy share several aspects [46]. Both the "wind-up" phenomenon induced by nerve damage and the "kindling" of hippocampal neurons in epilepsy, may be related to activation of N-methyl-D-aspartate (NMDA) receptors [47, 48]. Moreover, pathological sodium channels function has been demonstrated in neuropathic pain models [49, 50]. This may be the reason that anti-epileptic drugs (AEDs) can be effective in the treatment of neuropathic pain. Furthermore, there is evidence that AEDs blocking calcium and sodium channels may improve immune function in HIV-positive subjects [51]. Nonetheless, such medications may produce significant unwanted side effects in HIV-positive persons and may negatively interact with protease inhibitor drugs such that they should be used with caution [52]. The evidence based medicine supporting the symptomatic treatment of DSP associated with HIV infection will be explored in greater detail.

Carbamazepine

Carbamazepine (CBZ) is a derivate of iminostilbene and is chemically related to the tricyclic anti-depressants. Its effect on neuropathic pain is probably due to both central and peripheral mechanisms. The ability of CBZ to block channel conductivity seems to be frequency dependent. This enables CBZ to suppress the activity of both A-delta and C fibers, which are responsible for pain transmission, without interfering with normal nerve conduction [53]. Its effectiveness in pain control is well documented in trigeminal neuralgia [54, 55]. However, there are no Class I or Class II studies that have reported CBZ to be effective in treating pain associated with HIV-related peripheral neuropathy. In addition to the well-known risk of leukopenia and hyponatremia, major adverse reactions have been reported in HIV-positive patients [56-58]. Therefore, there is no evidence based medicine to support the use of CBZ in HIV-related painful neuropathy.

Gabapentin

There is only one controlled study on gabapentin (GBP) use in HIV-related painful neuropathy [59]. GBP was titrated up to a maximum of 2400 mg/daily. While this study reported an initial response in patients treated with the active drug compared to those taking placebo at four weeks, no statistically significant difference in primary outcome (e.g. a decrease in VAS pain score) was noted between the two study arms. Therefore, GBP has not been proven effective for the treatment of HIV-related painful neuropathy (HRPN).

Pregabalin

A large controlled trial was carried out to evaluate efficacy of pregabalin in HRPN [60]. The drug was titrated up to either the maximum tolerated dose or to 1200mg/daily. No statistically significant differences were reported.

Lamotrigine

Lamotrigine (LTG) is a phenyltriazine derivative able to block voltage-gated sodium channels and to inhibit the release of glutamate and aspartate. At a dosage of 50-400 mg/daily, LTG was shown to be effective in reducing pain in both subjects with trigeminal neuralgia refractory to other treatments [61]. It was also useful in reducing central post-stroke pain [62]. The same group conducted two controlled trials in HIV-related painful neuropathy [63, 64]. These studies' results are difficult to interpret but two salient points emerged. The first is that a significant pain reduction was only achieved in patients who were using concomitant anti-retroviral (ARV) therapy. The second is that there were a high number of drop-outs in the LTG treated group, which implies a narrow therapeutic index. As such, LTG likely has a limited role in the treatment of pain associated with HIV infection that should be used only in patients using concomitant ARV therapy.

Amitriptyline and Mexiletine

Two controlled studies assessing the efficacy in pain control of amitriptyline versus placebo in HIV-related painful neuropathy were performed. In both studies, another treatment arm was included; acupuncture [65] in one, mexiletine in the other [66]. The complex design of these two studies limited the conclusions. Nonetheless, both studies failed to demonstrate a statistically significant difference in the Gracely pain score when comparing either amitriptyline or mexiletine versus placebo. Duloxetine, which is approved for treatment of diabetic neuropathic pain, has not been tested in a similar manner.

Recombinant human Nerve Growth Factor (NGF)

NGF is a neurotrophin that plays a key role in the development and maintenance of small unmyelinated fibers [67]. While it was reported to be effective in painful HIV-related neuropathy in a clinical trial [68], it has limited practical use [69]. One significant limitation of the systemic administration of neurotrophic factors (NF) is their poor bioavailability due to their short half-life. Alternative transport models, such as "muscle-based" gene therapy, which would allow constant availability of significant circulating levels of NF, have been used effectively on animal models of sensorimotor polyneuropathy [70].

Prosaptide and P-Peptide

Two controlled studies analyzed the efficacy of these two agents with the Gracely pain score in HIV-related painful neuropathy and found no significant differences when compared to placebo [71, 72].

Acetyl –L-Carnitine

The efficacy of acetyl-L-carnitine in HIV-related painful neuropathy was assessed in six studies, only one of which was placebo controlled [73-78]. In this study, the analysis of the efficacy-evaluable (EE) population demonstrated a slight superiority of acetyl-L-carnitine when compared to placebo, whereas no difference was found after analyzing the intention to treat (ITT) population [77].

Smoked Cannabis

Two controlled studies suggest that smoked cannabis were superior to placebo in HIV-related painful neuropathy [79, 80]. The first cited study evaluated a maximum tolerated dose of 1 to 8% D-9-tetrahydrocannabinol administered four times per day whereas the second evaluated 3.56% D-9-tetrahydrocannabinol three times daily The limitations of these two studies include the short observation period (5 days) and the number of unblinded subjects in the active treatment arm. Therefore, it is not possible to draw any definite conclusions from these data.

Topical Capsaicin

Topical Capsaicin is used in patch forms containing different drug concentrations in the treatment of localized neuropathic pain. In a controlled study with low dose capsaicin (0.075%), there was no significant difference from placebo [81]. However, a higher concentration (8%) was reported to be more effective [82]. Nonetheless, it should be noted that topical capsaicin induces a burning sensation when applied to the skin whereas the placebo agent likely did not. Therefore, no definite conclusions may be inferred from these data. Moreover, there are no data on long term capsaicin treatment for patients with HIV-related painful neuropathy.

Opioids

In the 2010 revision, the EFNS Task Force revised its 2006 guidelines [83] on the pharmacological treatment of neuropathic pain [84]. Medications recommended as first line agents for neuropathic pain conditions such as diabetic neuropathy include tricyclic antidepressants, selective serotonin and norepinephrine reuptake inhibitors (SNRIs) such as duloxetine and venlafaxine as well as gabapentinoids that act on calcium channel alpha 2 delta ligands (e.g. gabapentin, pregabalin) [84]. Tramadol and opioids are reserved as second or third line agents [84]. The use of opioids in pain management in HIV-positive patients requires special considerations.

Opioids prescribed to HIV-positive patients may have potential interactions with other medications used to treat HIV disease. Ritonavir and lopinavir/ritonavir greatly increase plasma concentrations of oral oxycodone in healthy volunteers, which enhances its effect. When oxycodone is used in patients during ritonavir and lopinavir/ritonavir treatment, concomitant reductions in the oxycodone dose may be needed [85]. There is experimental evidence that morphine increases the expression of CCR5 receptors on microglial cells infected with HIV [86] and that heroin promotes HIV viral replication in cultured astrocytes [87]. Experimental data on animals [88] and post-mortem examination on humans also provide data indicating a more rapid course of HIV infection in people exposed to opioids [89].

Opioids may also augment the discomfort of painful HIV-related neuropathy [90]. Moreover, in some forms of neuropathic pain not related to HIV, opioids may exhibit pronociceptive actions through various interactive mechanisms between the immune system and the glia [89, 91-97]. However, not all opiates act in the same way. It appears that buprenorphine has no significant interaction with the immune system. Experimental data indicate that it has no interaction with the gp-120 protein such that it acts through a mechanism different from other analgesic opiates. Therefore, buprenorphine may be the preferred opioid agent for pain management in HIV-infected subjects [98-103].

In summary, the only analgesic agents with proven efficacy in HIV-related neuropathy are capsaicin 8%, smoked cannabis and rhNGF. However, rhNGF is clinically unavailable whereas smoked cannabis cannot be recommended as routine therapy. In clinical practice, when treating patients with HIV-associated neuropathy, it is important to try and maintain sustained virologic control while minimizing the use of potentially neurotoxic drugs.

Drug Induced Peripheral Neuropathy: Anti-Retroviral Drugs

While HAART therapy improves survival, it also exposes patients to the potential side effects of chronic drug administration. This has important implications for the risk of developing peripheral neuropathy. Furthermore, many patients already have an HIV-related neuropathy, which decreases the neural reserve of the peripheral nervous system [PNS], such that a drug induced neuropathy may develop earlier and with lower drug doses.

Although the incidence of DSP has been decreasing, drug-induced neuropathy is becoming more frequent [105]. This was more notable after the introduction of nucleoside reverse transcriptase inhibitors (NRTI) [8, 106]. The antiretroviral drugs zalcitabine (ddC), didanosine (ddI) and stavudine (d4T) have all been shown to favor the development of peripheral neuropathy. This occurs with variable frequency and is related to the dosage and treatment duration [12] as well as the number of patient years. Of these agents, ddC is the most frequently prescribed, followed by d4T and ddI [107]. It was reported that dideoxyribonucleotides display a synergistic neurotoxic effect when used in combination [107-109]. The incidence of polyneuropathy is also influenced by the administration of other potentially neurotoxic drugs, such as hydroxyurea. The combination of hydroxyurea and didanosine was reported to inhibit HIV-1 both in vitro and in vivo when administered to patients with CD4 counts lower than 300 cells/mm^3 [110]. These agents inhibit ribonucleic reductase and therefore impair DNA synthesis [110]. Other risk factors include the presence of pre-existing neuropathy from other causes (e.g. diabetes, vitamin B12 deficiency, chronic alcohol abuse), increased age, poor nutritional status and advanced HIV infection [12, 111, 112]. A "double hit" theory has been proposed in order to explain the mechanism by which HIV infection predisposes to antiretroviral drug induced neuropathy. Initially, neurons in the dorsal root ganglion (DRG) are injured during the inflammatory reaction triggered by HIV infection followed by a second phase in which they sustain mitochondrial damage due to NRTI toxicity. Restated, the development of peripheral neuropathy would represent the unmasking of previous subclinical neural injury induced by HIV infection.

The frequency of antiretroviral drug induced neuropathy varies between 15 to 40% with an onset that begins after 6-20 weeks of treatment [106, 112]. Clinical features are similar to that of DSP. The only distinctive feature is the temporal association between the administration of one or more NRTI and the acute appearance of a new or progressive sensory predominant neuropathy. Approximately half the patients report pain as the first and often only symptom, especially when higher doses are prescribed [112].

Neurophysiological studies typically demonstrate axonal features, although in some cases only a decreased amplitude of the sural nerve sensory potential or even normal findings may be evident [52]. The pathology demonstrates axonal degeneration, marked loss of unmyelinated nerve fibers [106, 113], myelin swelling, and alterations of mitochondrial morphology [111, 114].

One hypothesis is that NRTI toxicity is mediated by mitochondrial dysfunction [115, 116]. This is because the drug side effects are reminiscent of hereditary mitochondrial diseases with features of peripheral neuropathy, hepatic steatosis, lipodystrophy, lactic acidosis, ragged red fiber myopathy and pancreatitis [12, 111]. It was reported that elevated serum lactate levels may be useful in differentiating NRTI induced neuropathy form DSP, specifically in the subgroup related to stavudine use, with a 90% sensitivity and specificity (P=0.001) [52]. In affected tissues, ultrastructural alterations of mitochondria were detected [113, 114]. T cell mitochondrial numbers, morphology and apoptosis were assessed in an HIV positive patient who presented severe lactic acidosis after treatment with stavudine, didanosine and indinavir [117]. T cell mitochondria were markedly decreased in number when compared to normal values along with an increased percentage of apoptotic T cells. The main structural alterations were the swelling and disruption of cristae and internal structures, which were more evident at higher lactate concentrations. Morphological assessments performed one week after lactic acid normalization revealed a marked increase in both the number of mitochondria and the disappearance of structural alterations. Moreover, the percentage of apoptotic cells was less than 5%. The authors hypothesized that increased lymphocytic apoptosis was related to the release of pro-apoptotic factors from damaged mitochondria [117].

All NRTI have been reported, in vitro, to inhibit DNA polymerase γ. This is an enzyme that is responsible for mitochondrial DNA (mtDNA) synthesis such that mitochondrial toxicity would then result from mtDNA depletion [118, 119]. Since not all patients exposed to NRTI develop a neuropathy, a role for potentially predisposing genetic variants of polymerase γ was proposed [120, 121]. Moreover, a significant association between NRTI use and a decrease of mtDNA in the subcutaneous fat was reported. Nonetheless, no association between neuropathy and either a decrease of mtDNA in subcutaneous fat or lipoatrophy was identified in another report [122]. Nonetheless, these findings may be provide a useful method to unravel pre-symptomatic mitochondrial toxicity and to monitor clinical status in patients exposed to antiretroviral therapy. Considering that some studies have failed to demonstrate mtDNA depletion in NRTI treatcd HIV-positive patients, alternative mechanisms of tissue specific mitochondrial damage have been suggested [123]. It was observed that zidovudine inhibits both NADH-related respiratory function and NADH-cytocrome c reductase activity in mitochondria from isolated murine skeletal muscle, brain and liver [124]. Moreover, zidovudine inhibits adenylate kinase and ADP/ATP translocase in mitochondria from isolated liver [125, 126] and decreases succinate dehydrogenase activity in human muscle cells [127]. Didanosine induces cardiac toxicity in rats, likely on the basis of decreased activity of respiratory complexes, but not on the basis of mtDNA depletion [128]. With respect to the effect of nucleoside analogues, no correlations between the ability to increase lactate production and mtDNA depletion were reported [129].

Other conditions have been reported to be associated to NRTI use. Stavudine administration can induce a syndrome characterized by rapidly ascending muscular weakness and respiratory failure mimicking GBS, even though in some cases increased serum lactate may be present [130]. Zidovudine may trigger acute porphyritic neuropathy in patients who already display underlying dysfunction in porphyrin metabolism, or alternatively, it may cause dysfunction in porphyrin metabolism with a resultant secondary neuropathy [131].

Our recommended clinical approach consists in the early identification and discontinuation of the responsible medications and the use of symptomatic drugs for pain control. After drug discontinuation, approximately two thirds of patients demonstrate symptomatic improvement in time but this is often preceded by an initial worsening, or "coasting" due to a residual drug effect [132].

Drug Induced Peripheral Neuropathy: Other Drugs

In addition to antiretroviral agents, there are other drugs commonly used in HIV-positive subjects that are known to cause neuropathy in immune competent subjects as well. The agents that deserve special consideration include vincristine, vinblastine, taxole, isoniazide, ethambutol, dapsone, talidomide, and HMG-CoA reductase inhibitors. Such agents should be employed only when the risk to benefit ratio is favorable.

Acute Inflammatory Demyelinating Polyneuropathy

Guillain-Barré syndrome (GBS) is an acute peripheral neuropathy characterized by symmetrical muscle weakness occurring in the absence of identifiable causes of genetic, metabolic, or toxic origin. The characteristic presentation of the syndrome involves symmetrical paresis and/or paresthesias with an ascending pattern, reduction or loss of deep tendon reflexes and variable autonomic dysfunction. Signs and symptoms observed in the course of GBS are highly variable. The CSF protein concentrations are often elevated, with fewer than 10 white blood cells (WBCs) per μL, but up to 50 WBCs per μL is acceptable for diagnosis in the context of HIV infection [133]. Restated, the presence of 10-50 WBCs in the CSF does not exclude the diagnosis of GBS. Furthermore, patients presenting with the GBS with these CSF findings should undergo HIV testing.

Neurophysiological findings may include delayed or absent F-wave responses, prolonged distal motor latencies, and slowed conduction velocities in the later stages of the condition; findings that are similar to those noted in patients with acute inflammatory demyelinating polyneuropathy who do not have HIV infection [52].

Approximately two-thirds of patients with GBS describe an antecedent illness followed by an ascending paralysis occurring days to weeks later. Since 1985, several cases of the disease among HIV infected patients have been reported, with GBS occurring concomitantly with HIV seroconversion or during the initial phases of infection [133, 134-140].

Current evidence indicates that HIV-GBS usually precedes overt AIDS and a state of immunosuppression [141-143]. Although a few patients with AIDS and GBS were reported [144-146], most authors concur that GBS occurs early in HIV infection, when the CD4 count is high (>500) [142, 143]. GBS in HIV infected patients with CD4 cell counts less than 50 should be treated presumptively for CMV infection [147].

HIV infection is one of the most common causes of GBS in African countries, India, and other developing countries.

In HIV-infected patients, GBS has been reported in association with the immune reconstitution syndrome, whereby there is a re-emergence of previously anergic lymphocytes upon viral suppression with highly active antiretroviral therapy (HAART) [148-152]. Nucleoside analogue reverse transcriptase inhibitors (NRTIs), a key component of HAART, have been associated with GBS in HIV infected individuals as part of the immune reconstitution syndrome [153, 154].

The mechanisms proposed for GBS in HIV-1-infected patients include a direct action of HIV-1 on the nerves by neurotropic strains or by autoimmune mechanisms mediated by the formation of antibodies directed against the myelin sheath secondary to abnormal immunoregulation induced by HIV infection [155].

Both plasmapheresis and intravenous immune globulin (IVIG) have been used to treat GBS in HIV-infected individuals [156, 157]. There is a wide range in reported benefit varying from ineffective to a good response [136, 158]. Nevertheless, IVIG currently remains the preferred choice in treating HIV associated GBS given that IVIG does not induce immunosuppression. Twenty-five percent of all GBS patients require some degree of ventilatory support many of whom require ICU admission [159]. Outcomes after ICU care were reported to be similar in HIV-positive and HIV-negative patients diagnosed with GBS [160]. Many deaths due to GBS are attributed to autonomic disturbances, most commonly cardiac arrest, which is responsible for 20–30% of deaths [161].

The recurrence rate in GBS in general is about 3% [162]. The second onset occurred 9 weeks to 4 years after symptom onset and persisted for at least 3 years. More experience is needed to determine whether GBS patients with HIV infection are more likely to develop CIDP after GBS.

Chronic Inflammatory Demyelinating Polyneuropathy

Chronic inflammatory demyelinating polyneuropathy (CIDP) frequently presents as a symmetrical, mainly motor neuropathy in which both proximal and distal weakness are more prominent than are sensory complaints. In some cases, CIDP can also evolve asymmetrically [162]. Tendon reflexes are reduced or absent. CIDP in HIV infection can occur early, but more frequently appears in moderately advanced disease [52].

In most instances, neurophysiological examination shows demyelinating features which are similar to those described for GBS. However, in other cases, the exam might demonstrate only subtle slowing of proximal conduction or even mixed demyelinating and axonal features.

Protein concentrations in the CSF are generally increased, with fewer than 50 cells per μL [162]. CSF analysis is useful in exclusion of infectious or neoplastic causes, especially when patients have fewer than 200 CD4+ cells per μL. Importantly, lymphoma and diffuse infiltrative lymphocytosis syndrome neuropathy can mimic chronic inflammatory demyelinating polyneuropathy [163].

From an immunological standpoint, it should be recalled that Fas mediated T cell apoptosis is one of the mechanisms used by HIV to induce immune suppression. It is also noteworthy that an inherited deficiency within the same pathway is a risk factor for acquiring CIDP in immunocompetent subjects [164].

Treatment of CIDP in HIV positive patients includes plasma exchange, intravenous immunoglobulins, or corticosteroids, and patients often have excellent responses [52, 162].

Initiation of combination antiretroviral therapy (cART) in patients presenting with an immune-mediated disorder might be an important component of treatment [52], even in those with normal CD4 cell counts. Responses to treatment in HIV-infected patients are similar to those in patients not infected with HIV.

Neuropathy Associated with HIV Seroconversion

Cranial and peripheral neuropathies, together or separately, may appear within 1-2 weeks after the acute febrile syndrome, which characterizes primary HIV infection [52]. The most frequent condition is facial nerve palsy [166], followed by a syndrome which resembles the Guillain-Barre syndrome (GBS) [134, 167]. Acute bilateral brachial neuropathy has also been reported [168, 169].

Mononeuritis Multiplex

Mononeuritis multiplex (MM) may present in early stages, when it is related to a dysimmune or vasculitic process [12], as well as in later stages, when it is usually due to opportunistic infections [12]. The most common opportunistic infection is CMV, especially when CD4 count is < 50 cell/uL [170] (Table 3).

The pathology may reveal only inflammatory infiltrates when the MM is related to a dysimmune process, whereas it shows immune-complexes in perineural vessels and local damage when vasculitic in nature. HIV, HBV and HCV are all able to induce immune-complex formation [52]. Fibular, lateral cutaneous nerve of the thigh, radial, intercostal and the recurrent laryngeal are the most frequently involved nerves. Clinical features are usually indistinguishable from non HIV-MM [171, 172]. Neurophysiological studies combined with a nerve/muscle biopsy are useful in establishing the diagnosis.

The pathology demonstrates perivascular inflammation involving the epineurium and endoneurium [172]. In some patients, a sural nerve biopsy may reveal signs of a necrotizing vasculitis [171]. Patients with milder forms may undergo a spontaneous remission. In patients with moderate to severe involvement, the treatment consists of intravenous immunoglobulins and prednisone [171, 173]. When the MM is due to CMV infection, CSF studies reveal increased leukocytes in only 15% of cases, while PCR for CMV DNA in the CSF is positive in 90% of patients [52]. Treatment with ganciclovir and foscarnet is usually effective [170, 174].

Less often, MM may be a manifestation of other opportunistic infections such as varicella/zoster virus (VZV), HBV or HCV, especially when associated with cryoglobulinemia, syphilis or lymphomatous infiltration [168].

Table 3. Differential diagnosis of Mononeuropathy Multiplex

	Cryoglobulins	CD4+ cells count	Blood - CSF	Nerve biopsy	Treatment
Mononeuropathy Multiplex	Yes		HCV positive	Vasculitis (not mandatory)	Plasma exchange (if HCV positive consider peg-INF and Ribavirine)
			HCV negative		
	No	<50 cells/mL	Positive for CMV infection	Not needed	Foscarnet Ganciclovir
			Negative for CMV infection	No Vasculitis	
				Vasculitis	IV Ig / prednisone
		>50 cells/mL	HBV – other infectious agents - ANCA – ENA - ANA	Vasculitis	
				No Vasculitis	Supportive therapy

Legend: CSF: cerebrospinal fluid; CMV Cytomegalovirus; HBV: Hepatitis B Virus; ANCA: Anti Neutrophil Cytoplasmic Antibodies; ENA: Extractable Nuclear Antigens; ANA: Anti Nuclear Antibodies; PEG-INF: pegylate interferon; IV Ig: Intravenous Immunoglobulins.

Progressive Polyradiculopathy

Progressive polyradiculopathy is most often caused by CMV infection, which usually appears in advanced stages of immunodeficiency, when the CD4 count is < 50 cell/uL. Although this syndrome became extremely rare after HAART introduction, it is a severe condition that requires early anti-CMV treatment in order to prevent a very poor outcome. The clinical presentation is characterized by lumbosacral pain, saddle anesthesia, rapidly progressive flaccid paraparesis and urinary retention [175, 176]. At the onset of neurological manifestations, at least 30% of patients already manifested signs of CMV infection in other organs, most often in the retina [177]. The symptom onset is usually subacute, with insidious lumbar pain, weakness and sensory complaints affecting the lower limbs. The fully developed syndrome occurs within several days when patients present with an areflexic paraparesis and distal anesthesia. About 60% of patients report urinary dysfunction. This syndrome may also present in patients administered chronic anti-CMV treatment when the dosage is insufficient or in the case of drug resistance. If untreated, most patients with CMV polyradiculopathy expire within days to weeks [52]. In about 30% of patients, spinal MRI demonstrates spinal cord thinning, and on occasion, contrast enhancement of the nerve roots [177]. CSF analysis demonstrates a predominantly neutrophilic pleocytosis in at least 90% of patients (200 cells/uL in 40% of cases) [12], markedly decreased glucose and increased protein. PCR for

CMV DNA in the CSF is positive in about 90% of patients [178]. Therapy consists of ganciclovir and foscarnet, either alone or in combination [12]. After the induction phase, all patients should undergo adequate maintenance treatment.

VZV infection, neurosyphilis and leptomeningeal lymphoma have been reported to cause a progressive polyradiculoneuritis [179, 180]. Finally, it has been reported, that in rare cases, HIV itself may induce a lumbosacral polyradiculopathy [176].

Syphilitic Polyradiculopathy

This is a rare manifestation that may appear in patients with a previous secondary syphilitic infection that is probably due to syphilitic meningitis with nerve root involvement [179]. The syndrome is characterized by bilateral and progressive lower extremity pain, sensory loss and asymmetric distal weakness. Symptoms develop within a few weeks. A CD4 cell count > 100 cell/uL effectively excludes the alternative diagnosis of CMV polyradiculopathy. CSF studies typically demonstrate a neutrophilic pleocytosis, increased protein and decreased glucose [52]. Treatment with penicillin G is recommended.

Peripheral Neuropathy in Diffuse Infiltrative Lymphocytosis

This is a condition that shares some similarities with Sjögren's syndrome, although it displays multivisceral involvement and a marked increase of CD8 lymphocytes (CD8 cell counts > $1000/mm^3$). The most common presentation is subacute distal symmetric sensory neuropathy [181], which develops within days or weeks during the intermediate stages of HIV infection. About 30% of patients present with an asymmetric onset, half of whom will eventually progress towards symmetric involvement [164]. Isolated cranial nerve involvement is reported, most often facial nerve palsy, associated with parotidomegaly [52].

Neurophysiological studies typically demonstrate axonal features, although demyelination is observed in 15% of cases [164]. CSF studies typically demonstrate a mild and non-specific increase of lymphocytes and a marked increase in protein (up to 2g/L). Pathological studies typically demonstrate angiocentric infiltration by CD8 cells and necrosis of vessel walls [182]. Increased expression of HIV antigen p24 has been detected in macrophages infiltrating peripheral nerves [164; 183; 184]. CD8 cells also display HIV antigens as well as a marked proviral load [183]. No evidence of a monoclonal component was found in infiltrates. HAART is effective, since it leads to complete recovery in 65% of patients. As a systemic increase of CD8 cells is likely the main pathogenic event, it is not important to administer a treatment that is able to cross the blood-nerve barrier. Patients who do not respond to this first line treatment may have benefit from prednisone.

HCV Related Neuropathy

HIV co-infection is likely to favor HCV related complications since it increases its viral load [185]. Two different forms of neuropathy have been described; a distal symmetric sensory form with axonal involvement with occasional conduction blocks and a rare mononeuritis multiplex [186, 187]. Approximately 30% of patients also display CNS involvement whereas a similar percentage of patients manifest nephrotic syndrome [186]. The presence of cryoglobulinemia may help support the diagnosis.

Alpha-interferon, the standard treatment for HCV infection, with ribavirin, should be used with caution as these treatments may induce a neuropathy [188]. There is insufficient data that address the toxicity of ribavirin therapy either alone or in combination with alpha interferon. Nonetheless, patients with more severe forms of HCV infection may benefit from immunosuppressive treatment [188]. In such cases, they should discontinue HAART due to significant synergistic toxicity.

HTLV-I /II Related Neuropathy

Although Human T-lymphotropic Virus type I (HTLV-I) usually causes a myelopathy, some patients also develop a distal symmetric sensory neuropathy [189]. In particular, patients with HIV and HTLV-I co-infection may have an increased incidence of neuropathy when compared to those with an isolated HIV infection [190]. The pathology typically demonstrates epineural inflammatory infiltration, which is more pronounced around blood vessels [191]. There are only anecdotal reports on the efficacy of steroid treatment [189, 191]. Some authors report that also patients with HIV-1 and HTLV-II co-infection display an increased risk of developing an axonal sensory polyneuropathy [192, 193].

Conclusion

The PNS is frequently involved during all stages of HIV infection. Given that the spectrum of pathological processes is quite broad, diagnostic and therapeutic approaches are necessarily complex. During the diagnostic process, it is very important to assess the patient's immunological status, consider possible opportunistic infections and concomitant diseases, the pharmacological regimen as well as the patient's lifestyle. Treatment of a neuropathy associated with HIV infection and its treatments, both causal and symptomatic, should also take into account interactions with HIV, co-infections, and the patient's immunological and metabolic status.

In the absence of definitive evidence based medicine guidelines, the patient has an even greater responsibility to render treatment decisions. Nonetheless, it should be recalled that immune mediated processes such as acquired demyelination and vasculitic processes tend to occur early in the course of HIV infection. GBS may be the first manifestation of HIV infection and should be suspected when the WBC count on CSF analysis is between 10 and 50 WBCs. While immunosuppressive therapy is often helpful, it should be used with caution especially in those patients with low CD4 counts. Axonal neuropathies, predominantly DSP, tend to occur later in the course of HIV infection. It is important to identify any potential coinfection, concomitant disease that can induce a neuropathy and to remove any medication that might be inducing a neuropathy. With the exception of infectious and immune mediated processes, the mainstay of therapy is symptomatic treatment.

References

[1] UNAIDS 2011 GLOBAL HIV/AIDS RESPONSE. Epidemic update and health sector progress towards Universal Access Progress Report2011. *http:www.uniaids.org. Accessed February 12, 2013.*

[2] Brinley FJ, Pardo CA, Verma A. Human immunodeficiency virus and the peripheral nervous system workshop. *Arch Neurol* 2001; 58:1561-1566.

[3] Manji H. Neuropathy in HIV infection. *Curr Opin Neurol* 2000; 13:589-592.

[4] Woolf CJ, Allchorne A, Safieh-Garabedian B, Poole S. Cytokines, nerve growth factor and inflammatory hyperalgesia: the contribution of tumour necrosis factor alpha. *Br J Pharmacol* 1997; 121:417-424.

[5] Verma A. Epidemiology and clinical features of HIV-1 associated neuropathies. *J Peripher Nerv Syst* 2001; 6:8-13.

[6] Goodkin K, Wilkie FL, Concha M, Hinkin CH, et al. Aging and neuro-AIDS conditions and the changing spectrum of HIV-1-associated morbidity and mortality. *J Clin Epidemiol* 2001; 54 Suppl 1:S35-43.

[7] Schifitto G, McDermott MP, McArthur JC, Marder K, Sacktor N, Epstein L, Kieburtz K; Dana Consortium on the Therapy of HIV Dementia and Related Cognitive Disorders. Incidence of and risk factors for HIV-associated distal sensory polyneuropathy. *Neurology* 2002; 58:1764-1768.

[8] Keswani SC, Pardo CA, Cherry CL, Hoke A and McArthur JC. HIV-associated sensory neuropathies. *AIDS* 2002; 16:2105-2117.

[9] Griffin JW CT, McArthur JC. Peripheral neuropathies associated with HIV infection. In: *The Neurology of AIDS*. Edited by Gendelman HE LS, Epstein L, Swindells S. New York: Chapman and Hall 1998; 275-291.

[10] Fuller GN, Jacobs JM, Guiloff RJ. Nature and incidence of peripheral nerve syndromes in HIV infection. *J Neurol Neurosurg Psychiatry* 1993; 56:372-381.

[11] Tagliati M, Grinnell J, Godbold J, Simpson DM. Peripheral nerve function in HIV infection: clinical, electrophysiologic, and laboratory findings. *Arch Neurol* 1999; 56:84-89.

[12] Brew BJ. Peripheral nerve involvement in early and moderately advanced HIV disease. In: Brew BJ, editor. *HIV neurology*. New York: Oxford University Press 2001; 183-193.

[13] Luciano CA, Pardo CA, McArthur JC. Recent developments in the HIV neuropathies. *Curr Opin Neurol* 2003; 16(3):403-409.

[14] Herrmann D, De Marcaida J, Akowah K. Epidermal nerve fiber density, quantitative sensory testing, and virologic and immunologic measures as predictors of symptomatic HIV associated distal symmetrical polyneuropathy. *Ann Neurol* 2001; 50:S33.

[15] Cornblath DR, McArthur JC. Predominantly sensory neuropathy in patients with AIDS and AIDS-related complex. *Neurology* 1988; 38:794-796.

[16] Araujo AP, Nascimento OJ, Garcia OS. Distal sensory polyneuropathy in a cohort of HIV-infected children over five years of age. *Pediatrics* 2000;106(3):E35.

[17] Ferrari LF, Levine JD. Alcohol consumption enhances antiretroviral painful peripheral neuropathy by mitochondrial mechanisms. *Eur J Neurosci* 2010; 32(5):811-818.

[18] Robinson-Papp J, Gelman BB, Grant I, Singer E, Gensler G, and Morgello S. Substance abuse increases the risk of neuropathy in an HIV-infected cohort. *Muscle Nerve* 2012; 45(4):471-476.

[19] England JD, Gronseth GS, Franklin G, Carter GT, Kinsella LJ, Cohen JA, Asbury AK, Szigeti K, Lupski JR, Latov N, Lewis RA, Low PA, Fisher MA, Herrmann DN, Howard JF, Jr, Lauria G, Miller RG, Polydefkis M, Sumner AJ. Practice Parameter: Evaluation of distal symmetric polyneuropathy: Role of laboratory and genetic testing (an evidence-based review). *Neurology* 2009; 72:185-192.

[20] De La Monte SM, Gabuzda DH, Ho DD, Brown RH Jr, Hedley-Whyte ET, Schooley RT, Hirsch MS, Bhan AK. Peripheral neuropathy in the acquired immunodeficiency syndrome. *Ann Neurol* 1988; 23:485-492.

[21] Chaunu MP,Ratinahirana H, Raphael M, Henin D, Leport C, Brun-Vezinet F, Leger JM, Brunet P, Hauw JJ. The spectrum of changes on 20 nerve biopsies in patients with HIV infection. *Muscle Nerve* 1989; 12:452-459.

[22] Rizzuto N, Cavallaro T, Monaco S, Morbin M, Bonetti B, Ferrari S, Galiazzo-Rizzuto S, Zanette G, Bertolasi L. Role of HIV in the pathogenesis of distal symmetrical peripheral neuropathy. *Acta Neuropathol* 1995; 90:244-250.

[23] Rance NE, McArthur JC, Cornblath DR, Landstrom DL, Griffin JW, Price DL. Gracile tract degeneration in patients with sensory neuropathy and AIDS. *Neurology* 1988; 38:265-271.

[24] Holland NR, Stocks A, Hauer P, Cornblath DR, Griffin JW, McArthur JC. Intraepidermal nerve fiber density in patients with painful sensory neuropathy. *Neurology* 1997; 48:708-711.

[25] Polydefkis M, Yiannoutsos CT, Cohen BA, Hollander H, Schi- fitto G, Clifford DB, Simpson DM, Katzenstein D, Shriver S, Hauer P, Brown A, Haidich AB, Moo L, McArthur JC. Reduced intraepidermal nerve fiber density in HIV-associated sensory neuropathy. *Neurology* 2002; 58:115-119.

[26] Mah V, Vartavarian LM, Akers MA, Vinters HV. Abnormalities of peripheral nerve in patients with human immunodeficiency virus infection. *Ann Neurol* 1988; 24:713-717.

[27] Yoshioka M, Shapshak P, Srivastava AK, Stewart RV, Nelson SJ, Bradley WG, Berger JR, Rhodes RH, Sun NC, Nakamura S. Expression of HIV-1 and interleukin-6 in lumbosacral dorsal root ganglia of patients with AIDS. *Neurology* 1994; 44:1120-1130.

[28] Nagano I, Shapshak P, Yoshioka M, Xin K, Nakamura S, Bradley WG. Increased NADPH-diaphorase reactivity and cytokine expression in dorsal root ganglia in acquired immunodeficiency syndrome. *J Neurol Sci* 1996; 136:117-128.

[29] Jones G, Zhu Y, Silva C, Tsutsui S, Pardo CA,Keppler OT, McArthur JC, Power C. Peripheral nerve-derived HIV-1 is predominantly CCR5-dependent and causes neuronal degeneration and neuroinflammation. *Virology* 2005; 334:178-193.

[30] Tyor WR, Wesselingh SL, Griffin JW, McArthur JC, Griffin DE. Unifying hypothesis for the pathogenesis of HIV-associated dementia complex, vacuolar myelopathy, and sensory neuropathy. *J Acquir Immune Defic Syndr Hum Retrovirol* 1995; 9:379-388.

[31] Ahmed F, McArthur L, De Bernardi MA, Mocchetti I. Retrograde and anterograde transport of HIV protein gp120 in the nervous system. *Brain Behav Immun* 2009; 23:355-364.

[32] Acharjee S, Noorbakhsh F, Stemkowski PL, Olechowski C, Cohen EA, Ballanyi K, Kerr B, Pardo C, Smith PA, Power C. HIV-1 viral protein R causes peripheral nervous system injury associated with in vivo neuropathic pain. *Faseb J* 2010; 24:4343-4353.

[33] Conti L, Fantuzzi L, Del Cornò M, Belardelli F, Gessani S. Immunomodulatory effects of the HIV-1 gp120 protein on antigen presenting cells: implications for AIDS pathogenesis. *Immunobiology* 2004; 209:99-115.

[34] Romani B, Engelbrecht S. Human immunodeficiency virus type 1 Vpr: functions and molecular interactions. *J Gen Virol* 2009; 90:1795-1805.

[35] Herzberg U, Sagen J. Peripheral nerve exposure to HIV viral envelope protein gp120 induces neuropathic pain and spinal gliosis. *J Neuroimmunol* 2001; 116:29-39.

[36] Zheng W, Ouyang H, Zheng X, Liu S, Mata M, Fink DJ, Hao S. Glial TNF-alpha in the spinal cord regulates neuropathic pain induced by HIV gp120 application in rats. Mol *Pain* 2011; 7:40.

[37] Wallace VC, Blackbeard J, Pheby T, Segerdahl AR, Davies M, Hasnie F, Hall S, McMahon SB, Rice AS. Pharmacological, behavioural and mechanistic analysis of HIV-1 gp120 induced painful neuropathy. *Pain* 2007a; 133:47-63.

[38] Wallace VC, Blackbeard J, Segerdahl AR, Hasnie F, Pheby T, McMahon SB, Rice AS. Characterization of rodent models of HIV-gp120 and antiretroviral-associated neuropathic pain. *Brain* 2007b; 130:2688-2702.

[39] Keswani SC, Polley M, Pardo CA, Griffin JW, McArthur JC, Hoke A. Schwann cell chemokine receptors mediate HIV-1 gp120 toxicity to sensory neurons. *Ann Neurol* 2003; 54:287-296.

[40] Bodner A, Toth PT, Miller RJ. Activation of c-Jun N-terminal kinase mediates gp120IIIB- and nucleoside analogue-induced sensory neuron toxicity. *Exp Neurol* 2004; 188:246-253.

[41] Hoke A, Morris M, Haughey NJ. GPI-1046 protects dorsal root ganglia from gp120-induced axonal injury by modulating store-operated calcium entry. *J Peripher Nerv Syst* 2009; 14:27-35.

[42] Melli G, Keswani SC, Fischer A, Chen W, Hoke A. Spatially distinct and functionally independent mechanisms of axonal degeneration in a model of HIV-associated sensory neuropathy. *Brain* 2006; 129:1330-1338.

[43] Hahn K, Robinson B, Anderson C, Li W, Pardo CA, Morgello S, Simpson D, Nath A. Differential effects of HIV infected macrophages on dorsal root ganglia neurons and axons. *Exp Neurol* 2008; 210:30-40.

[44] Lehmann HC, Chen W, Borzan J, Mankowski JL, Hoke A. Mitochondrial dysfunction in distal axons contributes to human immunodeficiency virus sensory neuropathy. *Ann Neurol* 2011; 69:100-110.

[45] Zhang K, Rana F, Silva C, Ethier J, Wehrly K, Chesebro B, Power C. Human immunodeficiency virus type 1 envelope-mediated neuronal death: uncoupling of viral replication and neurotoxicity. *J Virol* 2003; 77:6899-6912.

[46] Thomas FP, Chalk C, Lalonde R, Robitaille Y, Jolicoeur P. Expression of human immunodeficiency virus type 1 in the nervous system of transgenic mice leads to neurological disease. *J Virol* 1994; 68:7099-7107.
[47] Coderre TJ, Melzack R. The role of NMDA receptor-operated calcium channels in persistent nociception after formalin-induced tissue injury. *J Neurosci* 1992; 12(9):3671-3675.
[48] McNamara JO. Analyses of the molecular basis of kindling development. *Psychiatry Clin Neurosci* 1995; 49(3):S175-178.
[49] England JD, Gamboni F, Ferguson MA, Levinson SR. Sodium channels accumulate at the tips of injured axons. *Muscle Nerve* 1994; 17(6):593-598.
[50] Pertin M, Ji RR, Berta T, Powell AJ, Karchewski L, Tate SN, Isom LL, Woolf CJ, Gilliard N, Spahn DR, Decosterd I. Upregulation of the voltage-gated sodium channel beta2 subunit in neuropathic pain models: characterization of expression in injured and non-injured primary sensory neurons. *J Neurosci* 2005; 25(47):10970-10980.
[51] Lee K, Vivithanaporn P, Siemieniuk RA, Krentz HB, Maingat F, Gill MJ, Power C. Clinical outcomes and immune benefits of anti-epileptic drug therapy in HIV/AIDS. *BMC Neurol* 2010; 10:44.
[52] Brew BJ. The peripheral nerve complications of human immunodeficiency virus (HIV) infection. *Muscle Nerve* 2003; 28:542-552.
[53] Backonja MM. Use of anticonvulsants for treatment of neuropathic pain. *Neurology* 2002; 59(5 Suppl 2):S14-17.
[54] Campbell FG, Graham JG, Zilkha KJ. Clinical trial of carbazepine (tegretol) in trigeminal neuralgia. *J Neurol Neurosurg Psychiatry* 1966; 29(3):265-267.
[55] Nicol CF. A four year double-blind study of tegretol in facial pain. *Headache* 1969; 9(1):54-57.
[56] Udawat H, Khandelwal V, D'Souza P, Goyal RK. Toxic epidermal necrolysis secondary to carbamazepine in a patient with human immunodeficiency virus infection. *J Assoc Physicians India* 2001; 49:918-919.
[57] Beltrán-Marín I, Mauri-Lledrá JA, Letona-Carbajo S, Flamarique-Pascual A. Carbamazepine intoxication in a HIV patient under artiretroviral therapy. Med Clin *(Barc)* 2006; 127(13):517-518.
[58] Bates DE, Herman RJ. Carbamazepine toxicity induced by lopinavir/ritonavir and nelfinavir. *Ann Pharmacother* 2006; 40(6):1190-1195.
[59] Hahn K, Arendt G, Braun JS, von Giesen HJ, Husstedt IW, et al. A placebo-controlled trial of gabapentin for painful HIV-associated sensory neuropathies. *J Neurol* 2004; 251:1260-1266.
[60] Simpson DM, Schifitto G, Clifford DB, Murphy TK, Durso-De Cruz E, Glue P, Whalen E, Emir B, Scott GN, Freeman R; 1066 HIV Neuropathy Study Group. Pregabalin for painful HIV neuropathy: a randomized, double-blind, placebo-controlled trial. *Neurology* 2010; 74:413-420.
[61] Zakrzewska JM, Chaudhry Z, Nurmikko TJ, Patton DW, Mullens EL. Lamotrigine (lamictal) in refractory trigeminal neuralgia: results from a double-blind placebo controlled crossover trial. *Pain* 1997; 73(2):223-30.
[62] Vestergaard K, Andersen G, Gottrup H, Kristensen BT, Jensen TS. Lamotrigine for central post stroke pain: a randomized controlled trial. *Neurology* 2001; 56(2):184-190.

[63] Simpson DM, Olney R, McArthur JC, Khan A, Godbold J, Ebel-Frommer K. A placebo-controlled trial of lamotrigine for painful HIV-associated neuropathy. *Neurology* 2000; 54(11):2115-2119.

[64] Simpson DM, McArthur JC, Olney R, Clifford D, So Y, Ross D, Baird BJ, Barrett P, Hammer AE; Lamotrigine HIV Neuropathy Study Team. Lamotrigine for HIV-associated painful sensory neuropathies: a placebo-controlled trial. *Neurology*. 2003; 60(9):1508-1514.

[65] Shlay JC, Chaloner K, Max MB, Flaws B, Reichelderfer P, Wentworth D, Hillman S, Brizz B, Cohn DL. Acupuncture and amitriptyline for pain due to HIV-related peripheral neuropathy: a randomized controlled trial. Terry Beirn Community Programs for Clinical Research on AIDS. *JAMA* 1998; 280:1590-1595.

[66] Kieburtz K, Simpson D, Yiannoutsos C, Max MB, Hall CD, Ellis RJ, Marra CM, McKendall R, Singer E, Dal Pan GJ, Clifford DB, Tucker T, Cohen B. A randomized trial of amitriptyline and mexiletine for painful neuropathy in HIV infection. AIDS Clinical Trial Group 242 Protocol Team. *Neurology* 1998; 51(6):1682-1688.

[67] Huang EJ, Reichardt LF. Neurotrophins: roles in neuronal development and function. *Annu Rev Neurosci* 2001; 24:677-736.

[68] McArthur JC, Yiannoutsos C, Simpson DM, Adornato BT, Singer EJ, Hollander H. A phase II trial of nerve growth factor for sensory neuropathy associated with HIV infection. AIDS Clinical Trials Group Team 291. *Neurology* 2000; 54:1080-1088.

[69] Schiffito G, Yiannoutsos C, Simpson D. Long-term treatment with recombinant nerve growth factor for HIV-associated sensory neuropathy. *Neurology* 2001; 57:1313-1316.

[70] Pradat PF. Treatment of peripheral neuropathies with neurotrophic factors: animal models and clinical trials. *Rev Neurol* (Paris) 2003; 159(2):147-161.

[71] Simpson DM, Dorfman D, Olney RK, McKinley G, Dobkin J, So Y, Berger J, Ferdon MB, Friedman B. Peptide T in the treatment of painful distal neuropathy associated with AIDS: results of a placebo-controlled trial. The Peptide T Neuropathy Study Group. *Neurology* 1996; 47(5):1254-1259.

[72] Evans SR, Simpson DM, Kitch DW, King A, Clifford DB, Cohen BA, McArthur JC; Neurologic AIDS Research Consortium; AIDS Clinical Trials Group. A randomized trial evaluating Prosaptide for HIV-associated sensory neuropathies: use of an electronic diary to record neuropathic pain. *PLoS One*. 2007; 2(6):e551.

[73] Hart AM, Wilson AD, Montovani C, Smith C, Johnson M, Terenghi G, Youle M. Acetyl-l-carnitine: a pathogenesis based treatment for HIV-associated antiretroviral toxic neuropathy. *AIDS* 2004; 18:1549-1560.

[74] Osio M, Muscia F, Zampini L, Nascimbene C, Mailland E, Cargnel A, Mariani C. Acetyl-L-carnitine in the treatment of painful antiretroviral toxic neuropathy in human immunodeficiency virus patients: an open label study. *J Peripher Nerv Syst* 2006; 11(1):72-76.

[75] Scarpini E, Sacilotto G, Baron P, Cusini M, Scarlato G. Effect of acetyl-L-carnitine in the treatment of painful peripheral neuropathies in HIV+ patients. *J Peripher Nerv Syst* 1997; 2(3):250-252.

[76] Herzmann C, Johnson MA, Youle M. Long-term effect of acetyl-L-carnitine for antiretroviral toxic neuropathy. *HIV Clin Trials* 2005; 6:344-350.

[77] Youle M, Osio M. ALCAR Study Group A double-blind, parallel-group, placebo-controlled, multicentre study of acetyl L-carnitine in the symptomatic treatment of

antiretroviral toxic neuropathy in patients with HIV-1 infection. *HIV Med* 2007; 8:241-250.

[78] Chiechio S, Copani A, Gereau RW, Nicoletti F. Acetyl-L-carnitine in neuropathic pain: experimental data. *CNS Drugs* 2007; 21 Suppl 1:31-8; discussion 45-6.

[79] Abrams DI, Jay CA, Shade SB, Vizoso H, Reda H, Press S, Kelly ME, Rowbotham MC, Petersen KL. Cannabis in painful HIV-associated sensory neuropathy: a randomized placebo-controlled trial. *Neurology* 2007; 68(7):515-521.

[80] Ellis RJ, Toperoff W, Vaida F, van den Brande G, Gonzales J, Gouaux B, Bentley H, Atkinson JH. Smoked medicinal cannabis for neuropathic pain in HIV: a randomized, crossover clinical trial. *Neuropsychopharmacology* 2009; 34(3):672-680.

[81] Paice JA, Ferrans CE, Lashley FR, Shott S, Vizgirda V, Pitrak D. Topical capsaicin in the management of HIV-associated peripheral neuropathy. *J Pain Symptom Manage* 2000; 19(1):45-52.

[82] Simpson DM, Brown S, Tobias J. NGX-4010 C107 Study Group Controlled trial of high-concentration capsaicin patch for treatment of painful HIV neuropathy. *Neurology* 2008; 70:2305-2313.

[83] Attal N, Cruccu G, Haanpää M, Hansson P, Jensen TS, Nurmikko T, Sampaio C, Sindrup S, Wiffen P; EFNS Task Force. EFNS guidelines on pharmacological treatment of neuropathic pain. *Eur J Neurol* 2006 Nov; 13(11):1153-1169.

[84] Attal N, Cruccu G, Baron R, Haanpää M, Hansson P, Jensen TS, Nurmikko T; European Federation of Neurological Societies. EFNS guidelines on the pharmacological treatment of neuropathic pain: 2010 revision. *Eur J Neurol* 2010; 17(9):1113-e88.

[85] Nieminen TH, Hagelberg NM, Saari TI, Neuvonen M, Neuvonen PJ, Laine K, Olkkola KT. Oxycodone concentrations are greatly increased by the concomitant use of ritonavir or lopinavir/ritonavir. *Eur J Clin Pharmacol* 2010; 66:977-985.

[86] Bokhari SM, Yao H, Bethel-Brown C, Fuwang P, Williams R, Dhillon NK, Hegde R, Kumar A, Buch SJ. Morphine enhances Tat induced activation in murine microglia. *J Neurovirol* 2009; 15:219-228.

[87] Reynolds JL, Mahajan SD, Sykes D, Nair MP. Heroin-induces differential protein expression by normal human astrocytes (NHA). *Am J Infect Dis* 2006; 2:49-57.

[88] Bokhari SM, Hegde R, Callen S, Yao H, Adany I, Li Q, Li Z, Pinson D, Yeh HW, Cheney PD, Buch S. Morphine potentiates neuropathogenesis of SIV infection in rhesus macaques. *J Neuroimmune Pharmacol* 2011; 6(4):626-639.

[89] Bell JE, Arango JC, Robertson R, Brettle RP, Leen C, Simmonds P. HIV and drug misuse in the Edinburgh cohort. *J Acquir Immune Defic Syndr* 2001; 31:S35-S42.

[90] Koeppe J, Armon C, Lyda K, Nielsen C, Johnson S. Ongoing pain despite aggressive opioid pain management among persons with HIV. *Clin J Pain* 2010; 26:190-198.

[91] Watkins LR, Hutchinson MR, Ledeboer A, Wieseler-Frank J, Milligan ED, Maier SF. Norman Cousins Lecture. Glia as the "bad guys": implications for improving clinical pain control and the clinical utility of opioids. *Brain Behav Immun* 2007; 21:131-146.

[92] Song P, Zhao ZQ. The involvement of glial cells in the development of morphine tolerance. *Neurosci Res* 2001; 39:281-286.

[93] Cui Y, Chen Y, Zhi JL, Guo RX, Feng JQ, Chen PX. Activation of p38 mitogen-activated protein kinase in spinal microglia mediates morphine antinociceptive tolerance. *Brain Res* 2006; 1069:235-243.

[94] Raghavendra V, Rutkowski MD, DeLeo JA. The role of spinal neuroimmune activation in morphine tolerance/hyperalgesia in neuropathic and sham-operated rats. *J Neurosci* 2002; 22:9980-9989.

[95] Tai YH, Wang YH, Wang JJ, Tao PL, Tung CS, Wong CS. Amitriptyline suppresses neuroinflammation and up-regulates glutamate transporters in morphine-tolerant rats. *Pain* 2006; 124:77-86.

[96] Johnston IN, Milligan ED, Wieseler-Frank J, Frank MG, Zapata V, Campisi J, Langer S, Martin D, Green P, Fleshner M, Leinwand L, Maier SF, Watkins LR. A role for proinflammatory cytokines and fractalkine in analgesia, tolerance, and subsequent pain facilitation induced by chronic intrathecal morphine. *J Neurosci* 2004; 24:7353-7365.

[97] Raghavendra V, Tanga FY, DeLeo JA. Attenuation of morphine tolerance, withdrawal-induced hyperalgesia, and associated spinal inflammatory immune responses by propentofylline in rats. *Neuropsychopharmacology* 2004; 29:327-334.

[98] Gomez-Flores R, Weber RJ. Differential effects of buprenorphine and morphine on immune and neuroendocrine functions following acute administration in the rat mesencephalon periaqueductal gray. *Immunopharmacology* 2000; 48:145-156.

[99] Martucci C, Panerai AE, Sacerdote P. Chronic fentanyl or buprenorphine infusion in the mouse: similar analgesic profile but different effects on immune responses. *Pain* 2004; 110:385-392.

[100] Franchi S, Panerai AE, Sacerdote P. Buprenorphine ameliorates the effect of surgery on hypothalamus-pituitary-adrenal axis, natural killer cell activity and metastatic colonization in rats in comparison with morphine or fentanyl treatment. *Brain Behav Immun* 2007; 21:767-774.

[101] Sacerdote P, Franchi S, Gerra G, Leccese V, Panerai AE, Somaini L. Buprenorphine and methadone maintenance treatment of heroin addicts preserves immune function. *Brain Behav Immun* 2008; 22:606-613.

[102] Palma J, Cowan A, Geller EB, Adler MW, Benamar K. Differential antinociceptive effects of buprenorphine and methadone in the presence of HIV-gp120. *Drug Alcohol Depend* 2011; 118(2-3):497-499.

[103] Adler MW, Geller EB, Chen X, Rogers TJ. Viewing chemokines as a third major system of communication in the brain, *AAPS J* 2006; 7:E865-E870.

[104] Benamar K, Palma J, Cowan A, Geller EB, Adler MW. Analgesic efficacy of buprenorphine in the presence of high levels of SDF-1α/CXCL12 in the brain. *Drug Alcohol Depend* 2011; 114:246-248.

[105] Sacktor N. The epidemiology of human immunodeficiency virus-associated neurological disease in the era of highly active antiretroviral therapy. *J Neurovirol* 2002; 8 (Suppl.2):115-121.

[106] Simpson DM, Tagliati M. Nucleoside analogue associated peripheral neuropathy in human immunodeficiency virus infection. *J AIDS* 1995; 9:153-161.

[107] Moore R, Wong W-M, Keruly J, McArthur JC. Incidence of neuropathy in HIV-infected patients on monotherapy versus those on combination therapy with didanosine, stavudine and hydroxyurea. *AIDS* 2000; 14:273-278.

[108] Scarsella A, Coodley G, Shalit P. Stavudine-associated peripheral neuropathy in zidovudine-naive patients: effect of stavudine exposure and antiretroviral experience. *Adv Ther* 2002; 19:1-8.

[109] Reliquet V, Mussini J, Chennebault J. Peripheral neuropathy during stavudine-didanosine antiretroviral therapy. *HIV Me* 2001; 2:92-96.

[110] Rossero M, Asmuth DM, Grady JJ, McKinsey DS, Green S, Andron L, Pollard RB. Hydroxyurea in combination with didanosine and stavudine in antiretroviral-experienced HIV-infected subjects with a review of the literature. *International Journal of STD and AIDS* 2003; 14:350-355.

[111] Moyle GJ, Sadler M. Peripheral neuropathy with nucleoside antiretrovirals: risk factors, incidence and management. *Drug Safety* 1998; 19:481-494.

[112] Fichtenbaum CJ, Clifford DB, Powderly WG. Risk factors for dideoxynucleoside-induced toxic neuropathy in patients with the human immunodeficiency virus infection. *J Acquir Immune Defic Syndr Hum Retrovirol* 1995; 10:169-174.

[113] Dalakas MC, Semino-Mora C, Leon-Monzon M. Mitochondrial alterations with mitochondrial DNA depletion in the nerves of AIDS patients with peripheral neuropathy induced by 2'3'-dideoxycytidine (ddC). *Lab Invest* 2001; 81:1537-1544.

[114] Lewis W, Dalakas MC. Mitochondrial toxicity of antiviral drugs. *Nature Med* 1995; 1:417-422.

[115] Kakuda TN. Pharmacology of nucleoside and nucleotide reverse transcriptase inhibitor-induced mitochondrial toxicity. *Clin Ther* 2000; 22:685-708.

[116] Brinkman K, Haldewych JM, Burger D, Smeitink JAM, Koopmans PP. Adverse effects of reverse transcriptase inhibitors: mitochondrial toxicity as a common pathway. *AIDS* 1998; 12:1735-1744.

[117] Tolomeo M, Mancuso S, Todaro M, Stassi G, Catalano M, Arista S, Cannizzo G, Barbusca E, Abbadessa V. Mitochondrial disruption and apoptosis in lymphocytes of an HIV infected patient affected by lactic acidosis after treatment with highly active antiretroviral therapy. *J Clin Pathol* 2003; 56:147-151.

[118] Feng JY, Johnson AA, Johnson KA, Anderson KS. Insights into the molecular mechanism of mitochondrial toxicity by AIDS drugs. *J Biol Chem* 2001; 276:23832-23837.

[119] Johnson AA, Ray AS, Hanes J Suo Z, Colacino JM, Anderson KS. Toxicity of antiviral nucleoside analogs and the human mitochondrial DNA polymerase. *J Biol Chem* 2001; 27:40847-40857.

[120] Chen D, Misra A, Garg A. Lypodystrophy in human immunodeficiency virus infected patients. *J Clin Endocrinol Metab* 2002; 87:4845-4856.

[121] Luzhansky JZ, Pierce AB, Hoy JF, Hall AJ. Leber's hereditary optic neuropathy in the setting of nucleoside analogue toxicity. *AIDS* 2001; 15(12):1588-1589.

[122] Cherry C, Gahan M, McArthur JC. Exposure to dideoxynucleosides is reflected in lowered mitochondrial DNA in subcutaneous fat. *J Acquir Immune Defic Syndr* 2002; 30:271-277.

[123] Pan-Zhou XR, Cui L, Zhou XJ, Sommadossi JP, Darley-Usmar VM. Differential effects of antiretroviral nucleoside analogs on mitochondrial function in HepG2 cells. *Antimicrob Agents Chemother* 2000; 44(3):496-503.

[124] Modica-Napolitano JS. AZT causes tissue-specific inhibition of mitochondrial bioenergetic function. *Biochem Biophys Res Commun* 1993; 194:170-177.

[125] Barile M, Valenti D, Passarella S, Quagliariello E. 3'-Azido-3'-deoxythmidine uptake into isolated rat liver mitochondria and impairment of ADP/ATP translocator. *Biochem Pharmacol* 1997; 53:913-920.

[126] Hobbs GA, Keilbaugh SA, Rief PM, Simpson MV. Cellular targets of 3'-azido-3'-deoxythymidine: an early (non-delayed) effect on oxidative phosphorylation. *Biochem Pharmacol* 1995; 50(3):381-390.

[127] Benbrik E, Chariot P, Bonavaud S, Ammi-Sai DM, Rey C, Gherardi R. Cellular and mitochondrial toxicity of zidovudine (AZT), didanosine (ddI) and zalcitabine (ddC) on cultured human muscle cells. *J Neurol Sci* 1997; 149:19-25.

[128] Skuta G, Fischer GM, Janaky T, Kele Z, Szabo P, Tozser J, Sumegi B. Molecular mechanism of the short-term cardiotoxicity caused by 2',3'-dideoxycytidine (ddC): modulation of reactive oxygen species levels and ADP-ribosylation reactions. *Biochem Pharmacol* 1999; 58(12):1915-1925.

[129] Chen CH, Vazquez-Padua M, Cheng YC. Effect of anti-human immunodeficiency virus nucleoside analogs on mitochondrial DNA and its implication for delayed toxicity. *Mol Pharmacol* 1991; 39:625-628.

[130] Wooltorton E. HIV drug stavudine (Zerit, d4T) and symptoms mimicking Guillain-Barrè syndrome. *Can Med Assoc J* 2002; 166(8):1067.

[131] Aramideh M, Koopmans RP, Koelman JH, Stam J. Rapidly progressing peripheral neuropathy with lactic acidosis and coproporphyria in a patient with HTLV-I associated T-cell leukaemia treated with zidovudine. *J Neurol* 2001; 248(7):621-622.

[132] Blum AS, Dal Pan GJ, Feinberg J, Raines C, Mayjo K, Cornblath DR. Low-dose zalcitabine-related toxic neuropathy: frequency, natural history, and risk factors. *Neurology* 1996; 46:999-1003.

[133] Brannagan TH 3rd, Zhou Y. HIV-associated Guillain-Barré syndrome. *J Neurol Sci* 2003; 208:39-42.

[134] Hagberg L, Malmvall BE, Svennerholm L, K. Alestig LK, Norkrans G. Guillain-Barré syndrome as an early manifestation of HIV central nervous system infection. *Scandinavian Journal of Infectious Diseases* 1986; 18(6):591-592.

[135] Thornton CA, Latif AS, Emmanuel JC. Guillain-Barré syndrome associated with human immunodeficiency virus infection in Zimbabwe. *Neurology* 1991; 41(6):812-815.

[136] Kumar SM, Markandeyulu AV, Gnanamuthu C. Guillain-Barré syndrome presenting in the anti-HIV seroconversion period. *Neurology India* 2003; 51(4):559.

[137] Ting SH, Yeh JH, and Chiu HC. Guillain-Barré syndrome with HIV infection: a case report. *Acta Neurologica Taiwanica* 2003; 12(3), 139-142.

[138] Millogo A. Sawadogo A, Lankoande D, Sawadogo AB. Guillain-Barré syndrome in HIV-infected patients at Bobo-Dioulasso Hospital (Burkina Faso). *Revue Neurologique* 2004; 160(5 Pt 1):559-562.

[139] Aggarwal HK, Chakrabarti D, Nand N, Bharti SK, Verma RP. HIV infection presenting as Guillain-Barré syndrome. *Journal, Indian Academy of Clinical Medicine* 2005; 6(4):341-342.

[140] De Castro G, Bastos PG, Martinez R, de Castro Figueiredo JF. Episodes of Guillain-Barrè syndrome associated with the acute phase of HIV-1 infection and with recurrence of viremia. Arquivos de Neuro-Psiquiatria 2006; 64(3A):606-608. Brannagan TH, McAlarney T, Latov N. Peripheral neuropathy in HIV-1 infection. In: Latov N, Wokke JHJ, Kelly JJ, editors. *Immunological and infectious diseases of the peripheral nerves.* Cambridge: Cambridge Univ. Press 1998; p. 285-307.

[141] Brannagan TH, McAlarney T, Latov N. Peripheral neuropathy in HIV-1 infection. In: Latov N, Wokke JHJ, Kelly JJ, editors. *Immunological and infectious diseases of the peripheral nerves*. Cambridge: Cambridge Univ. Press 1998; p. 285-307.

[142] Cornblath DR, McArthur JC. Peripheral neuropathies in human immunodeficiency virus type 1 infection. In: Asbury AK, Thomas PK, editors. *Peripheral Nerve Disorders*, vol. 2. Oxford: Butterworth 1995; p. 223-237.

[143] Simpson DM, Tagliati M. Neurologic manifestations of HIV infection. *Ann Intern Med* 1994; 121:769-785.

[144] Mishra BB, Sommers W, Koski CL, Greenstein JI. Acute inflammatory demyelinating polyneuropathy in the acquired immune deficiency syndrome. *Ann Neurol* 1985; 18:131-132.

[145] Parry O, Mielke J, Latif AS, Ray S, Levy LF, Siziya S. Peripheral neuropathy in individuals with HIV infection in Zimbabwe. *Acta Neurol Scand* 1997; 96:218-222.

[146] Qureshi AI, Cook AA, Mishu H, Krendel DA. Guillain-Barre syndrome in immunocompromised patients: a report of three patients and review of the literature. *Muscle Nerve* 1997; 20:1002-1007.

[147] Morgello S, Simpson DM. Multifocal cytomegalovirus demyelinative polyneuropathy associated with AIDS. *Muscle Nerve* 1995; 17:176-182.

[148] Hirsch HH, Kaufmann G, Sendi P, Battegay M. Immune reconstitution in HIV-infected patients. *Clin Infect Dis* 2004; 38:1159-1166.

[149] Makela P, Howe L, Glover S, Ferguson I, Pinto A, Gompels M. Recurrent Guillain-Barré syndrome as a complication of immune reconstitution in HIV. *Journal of Infection* 2002; 44(1):47-49.

[150] Piliero PJ, Fish DG, Preston S, Cunningham D, Kinchelow T, Salgo M, Qian J, Drusano GL. Guillain-Barré syndrome associated with immune reconstitution. *Clin Infect Dis* 2003; 36(9):e111-114.

[151] Puthanakit T, Oberdorfer P, Akarathum N, Wannarit P, Sirisanthana T, Sirisanthana V. Immune reconstitution syndrome after highly active antiretroviral therapy in human immunodeficiency virus-infected Thai children. *Pediatr Infect Dis J* 2006; 25:53-58.

[152] Teo EC, Azwra A, Jones RL, Gazzard BG, Nelson M. Guillain-Barré syndrome following immune reconstitution after antiretroviral therapy for primary HIV infection. *J HIV Ther* 2007; 12:62-63.

[153] Shah SS, Rodriguez T, McGowan JP. Miller Fisher variant of Guillain-Barré syndrome associated with lactic acidosis and stavudine therapy. *Clin Infect Dis* 2003; 36:e131-e133.

[154] Wooltorton E: HIV drug stavudine (Zerit, d4T) and symptoms mimicking Guillain-Barré syndrome. *Cmaj* 2002; 166(8):1067.

[155] Dalakas MC, Pezeshkpour GH. Neuromuscular diseases associated with human immunodeficiency virus infection. *Ann Neurol* 1988; 23(1):S38-S48.

[156] Kleyweg RP, van der Meche FGA, Meulstee J. Treatment of Guillain-Barré syndrome with high-dose gamma globulin. *Neurology* 1988; 38(10):1639-1641.

[157] Hassan KM, Mathew I. Guillain-Barré syndrome in an HIV seropositive subject. The *Journal of the Association of Physicians of India* 2000; 48(12):1214.

[158] Berger JR, Difini JA, Swerdloff MA, Ayyar DR. HIV seropositivity in Guillain-Barrè syndrome. *Annals of Neurology* 1987; 22(3):393-394.

[159] Seneviratne U. Guillain-Barré syndrome. *Postgraduate Medical Journal* 2000; 76(902):774-782.

[160] Schleicher GK, Black A, Mochan A, Richards GA. Effect of human immunodeficiency virus on intensive care unit outcome of patients with Guillain-Barré syndrome. *Critical Care Medicine* 2003; 31(6):1848-1850.

[161] McClellan K, Armeau E, Parish T. Recognizing Guillain-Barré syndrome in the primary care setting. *The Internet Journal of Allied Health Sciences and Practice* 2007; vol 5 n°1.

[162] Arnason BGW, Soliven B. Acute inflammatory demyelinating polyradiculoneuropathy. In: Dyck PJ, Thomas PK, Griffin JW, Low PA, Poduslo JF, editors. *Peripheral neuropathy. 3rd ed.* Philadelphia: Saunders 1993; p. 1437-1497.

[163] Miller RG, Parry GJ, Pfaeffl W, Lang W, Lippert R, Kiprov D. The spectrum of peripheral neuropathy associated with ARC and AIDS. *Muscle Nerve* 1988; 11:857-863.

[164] Moulignier A, Authier FJ, Baudrimont M, Pialoux G, Belec L, Polivka M, Clair B, Gray F, Mikol J, Gherardi RK. Peripheral neuropathy in human immunodeficiency virus-infected patients with the diffuse infiltrative lymphocytosis syndrome. *Ann Neurol* 1997; 41:438-445.

[165] Comi C, Fleetwood T, Dianzani U. The role of T cell apoptosis in nervous system autoimmunity. *Autoimmun Rev* 2012; 12:150-156.

[166] Piette AM, Tusseau F, Vignon D, Chapman A, Parrot G, Leibowitch J, Montagnier L. Acute neuropathy coincident with seroconversion for anti-LAV/HTLV-III. *Lancet* 1986; 1(8485):852.

[167] Vendrell J, Heredia C, Pujol M, Vidal J, Blesa R, Graus F. Guillain-Barré syndrome associated with seroconversion for anti-HTLV-III. *Neurology* 1987; 37(3):544.

[168] Brew BJ, Perdices M, Darveniza P, Edwards P, Whyte B, Burke WJ, Garrick R, O'Sullivan D, Penny R, Cooper DA. The neurological features of early and 'latent' human immunodeficiency virus infection. *Aust N Z J Med* 1989; 19(6):700-705.

[169] Elder G, Dalakas M, Pezeshkpour G, Sever J. Ataxic neuropathy due to ganglioneuronitis after probable acute human immunodeficiency virus infection. *Lancet* 1986; 2(8518):1275-1276.

[170] Roullet E, Assuerus V, Gozlan J, Ropert A, Said G, Baudrimont M, El Amrani M, Jacomet C, Duvivier C, Gonzales-Canali G. Cytomegalovirus multifocal neuropathy in AIDS: analysis of 15 consecutive patients. *Neurology* 1994; 44:2174-2182.

[171] Bradley WG, Verma A. Painful vasculitic neuropathy in HIV-1 infection: relief of pain with prednisone therapy. *Neurology* 1996; 47:1446-1451.

[172] Leger JM, Bouche P, Bolgert F, Chaunu MP, Rosenheim M, Cathala HP, Gentilini M, Hauw JJ, Brunet P. The spectrum of polyneuropathies in patients infected with HIV. *J Neurol Neurosurg Psychiatry* 1989; 52:1369-1374.

[173] Said G, Saimot AG, Lacroix C, Tardieu M. Peripheral nerve disease in HIV infected patients. In: Said G, Saimot AG, Lacroix C, Tardieu M, editors. *Neurological complications of HIV and AIDS*. Philadelphia: Saunders 1997; p 159.

[174] Said G, Lacroix C, Chemouilli P, Goulon-Goeau C, Roullet E, Penaud D, de Broucker T, Meduri G, Vincent D, Torchet M. Cytomegalovirus neuropathy in acquired immunodeficiency syndrome: a clinical and pathological study. *Ann Neurol* 1991; 29(2):139-146.

[175] Eidelberg D, Sotrel A, Vogel H, Walker P, Kleefield J, Crumpacker CS 3rd. Progressive polyradiculopathy in acquired immunodeficiency syndrome. *Neurology* 1986; 36:912-916.
[176] So YT, Olney RK. Acute lumbosacral polyradiculopathy in acquired immunodeficiency syndrome: experience in 23 patients. *Ann Neurol* 1994; 35:53-58
[177] Kim YS, Hollander H. Polyradiculopathy due to cytomegalovirus: report of two cases in which improvement occurred after prolonged therapy and review of the literature. *Clin Infect Dis* 1993; 17:32-37.
[178] Cinque P, Scarpellini P, Vago L, Linde A, Lazzarin A. Diagnosis of central nervous system complications in HIV infected patients: CSF analysis by the polymerase chain reaction. *AIDS* 1997; 11:1-17.
[179] Lanska MJ, Lanska DJ, Schmidley JW. Syphilitic polyradiculopathy in a HIV-positive man. *Neurology* 1988; 38:1297-1301.
[180] Léger JM, Hénin D, Bélec L, Mercier B, Cohen L, Bouche P, Hauw JJ, Brunet P. Lymphoma-induced polyradiculopathy in AIDS: two cases. *J Neurol* 1992; 239:132-134.
[181] Itescu S, Brancato LJ, Winchester RA. Sicca syndrome in HIV infection: association with HLA-DR5 and CD8 lymphocytosis. *Lancet* 1989; 2(8661):466-468.
[182] Pardo CA, McArthur JC, Griffin JW. HIV neuropathy: insights in the pathology of HIV peripheral nerve disease. *J Peripher Nerv Syst* 2001; 6:21-27.
[183] Gherardi RK, Chretien F, Delfau-Larue M-H, Authier F-J, Moulignier A, Roulland-Dussoix D, Belec L. Neuropathy in diffuse infiltrative lymphocytosis syndrome. *Neurology* 1998; 50:1041-1044.
[184] Price RW. Neuropathy complicating diffuse infiltrative lymphocytosis. *Lancet* 1998; 352(9128):592-594.
[185] Thomas DL, Shih JW, Alter HJ, Vlahov D, Cohn S, Hoover DR, Cheung L, Nelson KE. Effect of human immunodeficiency virus on hepatitis C virus infection among injecting drug users. *J Infect Dis* 1996; 174(4):690-695.
[186] Authier FJ, Pawlotsky JM, Viard JP, Guillevin L, Degos JD, Gherardi RK. High incidence of hepatitis C virus infection in patients with cryoglobulinemic neuropathy. *Ann Neurol* 1993; 34(5):749-750.
[187] Tembl JI, Ferrer JM, Sevilla MT, Lago A, Mayordomo F, Vilchez JJ. Neurologic complications associated with hepatitis C virus infection. *Neurology* 1999; 53(4):861-864.
[188] Vassilopoulos D, Calabrese LH. Hepatitis C infection and vasculitis. *Arthr Rheum* 2002; 46:585-597.
[189] Said G, Goulon-Goeau C, Lacroix C, Feve A, Descamps H, Fouchard M. Inflammatory lesions of peripheral nerve in a patient with human T-lymphotropic virus type I associated myelopathy. *Ann Neurol* 1988; 24(2):275-277.
[190] Harrison LH, Vaz B, Taveira DM, Taveira DM, Quinn TC, Gibbs CJ, de Souza SH, McArthur JC, Schechter M. Myelopathy among Brazilians coinfected with human T-cell lymphotropic virus type I and HIV. *Neurology* 1997; 48:13-18.
[191] McArthur JC, Griffin JW, Cornblath DR, Griffin DE, Tesoriero T, Kuncl R, Gibbs CJ, Farzadegan H, Johnson RT. Steroid responsive myeloneuropathy in a man dually infected with HIV-1 and HTLVI. *Neurology* 1990; 40:938-944.

[192] Zehender G, Colasante C, Santambrogio S, De Maddalena C, Massetto B, Cavalli B, Jacchetti G, Fasan M, Adorni F, Osio M, Moroni M, Galli M. Increased risk of developing peripheral neuropathy in patients coinfected with HIV-1 and HTLV-2. *J Acquir Immune Defic Syndr* 2002; 31(4):440-447.

[193] Zehender G, De Maddalena C, Osio M, Cavalli B, Parravicini C, Moroni M, Galli M. High prevalence of human T cell lymphotropic virus type II infection in patients affected by human immunodeficiency virus type 1-associated predominantly sensory polyneuropathy. *J Infect Dis* 1995; 172(6):1595-1598.

In: Contemporary Issues in Peripheral Neuropathy
Editor: Daniel L. Menkes
ISBN: 978-1-62948-681-9

Chapter IX

Familial Amyloid Polyneuropathy (FAP): Clinical Features, Pathophysiology, and Treatment

Mª Teresa Tomás[1,2], **Helena Santa-Clara**[1], **Élia Mateus**[3] **and Estela Monteiro**[3]*

[1]Exercise and Health Laboratory, Interdisciplinary Center for the Study of Human Performance; Faculty of Human Kinetics, Technical University of Lisbon
[2]Lisbon Higher School of Health Technology, Polytechnique Institut of Lisbon
[3]Hepatobiliopancreatic and Transplantation Center, Hospital Curry Cabral, Lisbon

Abstract

In the literature, concepts of "polyneuropathy", "peripheral neuropathy" and "neuropathy" are often mistakenly used as synonyms. Polyneuropathy is a specific term that refers to a relatively homogenous process that affects multiple peripheral nerves. Most of these tend to present as symmetric polyneuropathies that first manifest in the distal portions of the affected nerves. Many of these distal symmetric polyneuropathies are due to toxic-metabolic causes such as alcohol abuse and diabetes mellitus. Other distal symmetric polyneuropathies may result from an overproduction of substances that result in nerve pathology such as is observed in anti-MAG neuropathy and monoclonal gammopathy of undetermined significance. Other "overproduction" disorders are hereditary such as noted in the Portuguese type of familial amyloid polyneuropathy (FAP). FAP is a manifestation of a group of hereditary amyloidoses; an autosomal dominant, multisystemic disorder wherein the mutant amyloid precursor, transthyretin, is produced in excess primarily by the liver. The liver accounts for approximately 98% of all transthyretin production. FAP is confirmed by detecting a transthyretin variant with a

* Address correspondence to: Mª Teresa Tomás; PT, PhD, Lisbon Higher School of Health Technology, Polytechnical Institute of Lisbon, Av. D. João II, Lote 4.69.01 1990 - 096 Lisbon, Portugal, Telephone number: +351 962528947; +351 218980400, Fax number: (351) 218 980 460, e-mail: teresa.tomas@estesl.ipl.pt; mteresa.tomas@netcabo.pt; teresa.tomas@fmh.utl.pt.

methionine for valine substitution at position 30 [TTR (Met30)]. Familial Amyloidotic Polyneuropathy (FAP) – Portuguese type, was first described by a Portuguese neurologist, Corino de Andrade in 1939 and published in 1951. Most persons with this disorder are descended from Portuguese sailors who sired offspring in various locations, primarily in Sweden, Japan and Mallorca. Their descendants emigrated worldwide such that this disorder has been reported in other countries as well. More than 2000 symptomatic cases have been reported in Portugal. FAP progresses rapidly with an average time course from symptom onset to multi-organ involvement and death between ten and twenty years. Treatments directed at removing this aberrant protein such as plasmapheresis and immunoadsorption proved to be unsuccessful. Liver transplantation has been the only effective solution as evidenced by almost 2000 liver transplants performed worldwide. A therapy for FAP with a novel agent, "Tafamidis" has shown some promise in ongoing phase III clinical trials.

It is well recognized that regular physical activity of moderate intensity has a positive effect on physical fitness as gauged by body composition, aerobic capacity, muscular strength and endurance and flexibility. Physical fitness has been reported to result in the reduction of symptoms and lesser impairment when performing activities of daily living. Exercise has been advocated as part of a comprehensive approach to the treatment of chronic diseases. Therefore, this chapter concludes with a discussion of the role of exercise training on FAP.

1. Introdution

Many different classification systems have been used to characterize polyneuropathies. For purposes of this chapter, the authors will use the system advocated by Schaumberg et al.[1]. The term "Hereditary motor and sensory neuropathy" or HMSN is used to describe a group of conditions in which both sensory and motor fibers are affected in a distal and symmetrical manner. Familial Amyloidotic Polyneuropathy (FAP) has some similarities to HMSN in that it presents with progressive weakness and wasting of the distal muscles of the lower extremities that subsequently affects the hands in concert with a similar pattern of sensory loss. Unlike other HMSNs such as Charcot-Marie–Tooth, FAP often manifests significant autonomic dysfunction as well. This chapter focuses on FAP, the role of orthotopic liver transplantation in limiting disease progression, and concludes with a discussion of the role of exercise training in liver transplanted FAP patients.

2. Familial Amyloidotic Polyneuropathy (FAP)

Familial Amyloidotic Polyneuropathy (FAP) or "Corino Andrade's disease", is an autosomal dominantly inherited systemic amyloidosis [2]. FAP usually manifests in the second to fifth decade of life or later as a mixed sensorimotor and autonomic neuropathy [3]. FAP is caused by the extracellular deposition of insoluble amyloid fibers, which result from the deposition of a mutant protein, transthyretin (TTR), located on chromosome 18 [4]. TTR or "pre-albumin" is a protein of 127 amino acids that is primarily synthesized in the liver (~ 98%). TTR's normal function is as the carrier of thyroxine (T4) and retinol [5, 6]. Many mutations affecting TTR that result in amyloidosis have been described subsequent to the identification of the mutation responsible for FAP-Portuguese type in 1984. FAP-Portuguese type results from the mutation TTRMet30, in which valine is substituted for methionine (V30M or Val30Met) on the thirtieth carbon in the TTR's polypeptide chain. This abnormal TTR is deposited in all extracellular connective tissues except for the brain and the liver parenchyma [7, 8]. For the remainder of this chapter, FAP will refer to this specific genetic abnormality known as "Familial Amyloidotic Polyneuropathy-Portuguese type."

Most cases of FAP occur in Portugal, mainly in the northern and central regions. Nevertheless, there are descriptions of FAP in other endemic areas such as Japan (second most common worldwide focus), Sweden, Mallorca (3rd most common European focus) and Brazil [3, 7, 9-11]. Other cases have been reported in some families living in Finland, Holland, France, Denmark and the United States [2, 12].

While the clinical manifestations of FAP are similar despite their location, Portuguese patients tend to manifest earlier in life at a median age of 34 years (range 20 to 78 years) [9]. On average, men tend to develop symptoms earlier than women [13]. It should be noted that not all patients with FAP develop symptoms and that the deposition of mutated TTR may be induced by a secondary process such as a chronic infection or inflammation [14].

One of the main features of FAP is the sensorimotor and autonomic neuropathy [7]. Without treatment, death occurs within 10 to 20 years after symptom onset. The disease process first affects the longer, thinner and less myelinated axons. Therefore, small fiber sensory and autonomic functions are first affected [15, 16]. Thus, erectile dysfunction tends to be one of the first symptoms reported in men [7].

Other manifestations include weight loss, cardiac arrhythmias, renal failure with proteinuria and visual impairment by deposition of amyloid within the vitreous humor. Motor manifestations such as atrophy and muscle weakness occur later in the course of the illness [7]. Other authors have reported a decrease in bone mineral density [17]. Muscle weakness tends to affect the lower extremities first but diminished handgrip strength as compared to normal controls has also been reported in patients who do not report hand weakness [18].

Secondary psychiatric complications include progressive anxiety and depression [19]. Pressure ulcers, dehydration, extensive burns, and orchitis in patients with permanent indwelling catheters or catheterization have also been reported [3]. Cardiomyopathy, nephropathy, vitreous opacity, and carpal tunnel syndrome can occur alone or in association with the polyneuropathy [4, 13].

3. Medical Treatment Strategies

The first therapies were directed at removing the abnormal TTR from the serum. Neither plasma exchange nor immunoabsorption proved effective [20]. At present, stabilization of TTR may be the best therapeutic strategy for preventing the formation of altered amyloid. Therapy with Difflunisal©, based on the thyroxine binding sites (an important stabilizer of TTR), was proposed, such as the administration of $Cr3^+$ (trivalent chromium) normally present in food [10, 21].

Some authors also reported that tissue acidosis (pH 7.4-6.5), which may be observed in inflammatory conditions or ischemia, may contribute to modified TTR formation [8]. Therefore, any treatment strategy that prevents inflammation or ischemia may attenuate disease progression [8, 14, 22]. Other medical strategies include gene replacement therapy, prevention of amyloid formation and the dissolution of amyloid fibrils [21].

There is a novel, first-in-class drug for the treatment of transthyretin familial amyloidotic polyneuropathy, Tafamidis meglumine (Vyndaqel ®). Tafamidis is a small-molecule inhibitor that binds selectively to TTR in human plasma and kinetically stabilizes the tetrameric structure of both wild-type TTR and a number of different mutants. Clinical trials indicate that tafamidis slows disease progression and reduces the disease burden. Preliminary data report improvement in small and large nerve fiber function, modified body mass index and lower extremity neurological examination [23]. Tafamidis has been granted marketing authorization by the European Commission. The United States' Federal Food and Drug Administration is currently reviewing this drug for the same indication.

4. Liver Transplantation and FAP

a. Orthotopic Liver Transplant Selection Criteria

Orthotopic liver transplantation as an effective treatment for FAP was first reported in 1990 as a means of removing of the organ responsible for the primary production of TTR, especially for patients carriers of the variant Val30Met [24]. The utility of this technique was subsequently confirmed in a Portuguese study [24]. Given the scarcity of donor organs, a new technique known as sequential transplantation (or domino liver transplantation) was developed [25]. In this method, a morphologically and functionally normal liver is removed from a patient with FAP and reimplanted in another patient aged 50 or more with a terminal chronic liver disease [CLD] [4]. While the transplanted FAP liver could, in theory, lead to the emergence of symptoms of FAP after 10 years, this can serve as a temporizing measure such that the patient with CLD could remain longer on a transplant waiting list.

At present, liver transplantation for FAP patients is considered the standard of care for the treatment of FAP as the liver is where the greatest amount of TTR is produced [7]. Therefore liver transplantation should be proposed in the early symptomatic phases of the disease [26].

Table 1. Multiple Organ Transplant (31-12-2010) (FAPWTR)

Liver + Kidney	41
Liver + Heart	26
Liver + Previous Heart	9
Liver + Sequential Heart	1
Liver + Kidney + Heart	1
Total	**78**

As of December 2010, 1917 patients with FAP have undergone orthotopic liver transplantation. These were performed at 73 transplant centers in 19 different countries (911 in Portugal), as reported by *Familial Amyloidotic Polyneuropathy World Transplant Registry* (FAPWTR). Of these 1917 individuals, 56% were male and 44% female. The mean age at transplantation was 41 ± 11 years (range 21-72 years) and time from symptom onset to transplantation was 3.9 ± 2.8 years (range 0-30 years) [27]. Of these 1917 patients, 78 underwent combined transplantation (liver and kidney, liver and heart or liver, heart and kidney) [27] as listed in Table 1. By December 2010, 977 sequential liver transplants (or domino liver transplants) were performed worldwide of which 494 occurred in Portugal [27]. On average, approximately 120 patients worldwide are transplanted each year for FAP. A summary of the surgical centers that perform liver transplants may be found at www.fapwtr.org.

Prognosis, and transplantation list priority, is calculated on the basis of three parameters: the polyneuropathy disability scoring system (score PND), the modified body mass index (mBMI = BMI × serum albumin in g / L) and modified MELD score (Model of End-stage Liver Disease) [5]. The modified MELD score is calculated by assuming a 15% risk of mortality at 3 months that increases by an additional 10% for every 3 month period that the patient remains on the waiting list [5]. Patients at greater risk for mortality are assigned a higher priority for transplantation. However FAP patients' mortality risk is not dependent on their liver disease and the MELD score *per se* is not reflective of their need for liver transplant [28].

The PND score classifies FAP patients into five levels of disability as noted in Table 2: Level I - sensory changes, but gait is preserved; Level II – abnormal gait without requiring an assistive device; Level IIIA – Ambulation possible only with an assistive device; Level IIIB – Ambulation possible only with the use of two assistive devices and Level IV – patient bedridden or otherwise wheelchair confined [29, 30]. In order to be considered for transplantation, the patient should have a PND score < IIIb and a modified body mass index (mBMI) > 700.

Table 2. PND score (polyneuropathy disability scoring system)

Level I	Sensory changes, but gait is preserved
Level II	Gait without requiring any walking auxiliary
Level III A	Walking with an auxiliary
Level III B	Walking with two auxiliary
Level IV	Patient bedridden or in wheelchairs

Although survival following liver transplantation in FAP patients is related to both the recipient's medical status and the quality of the donor organ, current survival rates are approximately 90% after five years and 75% after ten years [31]. Causes of death after transplantation include cardiac complications (24%), sepsis (23%), donor liver malfunction (14%) and perioperative death (3%) [10, 27]. Domino liver transplantation or "sequential transplantation" survival rates were 91.8% at one year and 88.4% at 5 years [5]. These survival rates may increase over time as immunosuppressant agents with fewer side effects are developed [32].

b. Clinical Improvements Noted After Transplantation

While orthotopic liver transplantation is the only treatment known to halt the progression of FAP, the best results are obtained in younger subjects with the shortest disease duration [3,

4, 12, 26, 33-37]. Moreover, the greatest degree of improvement occurs within the first 12 months after which little to no improvement occurs [34]. Other authors opine that the post-operative improvements are augmented by concurrent rehabilitation programs [36]. Liver transplantation results in decreased levels of mutated TTR in the gut and blood [38-41]. However, mutated TTR remains in both the cerebrospinal fluid (CSF) and in the eye. As such, it is responsible for an increased risk of developing ocular symptoms including vitreous opacity [12, 42]. Despite the fact that mutated TTR remains in the CSF, no central nervous system complications have been reported [42].

Many transplanted patients report other clinical improvements including improved mood, weight gain with an improved mBMI, as well as lesser degrees of dysautonomia and neuropathic pain [34, 39, 43]. Sensory function returns in the order in which it was lost, (i.e. the last lost is the first to recover). Most of this improvement occurs within the first 12 months after transplantation, after which no further improvement tends to occur [34]. Notably, these authors reported that there is no significant improvement in motor function. FAP patients who undergo a liver transplantation often report an improvement in neurological function wherein the best results are observed in subjects with the shortest disease duration [44, 45].

Liver transplantation has not been demonstrated to improve cardiac function [34, 42, 43, 46]. Nonetheless, patients who undergo a liver transplantation report an improvement in many disease-associated symptoms except for diarrhea and male erectile dysfunction [3, 4, 12, 24, 33, 37, 41].

Transplantation is one of the most complex and challenging fields in medicine. Of all the advances, the most important ones have been in the field of immunosuppression. During the last decade, one-year survival rates have reached 95% in certain patient subgroups. These remarkable results can be attributed to multiple factors including improvement in organ preservation techniques, advances in intraoperative anesthetic management, refinement of surgical techniques, the introduction of new agents to treat the post-transplantation infectious complications, and a better understanding of immunosuppressive management [32, 47].

The standard immunosuppressive regimen consists of a combination of three types of agents. A calcineurin inhibitor, (e.g. cyclosporine or tacrolimus), is the mainstay of immunosuppressive therapy. Calcineurin inhibitors are typically combined with antimetabolites (e.g. mycophenolate mofetil or mycophenolic acid) and corticosteroids. This triple therapy combination results in therapeutic synergy while minimizing dose-related side effects [48-50].

Several adverse effects common to both calcineurin inhibitors are recognized, most notably nephrotoxicity and neurotoxicity although each has its own idiosyncratic side effects. Tacrolimus is more diabetogenic, whereas cyclosporine is more likely to induce dyslipidemia and hypertension [51]. Corticosteroids such as prednisone have numerous side effects including insulin resistance, weight gain, sodium and fluid retention, hypertension, hyperlipidemia, osteoporosis, aseptic bone necrosis, myopathy, cataracts, glaucoma, cushingoid appearance, peptic ulcer, dermatological issues (e.g. acne, hirsutism, skin fragility), susceptibility to infections, impaired wound healing, amenorrhea in women, and neuropsychiatric symptoms such as depression, mania, psychosis, and insomnia [47, 50, 52, 53].

The current range of available immunosuppressive agents allows for individualization of the treatment regimen. Nonetheless, significant adverse effects continue to complicate the post transplant period that affect survival and quality of life [53]. Thus, the preferred course of action is to balance the need for immunosuppression against these medications' potential side effects.

Liver transplantation improves both survival and quality of life [54]. These outcomes are correlated with the recipient's current health status, (e.g. presence of graft rejection, infection or surgical complication influences), as well as by the health care provided such as medication, patient education and mental support [54, 55]. The individual's ability to adhere to physical therapy and medical regimens plays a major role in post-transplantation recovery. Other factors that affect health related quality of life (HRQoL) include the patient's emotional state, degree of social interaction as well as physical and cognitive function [56].

c. Clinical Electrophysiological Improvements After Transplantation

Improved dysautonomia (e.g. diarrhea, orthostatic hypotension, neurogenic bladder) has been attributed to the regeneration of small fibers in the peripheral nervous system [34, 36, 41, 43]. Some authors reported that the nerve conduction studies remain unchanged after liver transplantation, which they attribute to halting the progression of large nerve fiber dysfunction [37, 39]. Other authors reported an improvement in post-transplant nerve conduction studies, an increased number of small myelinated fibers, and a reduced degree of myelinated axon loss [40, 41]; Another publication reported that FAP patients who underwent liver transplantation continue to demonstrate evidence of FAP associated neuropathy progression [57]. Therefore, the reviewers conclude that nerve conduction studies may not necessarily improve post-transplantation and should not be used as a means of assessing clinical improvement.

Nonetheless, clinical neurological deficits did not appear to progress in most patients characterized as having a "mild neuropathy" at the time of liver transplantation.[36, 39, 58] This differs markedly from the natural history of the disease, which tends to be progressive and unremitting. However, we have not observed any ambulatory improvement, even in those patients with moderate weakness before transplantation. In contrast, a reversal of sensory deficits was observed in some patients with a mild sensorimotor neuropathy or a pure sensory neuropathy [41, 59]. Other studies examined the maximal motor and sensory conduction velocities (MCV and SCV) of the ulnar and tibial nerves [37]. These authors reported that the recovery of peripheral nerve function in FAP patients after a liver transplant seems to be very slow and limited, especially the function of large diameter myelinated fibers. In one case report, there was biopsy-proven evidence of sensory nerve regeneration post liver transplantation as the number of myelinated fibers in a left sural nerve biopsy specimen obtained before and 3 years after transplantation demonstrated an interval increase in number of myelinated fibers [40]. Therefore, longitudinal studies of clinical electrophysiological progression after liver transplant are needed in order to determine the specificity and sensitivity of these studies with respect to nerve regeneration.

5. Exercise Training in FAP Patients after a Liver Transplant

Moderate physical exertion has been reported to improve body composition, aerobic capacity, muscular strength, endurance and flexibility [60]. Such exercise has been reported to lessen disease symptoms and to improve the patient's ability to perform activities of daily living [61]. Therefore, many authors recommend moderate exercise as part of a multifaceted treatment plan [60-64].

Exercise programs should be designed to reduce both the functional consequences of inactivity and the disease process itself; especially the loss of strength and muscle mass [65, 66]. With respect to peripheral neuropathy, it has been published that exercise improves peripheral nervous system function as measured on electrodiagnostic studies. These changes include greater degrees of axonal regeneration, increased conduction velocities and increased amplitudes of both of the motor and sensory responses [67]. Another review of exercise's effect on motor function in peripheral neuropathies reported that endurance training can increase muscle strength in affected muscles [68].

Many patients waiting for an organ transplant demonstrate impaired physical fitness when compared to healthy controls. Impaired performance measures included decreased muscle strength, reduced HRQoL values, decreased oxygen consumption (VO_2) and a reduced exercise capacity on a six minute walk test (6MWT) [69-72].

There are fewer studies that assessed these measures in FAP patients before transplantation, although there is some evidence that such patients have decreased lower extremity muscle strength along with reduced grip strength [18, 73]. One study reported on 48 FAP patients with a mean age of 34 ± 7 years (range 23-59 years) who were examined an average of 4 months after liver transplantation (range 2 - 12 months). This study reported decreased handgrip strength with values lower than 42 kg [18]. Notably, this is the cutoff value that indicates a "moderate risk" of functional limitation and disability [74]. Also, when body composition was assessed, this group demonstrated values consistent with reduced bone mineral density (BMD) at the proximal femur but not on total BMD as compared to normal controls [18].

All the improvements were positively correlated with levels of physical activity [75-78]. These data seem to indicate that patients who are physically fit after liver transplantation may undertake high-intensity exercise. Such patients have also been reported to tolerate high altitude hypoxia [79, 80], increased levels of exercise [81, 82] and an ability to return to work with minimal physical limitations [83].

To our knowledge, only five studies have analyzed the impact of an exercise training program on physical fitness of individuals undergoing liver transplantation [52, 84-87]. Of these five reports, only one addressed the diagnosis of FAP [87]. This case study reported on a patient who underwent a liver transplant ten years earlier who undertook an exercise program that resulted in increased muscle mass and aerobic capacity. Since that this was a case report, no specific guidance can be given regarding exercise programs for patients with FAP who undergo liver transplantation.

Given the rarity of this disorder and the restrictions associated with the use of immunosuppressive agents, such patients may not be able to perform aerobic exercises in locations readily accessible to the general public (e.g. fitness centers) for the first 6 to 12 months post-transplantation. As such, a home-based exercise program is what is usually recommended.

Two studies have been published on home-based exercise in patients with sensorimotor polyneuropathies [88, 89]. However, there are no reports that specifically addressed home-based exercise programs designed for patients with FAP.

A three-year Portuguese study was performed between 2006 and 2008 by the Hepatobiliopancreatic and Liver Transplantation Center of Hospital Curry Cabral (one of three centers and the most active for liver transplantation in Portugal) and the Exercise and Health laboratory from Faculty of Human Kinetics at Technical University of Lisbon. This study was conducted in order to assess how exercise training will change physical condition, health related quality of life and fatigue in those FAP patients. One-third of all patients with FAP, who underwent liver transplantation between 2006 and 2008, enrolled in the study and signed an informed consent. These patients were assigned to one of three exercise groups; supervised, home-based or control. These volunteers assigned to the exercise groups were asked to perform a one hour moderate intensity three times per week for six months. The parameters assessed included body composition (lean mass, fat mass and bone mass), functional capacity (six-minute walk test), muscular strength (handgrip strength and knee isometric strength), HRQoL and levels of fatigue.

The effect of ceasing exercise was performed after the study on 47% of the exercising patients in a third assessment 24 weeks after the study's conclusion.

There was a significant increase in patients who engaged in exercise in lean body mass, muscle strength and exercise capacity but not in HRQoL or fatigue reduction as compared to the controls. Those patients who performed a supervised exercise training program had better results than those who performed home-based exercise training. The decrements in these parameters observed after six months of not engaging in exercise were not statistically significant (data in press).

Conclusion

Familial Amyloidotic Polyneuropathy (FAP) or "Corino Andrade's disease," is an autosomal dominantly inherited systemic amyloidosis that results from the extracellular deposition of insoluble amyloid fibers. These amyloid fibers are created by a mutant protein, *transthyretin*, which is mainly produced in the liver. FAP presents as a sensorimotor and autonomic neuropathy with weight loss, cardiac arrhythmias, renal failure, visual impairment and clinical deterioration in several parameters of physical fitness.

Liver transplantation is at the moment the only non-experimental intervention that attenuates disease progression. Untreated patients tend to expire between 10 and 20 years after symptom onset. Early treatment leads to improved outcomes such that liver transplant should be proposed as early as possible after symptom onset. In addition to the operative risks inherent in liver transplantation and the post-operative risks associated with immunosuppression, these patients may present even greater losses in different components of physical fitness such as body composition, muscle strength, exercise capacity, as well as levels of perceived Health Related Quality of Life. However, the available literature indicates that a combined regular exercise program of moderate intensity demonstrates benefits in body composition (significant increases in weight, lean mass and skeletal muscle mass), muscle strength (significantly to grip strength) and exercise capacity (especially the ability to walk) in liver transplant FAP patients. The improvements observed in patients who maintained a prescribed exercise regimen translate into a decreased risk of future disability. Home-based programs may be a good option for these patients.

Clinical recommendations on participation in exercise training programs of moderate intensity should be part of a global intervention and routine care with this specific population (FAP patients undergoing liver transplantation). These recommendations should also be provided to FAP patients on a waiting list for liver transplant in order to improve their functional capacity and reduce the risk of future disability.

References

[1] Schaumberg HH, Berger AR, Thomas PK. *Disorders of peripheral nerves:* Davis Company 1992.

[2] Sales-Luís ML. Polineuropatia Amiloidótica Familiar do Tipo Português: do artigo original ao futuro. *Sinapse* 2006;6(Suplemento):40-42.

[3] Munar-Ques M. [Corino Andrade disease]. *An R Acad Nac Med (Madr)* 1999;116(3):667-680; discussion 681-662.

[4] Munar-Ques M. [Familial amyloid polyneuropathy 2003]. *Med Clin (Barc)* 2003;121(3):100-101.

[5] Pomfret E, Gish RG, Brandhagen D. Model for End-Stage Disease (MELD) Exception for Familial Amyloidotic Polyneuropathy. *Liver Transpl* 2006;12:S100-S101.

[6] Saraiva MJ, Sousa MM, Cardoso I, *et al.* Familial Amyloidotic Polyneuropathy. Protein Aggregation in the Peripheral Nervous System. *Journal of Molecular Neuroscience* 2004;23:35-40.

[7] Conceicao I. Clinica e história natural da polineuropatia amiloidotica familiar. *Sinapse* 2006;12 (2)(Maio, suplemento 1):86-90.

[8] Altland K, Richardson S. Histidine 31: The Achilles' Heel of Human Transthyretin. Microheterogeneity is Not Enough to Understand the Molecular Causes of Amyloidogenicity. In: Richardson SJ, Cody V, eds. *Recent Advances in Transthyretin Evolution, Structure and Biological Functions*. Berlin Heidelberg: Springer-Verlag 2009:201-214.

[9] Sousa A. Epidemiologia genética da polineuropatia amiloidotica familiar. *Sinapse* 2006;6(1, suppl 1, Maio):74-79.

[10] Ando Y, Nakamura M, Araki S. Transthyretin-Related Familial Amyloidotic Polyneuropathy. *Arch Neurol* 2005;62:1057-1062.

[11] Perdigoto R, Monteiro E. *Hepatologia de transplante: Minerva Coimbra* 2003.

[12] Coelho T. Familial amyloid polyneuropathy: new developments in genetics and treatment. *Curr Op Neurology* 1996;9:355-359.

[13] Hund E, Linke RP, Willig F, *et al.* Transthyretin-associated neuropathic amyloidosis. Pathogenesis and treatment. *Neurology* 2001;56:431-435.

[14] Villaplana GH, Rosino EH, Cubillana PL, *et al.* Corino-Andrade Disease (Familial Amyloidotic Polineuropathy Type I) in Spain: Urological and Andrological Disorders. *Neurology and Urodynamics* 1997;16:55-61.
[15] Barbosa AR, Barros P, Silva PG, *et al.* Paramiloidose, sistema autonómico e exercício. *Arq Fisiatria* 2003;10:93-102.
[16] Conceicao IM, Castro JF, Scotto M, *et al.* Neurophysiological markers in familial amyloid polyneuropathy patients: early changes. *Clin Neurophysiol* 2008;119(5):1082-1087.
[17] Conceição IM, Miranda LC, Simões E, *et al.* Bone mineral density in familial amyloid polyneuropathy and in other neuromuscular disorders. *European Journal of Neurology* 2005;12:480-482.
[18] Tomás MT, Santa-Clara H, Monteiro E, *et al.* Body composition, muscle strength, functional capacity, and physical disability risk in liver transplanted familial amyloidotic polyneuropathy patients. *Clin Transplant* 2011;25:E406-E414.
[19] Lopes A. Aspectos Psiquiátricos e Psico-Sociais nos Doentes com PAF. *Sinapse* 2006;6(1. Suplemento 1):129-133.
[20] Monteiro E, Perdigoto R, Furtado AL. Liver transplantation for familial amyloid polyneuropathy. *Hepatogastroenterology* 1998;45(23):1375-1380.
[21] Ando Y. Liver transplantation and new therapeutic approaches for familial amyloidotic polyneuropathy (FAP). *Med Mol Morphol* 2005;38:142-154.
[22] Adachi N. Current and Proposed Treatment of Familial Amyloidotic Polyneuropathy. *Clinical Neuropharmacology* 1989;12(6):506-513.
[23] de Lartigue J. Tafamidis for transthyretin amyloidosis. *Drugs Today (Barc)* 2012;48(5):331-337.
[24] Furtado E. Transplantação Hepática na Polineuropatia Amiloidótica Familiar. *Sinapse* 2006;6(1. Suplemento 1):151-153.
[25] Furtado A, Tomb L, Oliveira FJ, *et al.* Sequential Liver Transplantation. *Transplantation Proceedings* 1997;29:467-466
[26] Monteiro E, Freire A, Barroso E. Familial amyloid polyneuropathy and liver transplantation. *J Hepatology* 2004;41:188-194.
[27] (FAPWTR) FAPWTRaDLTR. *http://www.fapwtr.org.*
[28] Freeman Jr. RB, Gish RG, Harper A, *et al.* Model for End-Stage Liver Disease (MELD) Exception Guidelines: Results and Recommendations From the MELD Exception Study Group and Conference (MESSAGE) for the Approval of Patients Who Need Liver Transplantation With Diseases Not Considered by the Standard MELD Formula. *Liver Transpl* 2006;12:S128-S136.
[29] Suhr O, Danielsson A, Rydh A, *et al.* Impact of gastrointestinal dysfunction on survival after liver transplantation for familial amyloidotic polyneuropathy. *Dig Dis Sci* 1996;41(10):1909-1914.
[30] Juneblad K, Naslund A, Olofsson BO, *et al.* Outcome of exercise electrocardiography in familial amyloidotic polyneuropathy patients, Portuguese type, under evaluation for liver transplantation. *Amyloid* 2004;11(3):208-213.
[31] Wilczek HE, Larsson M, Ericzon B-G. Current Status of Liver Transplantation (LTx) for Hereditary Amyloidoses and Domino Liver Transplantation (DLT):The Familial Amyloidotic Polyneuropathy World Transplant Registry (FAPWTR) and the Domino

Liver Transplant Registry (DLTR) Perspective. *Transpl Int* 2009;22(4 Suppl (Meeting Abstract)):4.

[32] McMaster P, Dousset B. The improved results of liver transplantation. *Transplant Int* 1992;5:125-128.

[33] Steen L, Holmgren G, Suhr O, *et al.* World-wide survey of liver transplantation in patients with familial amyloidotic polyneuropathy. *Amyloid* 1994;1:138-142.

[34] Tashima K, Ando Y, Terazaki H, *et al.* Outcome of liver transplantation for transthyretin amyloidosis: follow-up of Japanese familial amyloidotic polyneuropathy patients. *J Neurol Sci* 1999;171(1):19-23.

[35] Jonsén E, Suhr O, Tashima K, *et al.* Early liver transplantation is essential for familial amyloidotic polyneuropathy patient's quality of life. *Amyloid* 2001;8:52-57.

[36] Parrilla P, Ramirez P, Andreu LF, *et al.* Long-term results of liver transplantation in familial amyloidotic polyneuropathy type I. *Transplantation* 1997;64(4):646-649.

[37] Kobayashi S, Morita H, Asawa T, *et al.* Peripheral nerve function in patients with familial amyloid polyneuropathy after liver transplantation. *Amyloid: J Protein Folding Disord* 2003;10:17-24.

[38] Rydh A, Suhr O, Hietala SO, *et al.* Serum amyloid P component scintigraphy in familial amyloid polyneuropathy: regression of visceral amyloid following liver transplantation. *Eur J Nucl Med* 1998;25:709-713.

[39] Parrila P, Lopes-Andreu FR, Ramirez P, *et al.* Familial Amyloidotic Polyneuropathy Type I (Andrade Disease): A New Indication for Liver Transplant. *Transplantation* 1994;57(3):473-475.

[40] Ikeda SI, Takei Y, Yanagisawa N, *et al.* Peripheral Nerves Regenerated in Familial Amyloid Polyneuropathy after Liver Transplantation. *Annals of internal medicine* 1997;127(8 (part 1)):618-620.

[41] Adams D, Samuel D, Goulon-Goeau C, *et al.* The course and prognostic factors of familial amyloid polyneuropathy after liver transplantation. *Brain* 2000;123(7):1495-1504.

[42] Hörnsten R, Wiklund U, Olofsson B-O, *et al.* Liver Transplantation Does Not Prevent the Development of Life-Threatning Arrhytmia in Familial Amyloidotic Polyneuropathy, Portuguese-Type (ATTR Val30Met) Patients. *Transplantation* 2004;78:112-116.

[43] Pomfret E, Lewis WD, Jenkins RL, *et al.* Effect of orthotopic liver transplantation on the progression of familial amyloidotic polyneuropathy. *Transplantation* 1998;65(7):918-925.

[44] Bergethon PR, Sabin TD, Lewis D, *et al.* Improvement in the polyneuropathy associated with familial amyloidotic polyneuropathy after liver transplantation. *Neurology* 1996;47:944-951.

[45] Takei Y, Ikeda SI, Hashikura Y, *et al.* Partial-Liver Transplantation to Treat Familial Amyloidotic Polyneuropathy: Follow-uo of 11 Patients. *Annals of internal medicine* 1999;131(8):592-595.

[46] Coutinho CA. Envolvimento Cardíaco na Polineuropatia Amiloidótica Familiar. *Sinapse* 2006;6, suplemento(1):92-98.

[47] Forman LM. Long-Term Metabolic Complications Posttransplantation. Controversies in Management. In: Everson GT, Trotter JF, eds. *Clinical Gastroenterology: Liver*

Transplantation: Challenging Controversies and Topics. Totowa: Humana press 2009:135-144.

[48] Levy GA. Long term immunosuppression and drug interactions. *Liver Transpl* 2001;7(11, Suppl 1):S53-S59.

[49] Muir AJ. Immunosuppressive Medications. In: Killenberg PG, Clavien P-A, eds. *Medical care of the Liver Transplant Patient*. Massachusetts: Blackwell Publishing Ltd 2006:505-521.

[50] López MM, Valenzuela JE, Álvarez FC, *et al.* Long-term problems related to immunosuppression. *Transpl Immunol* 2006;17:31-35.

[51] Åberg F. Long-term clinical outcome after liver transplantation. *Transplantation and Liver Surgery Clinic, Department of Surgery, Helsinki University Central Hospital*. Helsinki: Faculty of Medicine, University of Helsinki 2010:88.

[52] Surgit O, Ersoz G, Gursel Y, *et al.* Effects of exercise training on specific immune parameters in transplant recipients. *Transpl Proc* 2001;33:3298.

[53] Renner EL, Dufour J-F. Medical Problems after Liver Transplantation. In: Killenberg PG, Clavien P-A, eds. *Medical Care of the Liver Transplant Patient*. Massachusetts: Blackwell Publishing Ltd 2006:397-418.

[54] Tome S, Wells J, Said A, *et al.* Quality of life after liver transplantation. A systematic review. *J Hepatology* 2008;48:567-577.

[55] Bownik H, Saab S. Health-Related Quality of Life After Liver Transplantation for Adult Recipients. *Liver Transpl* 2009;15:S42-S49.

[56] Forsberg A, Persson L-O, Nilsson M, *et al.* The Organ Transplant Symptom and Well-Being Instrument – Psychometric Evaluation. *The Open Nursing Journal* 2012;6:30-40

[57] Bentes C, Conceição I, Carvalho M, *et al.* Liver transplantation in familial amyloidotic polyneuropathy (FAP) type I. Clinical and electromyographic evaluation. In: Editore M, ed. *ECCN 98 9th European Congress of Clinical Neurophysiology*. Ljubljana. Slovenija 1998:675-678.

[58] de Carvalho M, Conceicao I, Bentes C, *et al.* Long-term quantitative evaluation of liver transplantation in familial amyloid polyneuropathy (Portuguese V30M). *Amyloid* 2002;9(2):126-133.

[59] Bergethon PR, Sabin TD, Lewis D, *et al.* Improvement in the polyneuropathy associated with familial amyloid polyneuropathy after liver transplantation. *Neurology* 1996;47(4):944-951.

[60] Pederson BK, Saltin B. Evidence for prescribing exercise as therapy in chronic disease. *Scan J Med Sci Sports* 2006;16(Suppl. 1):3-63.

[61] Kujala UM. Is it really important for sick people to perform exercise? . *Scan J Med Sci Sports* 2006;16:145-146.

[62] Vuori I. Physical activity and health: Metabolic and cardiovascular issues. *Advances in Physiotherapy* 2007;9:50-64.

[63] Suominen H. Physical activity and health: Musculoskeletal issues. *Advances in Physiotherapy* 2007;9:65-75.

[64] Donaghy M. Exercise can seriously improve your mental health: Fact or fiction? *Advances in Physiotherapy* 2007;9:76-88.

[65] McDonald CM. Physical activity, health impairments, and disability in neuromuscular disease. *Am J Phys Med Rehabil* 2002;81(11 Suppl):S108-120.

[66] Kilmer DD. The Role of Exercise in Neuromuscular Disease. *Physical Medicine And Rehabilitation Clinics of North America* 1998;9(1):115-125.
[67] Isojärvi H, Keinänen-Kiukaanniemi S, Kallio M, *et al.* Exercise and Fitness are Related to Peripheral Nervous System Function in Overweight Adults. *Medicine & Science in Sports & Exercise* 2010;42(7):1241-1245.
[68] White CM, Pritchard J, Turner-Stokes L. Exercise for people with peripheral neuropathy. *Cochrane Database Syst Rev* 2004(4):CD003904.
[69] Leitao AV, Castro CL, Basile TM, *et al.* [Evaluation of the nutritional status and physical performance in candidates to liver transplantation]. *Rev Assoc Med Bras* 2003;49(4):424-428.
[70] Kjaer M, Beyer N, Secher NH. Exercise and organ transplantation. *Scand J Med Sci Sports* 1999;9(1):1-14.
[71] Wiesinger GF, Quittan M, Zimmermann K, *et al.* Physical performance and health-related quality of life in men on a liver transplantation waiting list. *J Rehabil Med* 2001;33(6):260-265.
[72] Haykowsky M, Taylor D, Kim D, *et al.* Exercise training improves aerobic capacity and skeletal muscle function in heart transplant recipients. *Am J Transplant* 2009;9(4):734-739.
[73] Tomás MT, Santa-Clara H, Monteiro E, *et al.* Alterações da força preensão em portadores de Polineuropatia Amiloidotica Familiar. . *Acta Médica Portuguesa* 2010;23:803-810.
[74] Rantanen T, Guralnik JM, Ferrucci L, *et al.* Coimpairments: strength and balance as predictors of severe walking disability. *J Gerontol A Biol Sci Med Sci* 1999:M172-176.
[75] Krasnoff JB, Vintro AQ, Ascher NL, *et al.* Objective measures of health-related quality of life over 24 months post-liver transplantation. *Clin Transplant* 2005;19(1):1-9.
[76] Painter P, Krasnoff J. Abdominal Organ Transplant (Kidney, Liver, Pancreas). In: Durstine JL, Moore GE, eds. *ACSM's Exercise Management for Persons with Chronic Diseases and Disabilities*: Human Kinetics 2003:180-185.
[77] Painter PL, Luetkemeier MJ, Moore GE, *et al.* Health-related fitness and quality of life in organ transplant recipients. *Transplantation* 1997;64(12):1795-1800.
[78] Painter P, Krasnoff J, Paul SM, *et al.* Physical activity and health-related quality of life in liver transplant recipients. *Liver Transpl* 2001;7(3):213-219.
[79] Pirenne J, Van Gelder F, Kharkevitch T, *et al.* Tolerance of liver transplant patients to strenuous physical activity in high-altitude. *Am J Transplant* 2004;4(4):554-560.
[80] Roi GS, Mosconi G, Capelli I, *et al.* Alpine Skiing and Anaerobic Performance in Solid Organ Transplant Recipients. *Transpl Proc* 2010;42:1029-1031.
[81] Tomczak CR, Warburton DE, Riess KJ, *et al.* Pulmonary oxygen uptake and heart rate kinetics during thc six-minute walk test in transplant recipients. *Transplantation* 2008;85(1):29-35.
[82] Maquirriain J. Fracturas em doentes activos com orgãos transplantados. *The Physician and sporstmedicine* 2002;4(6):37-41.
[83] Robinson LR, Switala J, Tarter RE, *et al.* Functional outcome after liver transplantation: a preliminary report. *Arch Phys Med Rehabil* 1990;71(6):426-427.
[84] Beyer N, Aadahl M, Strange B, *et al.* Improved physical performance after orthotopic liver transplantation. *Liver Transpl Surg* 1999;5(4):301-309.

[85] Krasnoff JB, Vintro AQ, Ascher NL, *et al.* A randomized trial of exercise and dietary counseling after liver transplantation. *Am J Transplant* 2006;6(8):1896-1905.

[86] Warburton DE, Sheel W, Hodges AN, *et al.* Effects of Upper Extremity Exercise Training on Peak Aerobic and Anaerobic Fitness in Patients After Transplantation. *The American Journal of Cardiology* 2004;93:939-943.

[87] Tomás MT, Santa-Clara H, Monteiro E, *et al.* Effects of an Exercise Training Program in Physical Condition After Liver Transplantation in Familial Amyloidotic Polyneuropathy: A Case Report. *Transplantation Proceedings* 2011;43:257-258.

[88] Wright N, Kilmer D, McCrory M, *et al.* Aerobic Walking in Slowly Progressive Neuromuscular Disease: Effect of a 12-Week Program. *Arch Phys Med Rehabil* 1996;77:64-69.

[89] Lindeman E, Leffers P, Spaans F, *et al.* Strength Training in Patients With Myotonic Dystrophy and Hereditary Motor and Sensor Neuropathy: A Randomized Clinical Trial. *Arch Phys Med Rehabil* 1995;76:612-620.

In: Contemporary Issues in Peripheral Neuropathy
Editor: Daniel L. Menkes
ISBN: 978-1-62948-681-9

Chapter X

Peripheral Neuropathy in Pelvic Floor Dysfunction

Consuelo Valles-Antuna[1] and Jesus M. Fernandez-Gomez[2]*
[1]Clinical Neurophysiologist, [2]Urologist, Associate Professor of Urology
Hospital Universitario Central de Asturias. Universidad de Oviedo

Abstract

Pelvic floor dysfunction [PFD] is a prevalent public health problem that undermines the quality of life in people of all ages that may require extensive, expensive and ongoing treatments. PFD predominantly affects women, particularly older women, such that its prevalence is likely to increase with an aging population. The currently available treatments for PFD tend to be inadequate and often require chronic therapy. A comprehensive understanding of the pathophysiology of PFD is essential for the proper management of this disorder as well as for the development of new therapies. One important cause of pelvic floor dysfunction is that of peripheral neuropathy. Therefore, it is imperative that all physicians who encounter PFD be well versed in the effects of peripheral nerve dysfunction on PFD. This knowledge will allow the physician to make an accurate diagnosis, render appropriate treatments, generate an accurate prognosis, and improve the affected patient's quality of life.

Introduction

The pelvic floor is formed by a dome-shaped striated muscular sheet or sling. As most pelvic floor dysfunction [PFD] occurs in women, this chapter will discuss these concepts with reference to female anatomy. This muscular sheet, along with the endopelvic fascia, supports the bladder, uterus and rectum. Thus, the pelvic floor includes all the structures lying between the peritoneum and the vulvar skin including the pelvic viscera, endopelvic fascia, levator ani

* Corresponding author: jmfernandezgomez23@gmail.com.

muscles, perineal membrane and superficial genital muscles. Functionally, the pelvic floor is a balanced system in which every component contributes to maintain normal function. This complex interplay requires an integrated coordination of the somatic and autonomic nervous systems. These systems are controlled by a complex circuitry of the central and peripheral nervous systems, which are under both voluntary and involuntary control.

Pelvic floor dysfunction is widely prevalent, especially in older women. It includes urinary incontinence, lower urinary tract dysfunction (LUTD), defecatory dysfunction, chronic pelvic pain syndromes, sexual disorders, and female pelvic organ prolapse. Given the complex neuroanatomical pathways and organs involved, two or more of these disorders often coexist in the same patient [1]. Pathophysiological mechanisms include dysfunction of the pelvic muscles, connective tissue or neural components.

Neurogenic PFD may result from lesions affecting the central nervous system, peripheral nervous system or both. Central lesions may affect cortical, subcortical, brainstem or spinal cord regions. Peripheral nerve lesions affect neural structures lying outside the pial membrane of the spinal cord and brainstem, including nerve roots, plexuses and peripheral nerves. In this chapter we focus on the clinical characteristics, electrodiagnostic findings and management of PFD associated with peripheral nerve disorders.

Neuroanatomy

At the central level, multiple structures are involved in the neural control of pelvic floor functions. The midbrain periaqueductal gray matter as well as the lateral (L) area of the ventral pons, medial (M) pontine micturition center region of the dorsomedial pons, hypothalamus, cingulate gyrus and the prefrontal cortex participate in micturitional control. Bowel control is less completely understood, although the literature indicates that the insula, prefrontal cortex and anterior cingulate cortex are associated with the conscious perception and processing of the intestinal environment [2]. Neural control of sexual responses involves much of the nervous system as well. The paragigantocelularis nucleus, some regions of the hypothalamus such as the medial preoptic area (MPOA) as well as the paraventricular nucleus (PVN) participate in the sexual response. Other areas that play a role in this response include the amygdala, the septal region, the cingulate gyrus, as well as the parietal, prefrontal and orbitofrontal cortices.

At the peripheral level, the pelvic floor is innervated by three main types of peripheral nerves; the sympathetic, parasympathetic and somatic nerves. Each of these has both efferent and afferent components. Somatic and visceral sensory inputs from pelvic floor are transmitted by myelinated and unmyelinated fibers. Sensory neurons, somatic or autonomic, are of the pseudounipolar type in that their cell bodies are located in the dorsal root ganglia of spinal nerves. The distal portions of these sensory nerves transmit the information towards the dorsal root ganglion whereas the central portion transmits information into spinal cord. These afferent segments either terminate segmentally or, in some cases, terminate after branching for reflex connections that may ascend as far as the brainstem [3]. The sympathetic fibers enter the spinal cord at the T10 to L2 spinal levels while the non-cranial nerve supplied parasympathetic fibers enter at S2 to S4. Both of these systems' afferents participate in pelvic reflex activity.

Efferent pathways also have both somatic and autonomic components. The sympathetic efferent fibers originate in the intermediolateral cell column of the spinal cord between vertebral T10 and L2. They exit the spinal cord through the anterior root, comingled with somatic efferent fibers, to form the spinal nerve root. Subsequently, as the white communicant rami, they synapse in the ganglia of the sympathetic paravertebral chain. These postganglionic efferent fibers travel coextensively with the somatic segmental fibers to reach the pelvic floor through the cavernosa, pelvic and pudendal nerves [4]. Alternatively, sympathetic preganglionic fibers destined for the pelvic organs may pass directly through the paravertebral ganglia and exit as preganglionic visceral or splanchnic nerves. These fibers may synapse on one of the prevertebral or collateral ganglia on the anterior aspect of the aorta or internal iliac vessels before continuing inferiorly as the right and left hypogastric nerves, which contain fibers that contribute to the pelvic plexus [3]. Other fibers pass through both the paravertebral and vertebral ganglia before reaching the pelvic plexus [5].

The preganglionic parasympathetic motor nerves to the bladder and other pelvic organs exit the sacral spinal cord in the anterior roots S2–S4 forming part of the spinal nerves. They continue in the anterior spinal rami through the pelvic splanchnic nerves to ganglion cells in the pelvic plexus; a dense complex of pre and postganglionic sympathetic and parasympathetic fibers and ganglia. The pelvic plexus gives rise to multiple subsidiary plexuses and nerves that supply visceral and somatic structures. Visceral structures are innervated in conjunction with the vascular supply. In contrast, somatic structures are segmentally innervated along with the somatic spinal nerves destined for the same location [5].

The somatic efferent fibers arise from motor neurons in the anterior cell column of lumbosacral spinal cord in order to innervate the skeletal muscles. Onuf's nucleus is a subgroup of alpha motor neurons located ventrolaterally within the anterior horn at S1 to S3. It provides innervation to the urethral and anal sphincters as well as to the levator ani muscle. While Onuf's nucleus' neurons are relatively resistant to polio and amyotrophic lateral sclerosis, they are often involved in multiple system atrophy. Thus, anal sphincter electromyography (EMG) may help to distinguish multiple system atrophy from other neurodegenerative disorders such as Parkinson disease [6]. Efferent motor axons traverse the anterior roots of the spinal cord at the lumbar, sacral, and coccygeal levels. The ventral divisions of the corresponding spinal nerves contribute to the lumbosacral plexuses, via the anterior root of the spinal cord at the lumbar, sacral, and coccygeal levels. The terminal branch of the sacral plexus is the pudendal nerve which divides into three major branches: the dorsal nerve of the penis/clitoris (to provide cutaneous supply to the clitoris/penis), the inferior rectal nerve (to the lower anal canal, the external anal sphincter and the skin around the anus) and the perineal nerve. The perineal nerve divides into sensory and motor branches. The sensory branches innervate the local skin surface and the distal urethra whereas the motor branches innervate the superficial and deep perineal muscles including the external urethral sphincter and parts of the levator ani muscle.

Overview of Neural Control of Pelvic Floor Function

Pelvic floor function requires a highly integrated degree of neuronal circuitry. Coordination strongly depends on a functioning muscle-elastic system composed of

Pelvic organ prolapse includes defects of the anterior vaginal wall (e.g. cystocele), vaginal apex (e.g. uterine prolapse, vaginal vault prolapse, and enterocele), and posterior vaginal wall (e.g. rectocele and enterocele). Similar to other pelvic floor disorders, the etiology tends to be multifactorial with childbirth as the main factor. Other contributing factors are due to conditions that result in chronic increased abdominal pressure, (e.g. multiple large uterine fibroids).

Chronic pelvic pain is a common and disabling condition in both genders. In women, it is defined as non-menstrual pain of at least 6 months duration. Its prevalence in women aged 18 to 50 has been estimated at 15% [15]. Pelvic pain may be caused by malignant and non-malignant conditions. Non-malignant causes may be lower urinary tract or pelvic organ dysfunction, neurological disease (e.g. peripheral neuropathy), orthopedic disease (e.g. lumbar disc prolapse), post bacterial/viral inflammation, post-surgery and others. Malignant conditions frequently associated with pelvic pain include urogenital cancer, lymph node metastases and bone metastases [16].

Erectile dysfunction (ED) is a common form of PFD which consists in the persistent inability to obtain and maintain an erection sufficient to permit satisfactory sexual performance [17]. A community based, random sample observational survey of non-institutionalized men aged 40 to 70 years old, conducted from 1987 to 1989, reported that combined prevalence of minimal, moderate and complete impotence was 52% [18]. ED disrupts physical and psychosocial health and is associated with a significant negative impact on the patient's quality of life. ED may result from either organic or psychological causes but may also be medication-related [19]. Pathophysiological mechanisms of PDF can be related to muscular, connective tissue and/or neurological dysfunction. Almost each type of PFD may result from a neurological disease or direct injury to the nervous system. Neurogenic PFD may result from dysfunction of either the central or peripheral nervous systems.

PFD in the Context of Neurological Disorders

The location, extent and evolution of neurological damage may all influence the clinical expression of PFD. Traditionally, the neurological pathology has been divided into suprapontine, suprasacral spinal cord and subsacral or peripheral lesions. Peripheral nervous system damage can correspond to one of the following syndrome patterns: radiculopathy, polyradiculopathy, plexopathy, polyneuropathy, multiple mononeuropathies (mononeuropathy, or mononeuritis multiplex) and mononeuropathies [20]. The causative pathology may disrupt somatic pathways, autonomic pathways or both, with preferential effects on small or large fibers.

Lumbosacral roots and cauda equina damage. Sacral radiculopathy may be the result of lumbosacral discopathy, orthopedic surgery or of other conditions that result in radiculopathy or pathology affecting the nerve roots. PFD from radiculopathies may result from infectious agents such as herpes zoster, cytomegalovirus, *Borrellia burgdorferi* or by infiltrative diseases such as sarcoidosis or lymphoma. [21]

Given the differential growth rates between the vertebral column and spinal cord, there is a discrepancy in spinal cord segments compared with vertebral segments with respect to the pelvis. The spinal cord terminates between the L1 and L2 vertebral levels. Thus, the ventral and posterior lumbosacral roots travel significant distances intradurally before reaching their respective neural foraminae. These roots are collectively referred as *cauda equina*. As dorsal root ganglion is located within the neural foramen at each level, lesions affecting the *cauda equina* are preganglionic for sensory fibers with respect to the dorsal ganglion. Therefore, the sensory nerve action potentials will be unaffected in these processes. As such, normal sensory nerve conduction studies do not exclude sensory dysfunction as a cause of PFD. Nonetheless, nerve conduction studies should be performed as part of this evaluation.

Although *cauda equina* lesions are uncommon, a central prolapse of L4-L5 and L5-S1 intervertebral discs is the most common cause. Other possible causes in order of descending frequency include anatomical disruptions (fractures and subluxation), spinal surgery, primary or metastatic tumors, spinal stenosis and spinal anesthesia [22].

The classical picture of complete acute *cauda equinopathy* includes bilateral sciatica, lower extremity weakness and sensory loss associated with bladder dysfunction. The most prominent features tend to be lower back pain, sacral sensory loss and urinary retention [23]. Sensory symptoms consist of numbness and tingling in the saddle region, the back of the thighs and legs and the soles of the feet. "Saddle region" sensory loss, usually implies dysfunction of the conus medullaris as well. Depending on the level involved, dorsiflexion (L5) or plantar flexion (S1) of the toes and feet may be affected.

Chronic *cauda equina* syndrome can present with a long history of chronic back pain, with or without sciatica, which may also be associated with slow progression to sensory loss and urinary symptoms [24]. Motor deficits strongly depend on the level of the injury. Lesions of the L5 root and below result in an inability to heel walk and perform dorsiflexion whereas inclusion of S1 root and roots below result in an inability to stand on the toes or to perform plantar flexion. Sensory loss, usually bilateral and asymmetric, typically indicates pathology affecting the sensory nerve roots. Pathology affecting the S2-S4 roots results in pelvic organ dysfunction without any impairment of lower extremity mobility.

With respect to the relationship between root damage and pelvic floor symptoms, Bindley's observations of the sacral root stimulation effect on the pelvic organ function are relevant. This author reported that stimulation of S3 had the greatest effect on detrusor pressure rise whereas the rectum responded equally to S2, S3 and S4 nerve root stimulation. Even with constant stimulation, the pelvic colon and rectum responded with waves of contraction that brought feces down into the rectum. S2 stimulation induced penile erection in men but without emission of semen. In some women, it was reported that sacral anterior root stimulation resulted in vaginal lubrication. [25]. Urinary retention is the most frequent symptom that indicates acute neurological dysfunction. While incontinence may be an initial symptom of cauda equina syndrome [CES], it tends to be more common in chronic conditions. Urgency and frequency were less commonly reported [26]. While fecal and flatus incontinence are very frequent in chronic lesions, constipation is the most common bowel symptom in acute neurological dysfunction in both genders [27]. Orgasmic dysfunction, which manifests as impaired genital sensation and erectile dysfunction, is the most common sexual complaint in men with CES [28]. Unfortunately, as cauda equina lesions are preganglionic for sensory fibers, no regrowth of axons into the spinal cord occurs. Therefore, sensory loss portends a poor prognosis. In women, diminished vaginal lubrication in response to psychogenic and local stimulation has been reported [29].

The lumbosacral plexus derives from the ventral primary rami of the twelfth thoracic through fourth sacral levels and is situated within the substance of the psoas major muscle. The lumbosacral plexus is the origin of the following nerves: the iliohypogastric nerve (T12-L1), the ilioinguinal nerve (L1), the genitofemoral nerve (L1-L2), the lateral femoral cutaneous nerve of the thigh (L2-L3), the femoral nerve (L2-L4), the obturator nerve (L2-L4), the superior gluteal nerve (L4-S1), the inferior gluteal nerve (L5-S2), the sciatic nerve (L4-S3), the posterior femoral cutaneous nerve (S1-S3) and the pudendal nerve (S1-S4) [30].
Lesions of the entire lumbosacral plexus are rare and tend to be incomplete. They result in paralysis or paresis of the entire lower extremity, with diminished or absent reflexes and sensory disturbance affecting the entire leg and perineal area. Most injuries to the lumbosacral plexus primarily involve the lumbar segments, sacral segments, or individual peripheral nerves.

Lesions of the sacral plexus are frequently incomplete and occur most commonly with neoplasms or surgical trauma. Lesions of the entire sacral plexus result in motor disturbances in the distribution of the superior gluteal, inferior gluteal, sciatic and pudendal nerves. Sensation may be lost in the distribution area of the pudendal nerve, sciatic nerve and in the distribution of the posterior femoral cutaneous nerve (posterior thigh and popliteal fossa). Difficulty with bladder or bowel control may also result from injury to the pudendal nerve.

During labor and delivery, the descending fetal head may compress the lumbosacral trunk [31]. Intrapartum maternal lumbosacral plexopathy presents with weakness of ankle dorsiflexion, eversion, and inversion, associated with sensory loss in the L5 dermatome [32]. It usually involves the upper plexus (L2–S1) with resultant obturator, femoral, or sciatic nerve palsies. Symptoms are usually unilateral and typically on the same side as the infant's brow during the descent. Urinary, anorectal, or sexual dysfunctions are rare and are due to autonomic involvement. Postpartum lumbosacral plexopathy may occur after vaginal delivery and may be limited to autonomic and perineal manifestations including urinary difficulty, anorectal impairment, and sexual dysfunction that involve only the S2-S4 nerve root distributions without limb sensory or motor signs [33].

Pudendal mononeuropathy. Pregnancy itself is a risk factor of neuropathy as it generates a continuous abnormal pressure on the weak area of the anterior perineum, which may result in damage to the pelvic muscles and the pudendal nerve. There is mounting scientific evidence that supports the association between vaginal childbirth and pudendal nerve injury. In 1994, Sultan recognized that the first delivery is the most deleterious to the integrity of the pelvic floor neural network [34]. Allen et al., in a prospective study published in 1990, found that vaginal delivery causes partial denervation of the pelvic floor, with subsequent re-innervation, in most women having their first child [35]. Pudendal nerve compression is the main mechanism of pelvic floor nerve damage in childbirth. Alcock's canal has been hypothesized as the potential site of compression by the fetal head during the second stage of labor.

Pudendal neuropathy would be the result of combination of direct compression injury of the pelvis and traction injury during elongation of the birth canal. Additionally, isolated lesions of pudendal nerve terminal rami and injury of pudendal branches of the sacral plexus are possible during labor [36]. Epidural anesthesia has been considered by some authors to be a risk factor for PFD associated with childbirth [37]. However, other authors reported found no such association [38].

In addition to pregnancy and childbirth, there are other causes of pudendal neuropathy. Compression of the pudendal nerve in Alcock's canal was first described by Amarenco in cyclists [39]. Pudendal neuropathy has also been described in patients having aberrant development and subsequent malpositioning of the ischial spine that appear to be associated with athletic activities during their youth [40]. Perineal descent, chronic straining and pelvic organ prolapse may also induce pudendal nerve damage. Other authors report pudendal nerve injury after pelvic floor surgery involving vaginal dissection [41], after TOT (transobturator tape) surgery for stress urinary incontinence [42] and in a few cases of classical Labat's posterior sciatic nerve block [43].

Pudendal neuralgia (PN) is defined as an idiopathic chronic pain syndrome in the perineal area that occurs in the absence of causative organic diseases [44]. Secondary causes of pudendal neuralgia include entrapment and injury to the pudendal nerve in the Alcock´s canal, herpetic neuropathy, stretch neuropathy, and post-radiotherapy neuropathy [45].

Some clinical characteristics of pudendal neuralgia have been proposed as diagnostic criteria [46]. The pain should be limited to the innervation territory of the pudendal nerve and is predominantly experienced while sitting; in accordance with the nerve compression etiology hypothesis. In long-standing pudendal neuralgia, the pain may become continuous, but it should be exacerbated while sitting. Less commonly reported symptoms mat include sensation of a rectal foreign body and the worsening of pain during defecation. Other possible symptoms include burning, numbness, increased sensitivity, electric shock, knife-like or aching pain, feeling of a lump or foreign body in the vagina, twisting or pinching, abnormal temperature sensations, hot poker sensation, straining or burning when urinating, painful intercourse, and sexual dysfunction. Notably, it may also present as a persistent genital arousal disorder (genital arousal without desire) or the opposite problem - loss of sensation. PN pain rarely awakens the patient at night. No objective sensory impairment should be found on clinical examination, even in the presence of paresthesias. Anesthetic infiltration of the pudendal nerve often relieves the pain. [46].

The pudendal nerve provides motor innervation to external anal sphincter and to the superficial and deep perineal muscles, including the external urethral sphincter and parts of the *levator ani* muscle. Therefore, PFD associated with pudendal neuropathy may include urinary and fecal incontinence as well as ejaculatory disorders. Lesions affecting the autonomic fibers in the pudendal nerve may result in erectile and bladder dysfunction, along with impaired sensation in distal urethra.

Pelvic Nerve injury. Pelvic surgery, direct injury and trauma may result in autonomic dysfunction. Bladder, bowel and sexual dysfunction are common following radical surgery for malignances arising from the cervix, bladder, prostate and rectum. The pelvic plexus, superior hypogastric plexus, hypogastric nerves or pelvic splanchnic nerves may be damaged depending on the surgical site and the extent of the surgery. Radiotherapy may have an additional effect on pelvic nerve damage. Nerve-sparing surgical techniques aim to minimize damage to autonomic function and may be associated with fewer pelvic floor disorders.

Urinary and sexual dysfunction is common following radical hysterectomy in patients with cervical cancer. The most frequent symptom is transient bladder atony [47]. Surgical complications may also include incontinence, pelvic floor weakness, fistula formation and bladder injury. Adjuvant pelvic irradiation may result in additional nerve and bladder wall damage that manifests as a smaller bladder capacity and detrusor overactivity. Negative impacts on sexual function include decreased sexual interest, diminished vaginal lubrication, narrow/short vagina, labial hypesthesia, dyspareunia and sexual dissatisfaction [48]. Techniques for nerve-sparing radical hysterectomy have evolved that aim to minimize damage to autonomic nerves to minimize post-operative bladder, bowel and sexual dysfunction.

Major pelvic urological surgery comprises radical prostatectomy and radical cystectomy in the male patient and radical cystectomy in the female. Nerve-sparing techniques are available both for prostatectomy and for male and female radical cystectomy in order to avoid post-surgical sexual dysfunction. Erectile dysfunction, decreased orgasm, insufficient lubrication, lack of sexual desire, and dyspareunia are prevalent problems after radical cystectomy [49]. Damage to the cavernosal nerves may result in erectile dysfunction following radical prostatectomy. Injury to the pelvic nerve supply to the internal sphincter may cause some cases of postsurgical incontinence.

Urogenital dysfunction is a common problem after abdominoperineal resection for rectal cancer treatment. More than half of patients experience deterioration in sexual function, consisting of ejaculatory problems and impotence in men and vaginal dryness and dyspareunia in women. Urinary dysfunction occurs in one-third of patients treated for rectal cancer. Surgically related nerve damage is the main cause of urinary dysfunction. In contrast, radiotherapy appears to contribute the development of sexual dysfunction without affecting urinary function [50, 51].

Polyneuropathy and multiple mononeuropathies are generalized processes affecting the peripheral nerves. It is important to determine the topographical pattern, whether the process is predominantly motor, sensory or autonomic, the time course (acute, subacute or chronic) and whether the pathological process is a primary myelinopathy or axonopathy.

The pathophysiology of pelvic floor dysfunction in the context of a generalized peripheral nerve disease includes alteration of the autonomic and somatic pathways. This results in alterations in pelvic neural control and an increased susceptibility of individual nerves to focal pathology such as compression, traction and ischemia.

Diabetes mellitus is the most common cause of peripheral neuropathy in the developed world. The common topographic pattern is that of a distal symmetrical axonal neuropathy. It commonly manifests as a painful sensory neuropathy due to damage of the thinly myelinated A-delta fibers as well as the unmyelinated C fibers. Small fiber symptoms include burning, sharp stabbing pain and a sensation of walking on pebbles. Involvement of the larger, thickly myelinated Aß-fibers results in numbness, "pins and needles" and a sensation of tightness.

Erectile dysfunction in diabetic men is very frequent with an estimated prevalence ranging between 9-95% [52]. It may be due to vessel arteriosclerosis, autonomic neuropathy, anxiety, depression and some medications. Diabetic men tend not to respond as well to phosphodiesterase inhibitors. In addition to ED, retrograde ejaculation may occur due to sympathetic denervation of the internal urethral sphincter. Impaired testicular pain sensation is considered to be a sign of autonomic neuropathy [21].

A study of sexual function in women reported that sexual function scores concerning the sexual drive, arousal, vaginal lubrication, orgasm and overall satisfaction domains were all lower in diabetic women. This study also reported that age but not body mass index, glycemic control, education or employment status were also determinants of function [53].

Bladder and bowel dysfunction in diabetic persons is multifactorial. The onset of bladder dysfunction in diabetes is usually insidious. It classically manifests as a loss of sensation of bladder filling, decreased frequency of voiding, slowing of urinary stream, and difficulty in voiding with incomplete emptying that often culminates in chronic retention [21]. The presence of a peripheral neuropathy and elevated glycosylated hemoglobin levels are risk factors for voiding dysfunction [54]. With respect to bowel dysfunction, it was reported that increased thresholds of conscious rectal sensation in incontinent patients with diabetes mellitus may contribute to fecal incontinence by impairing the recognition of impending defecation [55].

Alcoholic Neuropathy. Chronic consumption of alcohol, especially to the exclusion of adequate nutritional intake, may induce a generalized axonal sensorimotor axonal polyneuropathy. In some patients, it may have an acute or subacute onset resembling the Guillain-Barre Syndrome. While autonomic dysfunction is common, it is usually often asymptomatic such that it is not routinely assessed. Ravaglia reported that among patients with autonomic symptoms (55%), erectile dysfunction is the most common symptom. Its presence indicates a higher degree of parasympathetic nervous system dysfunction [56].

Guillain-Barré Syndrome is an acute, symmetrical, ascending polyradiculoneuropathy with predominantly motor symptoms. Although autonomic dysfunction is present in about 2/3 of patients, PFD has not been systematically evaluated. Notably, bladder dysfunction has been proposed as an exclusionary criterion so that it may be distinguished from an acute myelopathy. Nonetheless, Sakakibara reported the presence of urinary dysfunction in 27.7% of patients with the Guillain-Barre Syndrome, 9.2% of whom presented with urinary retention [57]. Underactive detrusor, overactive detrusor, and to a lesser extent, hyperactive sphincter were the major urodynamic abnormalities. The underlying mechanisms of urinary dysfunction appear to involve both hypo and hyperactive lumbosacral nerves. Male erectile dysfunction may also occur as part of autonomic dysfunction in GBS, but this has not been prospectively evaluated.

Chronic inflammatory polyneuropathy (CIDP). Although autonomic dysfunction is uncommon in CIDP, voiding difficulty, urinary urgency and evidence of both bladder evacuation and storage disorders have been described. Micturition symptoms were more frequently found in cases presenting with severe weakness [58].

Acute idiopathic autonomic neuropathy is a condition characterized by acute onset of autonomic dysfunction. This likely results from dysfunction of the pre- and postganglionic autonomic fibers. Urinary retention and voiding difficulty are common such that cystometry often demonstrates detrusor areflexia. ED and constipation are common as well [59].

Autoimmune autonomic ganglionopathy is an acquired neurological disorder characterized by diffuse autonomic failure. The clinical manifestations reflect impairment in sympathetic function (orthostatic hypotension, anhidrosis), parasympathetic function (reduced lacrimation, salivation and pupil constriction) and enteric function (ileus, abdominal colic, diarrhea, and constipation [60]. Ganglionic acetylcholine receptor antibodies, which impair synaptic transmission in autonomic ganglia, are found in many patients.

Pure autonomic failure is a degenerative postganglionic autonomic disorder in which nocturia and voiding dysfunction are frequent. Bladder emptying is often affected. ED and constipation are also common [21].

HIV Neuropathy. PFD in patients with AIDS may be related both to any of the neurological manifestations of AIDS including encephalitis, meningitis, cerebral toxoplasmosis, myelitis, polyradiculoneuritis, tumors, HIV related peripheral neuropathy or neuropathy related to antiretroviral therapy [61]. Urge incontinence and detrusor external sphincter dyssynergia may occur in the context of HIV related vacuolar myelopathy.

Familial amyloid polyneuropathies (FAPs) form a group of multisystem disorders transmitted as an autosomal dominant trait. Nerve pathology results from amyloid deposition. The earliest manifestations are related to the preferential involvement of small-diameter sensory and autonomic nerves. The symptomatology and clinical course can be highly variable. The most common presentation is that of a distal, symmetric length-dependent polyneuropathy that starts in the feet with loss of temperature and pain sensation along with autonomic dysfunction. Autonomic neuropathy occurs in most people with early-onset FAP. The cardiovascular, gastrointestinal, and genitourinary systems are commonly affected in these patients. In men, erectile dysfunction is an early feature that may precede the sensory symptoms of FAP neuropathy. Urinary symptoms including dysuria and urinary retention occur later in the course of this illness [62].

PFD may also occur with other hereditary polyneuropathies such as familial dysautonomia, Charcot-Marie-Tooth disease and the porphyrias.

Diagnosis

A pelvic floor disorder should be viewed as a symptom rather than as a diagnosis. Therefore, the initial course of action is to establish the underlying cause. This may require ancillary testing or a referral to a specialist.

Nonetheless, there are certain specific data that should be recorded in each patient presenting with PFD. This data set should include at least five domains: the subject's observations, quantification of symptoms; the clinician's observations (anatomic and functional), quality of life and socioeconomic measures [63].

The importance of a comprehensive history cannot be overemphasized. It must include questions about congenital abnormalities, cardiovascular, endocrine and neurological diseases, psychological and psychiatric disturbances, local genital or pelvic alterations, prior trauma, relevant surgery or radiation history and general health. In women, the general history must also include assessment of menstrual history, obstetric history and hormonal status. Detailed questions regarding LUTD, incontinence, bowel and sexual function are relevant. As it is important to define the cause of PFD, a comprehensive and compassionate inquiry is required in order to obtain accurate information. Formal questionnaires may be used to obtain standardized information. These include the International Index of Erectile Function (IIEF) [64], the Female Sexual Function Index (FSFI) [65], the Incontinence Impact Questionnaire, the Urogenital Distress Inventory [66] and the American Urological Association symptom index for benign prostatic hyperplasia [67]. Voiding and Bowel Diaries are simple and useful for initial assessment as they provide information regarding voiding and bowel patterns.

Objective evaluation of pelvic floor functioning should be performed in order to determine their quality. Various techniques such as monitoring nocturnal penile erection and pad tests may be used in daily practice in order to obtain an objective quantification of symptoms. However, their utility has not been evaluated within the context of evidence based medicine.

Physical examination techniques must be focused on all organ systems that may be implicated in PFD. An initial assessment includes general observation for mobility, cognitive status, peripheral edema and body habitus. A discussion of a complete urogynecological examination is beyond the scope of this chapter. However, a focused neurological examination might be performed if nervous system involvement is suspected. In these patients, the basic physical examination of the nervous system should be supplemented to include sensory evaluations of the lower abdomen, perineum and lower extremities. Reflex tests include the cremasteric reflex in men, the anal wink and the bulbocavernosus or clitoroanal reflex in women. In the lower extremities, the knee and ankle reflexes should be examined bilaterally. An adequate assessment of pelvic floor muscle function should include testing of the perianal and paravaginal muscles. This should include documentation of their initial resting tone, presence of contraction and lift of the pelvic floor, as well as their subsequent relaxation [5]. Other regions to be inspected include the lower back (for nevi and hypertrichosis) and the lower extremities for evidence of deformities or muscle atrophy.

Neurophysiological tests extend the neurological examination and assist clinicians in diagnosing neurological diseases or injuries that result in PFD. In general, neurophysiological tests are used to study afferent, efferent and reflex pathways, both in the somatic and autonomic nervous systems. Although the pelvic neuroanatomy imposes some restrictions to neurophysiological techniques, these can be helpful in detecting the presence of an underlying polyneuropathy in the genesis of different types of PFD.

Needle electromyography (EMG) is performed by means of surface, concentric needle or fine wire electrodes that record the bioelectrical activity from muscle in order to detect diseases of the muscle fibers themselves or changes in their innervation. Neurogenic changes may be due to injury at any level along the peripheral motor pathway supplying pelvic floor muscles from the alpha motor neuron to the terminal rami of the peripheral motor nerves. In pelvic floor muscles, only neurogenic changes are routinely evaluated. The concentric needle electrode consists of a central insulated platinum wire inserted through a steel cannula and the tip ground to provide an elliptical recording area that can detect spike or other muscle electrical activity from approximately 20 muscle fibers [68].

The use of concentric needle electrodes a permits the investigation of insertional and spontaneous activity, motor unit action potential (MUAP) morphology as well as recruitment and interference patterns. MUAP measurements should include quantitative analysis of amplitude, duration, as well as the number of phases and turns. Electrode repositioning allows a more accurate examination. Although almost all pelvic floor muscles may be examined, the selection of muscles for examination is determined by their accessibility and the amount of information to be gained. EMG interpretation of pelvic floor muscles (particularly of the sphincters) is difficult, given the morphology of pelvic muscle MUAPs and the inherent difficulty for many patients to achieve complete relaxation. The bulbocavernosus muscle is useful because it is easily accessible, has no tonic activity at rest and can be easily activated [69]. However, once an abnormality is identified, additional studies are required. These additional studies should evaluate both pudendal- and non-pudendal innervated muscles in order to determine the extent of involvement.

Alternative strategies may be appropriate for the selection of muscles in other clinical settings. For example, the external anal sphincter is often selected for the assessment of sphincter involvement in atypical Parkinsonism [5]. The external urethral sphincter might also be included in the evaluation of urinary retention in a woman with possible Fowler's syndrome; a cause of urinary retention in young women [70].

Gross changes of denervation and reinnervation may be observed following conus medullaris, cauda equina or peripheral motor nerve lesions. Definitive neurogenic changes may be observed in anal and urethral sphincters in patients with multiple system atrophy (MSA); this feature being helpful in distinguishing MSA from Parkinson disease and progressive supranuclear palsy [71]. In contrast, EMG is normal in patients with acute idiopathic autonomic neuropathy [58].

Pelvic floor denervation is implicated in the pathophysiology of genitourinary prolapse and genuine stress incontinence [72]. Numerous complex repetitive discharges have been described in the external urethral sphincter of patients with idiopathic urinary retention [73]. A neurogenic EMG pattern in the external anal sphincter probably reflects involvement of the inferior rectal branch or of an intrasphincteric branch of the pudendal nerve.

Surface EMG is useful for monitoring the presence or absence of contraction and may provide kinesiological data but its specificity is limited by volume conduction. Kinesiological EMG is used to assess patterns of individual muscle activity/inactivity during defined maneuvers commonly performed during urodynamic exploration. Although little is known about the complex activity patterns of pelvic floor muscles, it is assumed that they function as one coordinated muscle. In normal persons, voiding is characterized by cessation of EMG activity in the urethral sphincters followed by detrusor contraction. Defecation requires increased rectal pressure coordinated with relaxation of the anal sphincter and pelvic floor muscles. Dyssynergia is described on the basis of the relationship between urethral sphincter and detrusor contraction and/or on the basis of paradoxical contraction of the puborectalis muscle during the defecation.

Nerve conduction studies (NCS) are used to distinguish between primary myelinopathies and primary axonopathies. They are performed according to Falck et al. [74] or Trojaborg [75], by means of surface or needle monopolar electrodes. Motor nerve conduction studies can identify features of demyelination and axon loss, defects of neuromuscular junction transmission, and they can reflect severe muscle fiber loss [76]. Motor nerve fibers are studied by applying electrical stimuli to the motor nerve and recording the compound muscle action potential (CMAP) from one or more muscles supplied by the nerve. Important measurements include the latency of the CMAP and the motor nerve conduction velocity (MNCV). The CMAP represents a summation in the volume conduction of all the individual muscle fiber action potentials activated by the stimulus and within the territory of the active recording electrode [76]. Sensory nerve conduction studies (SNCS) provide useful and direct information of the population and function of the sensory axons and their involvement in disease processes. Electrophysiological studies of sensory fibers differ from motor fibers in that the sensory action potential (SNAP) is recorded directly from the nerve and has a much smaller amplitude than its motor counterpart, the CMAP. The parameters of NCS that provide meaningful information in clinical evaluation include sensory conduction velocity (SNCV), the amplitude, and the latency of SNAP. The sensory fibers that contribute to the SNAP have a diameter greater than 7–8 mm [77]. The sensory nerves also contain small myelinated and unmyelinated fibers [78], but they are not assessed with conventional NCS. Physiological factors such as age, height and cutaneous temperature may also influence NCS results. Nonetheless, NCS may help detect pathology such as loss of large diameter fibers, abnormalities in myelin function or axon loss.

The distal motor latency of the pudendal nerve can be measured by recording, with a concentric needle electrode, responses from the bulbocavernosus or the external anal sphincter muscles after electrical stimulation of the nerve at the ischial spine. The most commonly used technique relies on the St Mark's stimulator. It consists of a bipolar stimulating electrode on the tip of the gloved finger inserted into the rectum or vagina, and a recording electrode pair placed proximally on the base of the finger [79]. Stimulation is applied close to the ischial spine. Because these studies are highly technique dependent, their validity in the assessment of pudendal nerve function is controversial. The same statement is applicable to sensory nerve conduction studies of the dorsal nerve of the penis.

In summary, given the unique anatomy of the pelvic floor, the usefulness of pelvic nerve conduction studies is limited. However, clinical neurophysiology studies of the lower extremities are often helpful in this context.

Somatosensory Evoked Potentials (SSEPs) are used to investigate conduction in the large fiber sensory pathways from the peripheral site of stimulation to the somatosensory cortex. They are recorded from surface electrodes placed over the scalp, spine, and peripheral nerves along the anatomical course of the large fiber sensory pathways. These electrical potentials are generated after the activation of large diameter afferent myelinated nerve fibers in a mixed peripheral nerve. SSEPs have been used in the assessment of sensory pathways in the brain, brain stem, spinal cord, and peripheral nerves [80].

SSEPs evoked by tibial nerve stimulation evaluate lumbosacral afferent pathways. Responses are elicited by electrical stimulation of the tibial nerve at the ankle. The sequence of negative and positive potentials recorded from the knee, low back and scalp can be recognized by their distribution time course and their relation with other peaks. Responses from posterior tibial or sciatic nerves (N8) are recorded by electrodes placed at popliteal fossa. The N20, recorded at T10-L2 level, represents the post-synaptic response in the gray matter of the lumbosacral spinal cord. The N30 wave, recorded at the C2 level, is likely generated at the cervical-medullary junction. The P40, which is the major positive cortical peak registered at scalp, is generated in the post-central somatosensory cortex. The latency from stimulus to cortical response (P40) is the total conduction time, the latency to the N20 wave is the peripheral nerve conduction time and N20 to P40 interpeak latency represents the central conduction time, which has two components. The intraspinal conduction time is calculated by subtracting N20 from N30 whereas the intracranial conduction time is calculated by subtracting N30 from P40 [81].

Pudendal somatosensory evoked potentials are elicited with stimulation of the dorsal nerve of the penis/clitoris and manifest a major positive peak (P40) generated from the somatosensory cortex and registered at scalp.

SSEP are used to evaluate both the peripheral and central nervous systems. SSEP abnormalities may demonstrate involvement of the large fiber sensory pathways, may help localize the lesion within these large fiber sensory pathways and may help render a prognosis. Nonetheless, SSEP abnormalities do not indicate a specific diagnosis. To the contrary, large fiber sensory pathology cannot be excluded even when the SSEP findings are normal [82].

The combination of pudendal and tibial evoked potentials is of value for topographical evaluation of somatosensory pathways. Cerebral SSEPs during penile/clitoral stimulation may be useful for intraoperative monitoring and have been used to study the mechanism of sacral neuromodulation [83]. It has been suggested that tibial SSEPs might have a role in the prognosis and efficacy of tibial neuromodulation [84].

Sacral reflexes are the contraction of pelvic floor muscles in response to stimulation of the perineum, urethra/bladder, or anus. The afferent pathways of the reflex may be somatic, sympathetic, or parasympathetic, depending on the site of stimulation. However, the efferent pathway is somatic and is usually monitored in muscles innervated by the pudendal nerve [5].

The bulbocavernosus reflex (BCR) has both afferent and efferent limbs in the pudendal nerve and is centrally integrated at S2-S4 spinal cord levels. It is a complex response, often forming two components. The first component (R1), generally accepted as the true BCR, is stable and does not habituate. The R1 is thought to be an oligosynaptic reflex response [85]. The R2 has a longer latency and higher thresholds in normal persons. The BCR is elicited in men by stimulating the dorsal nerve of the penis with electrical pulses on the shaft of the penis and recorded responses from the left and right bulbocavernosus muscles with concentric needle electrodes according to Ertekin's method [86]. Similar studies may be performed in women by having the subject stimulated her own clitoris with a pediatric stimulator. Testing of the sacral reflexes assesses the integrity of the sacral spinal cord at S2 to S4 as well as the associated afferent and efferent pathways. With a complete lesion, the reflex is absent. An incomplete lesion may be associated with a prolonged latency and a diminished or absent response. Markedly prolonged latencies have been documented in patients with hereditary motor and sensory dysmyelinating neuropathies, (e.g. HMSN-I) [87].

The previously discussed neurophysiological methods assess myelinated fibers but not unmyelinated C and thin myelinated A-delta fibers, which encompass thermal and nociceptive sensation and as well as autonomic functions. Specific diagnostic tests for small fiber neuropathy are skin biopsy, including a count of the intra-epidermal small nerve fibers that cross the basal membrane, quantitative sensory tests and autonomic testing. Direct methods for evaluating the autonomic nerves innervating the pelvic viscera are not available. Nonetheless, specific autonomic tests as thermoregulatory sweat test, quantitative sudomotor axon reflex testing, sympathetic skin response testing and quantitative sensory testing are all capable of assessing autonomic function.

Sympathetic Skin Response (SSR) is generated in the deeper layers of the skin by a reflex, sympathetically mediated activation of sweat glands. It is a multisynaptic reflex that requires integrity of hypothalamic, brainstem and spinal circuits. The efferent limb of the reflex arc involves sympathetic neurons at intermediolateral cell column of the spinal cord. Preganglionic fibers for upper extremity arise from spinal cord at T5-7 segments whereas those for pelvic floor and lower extremity arise at T10-12 spinal levels. Postganglionic C fibers have sudomotor function such that their activation induces a decrement in electrical resistance of skin by increasing sweat gland secretion [88, 89]. Evaluation of the SSR must be performed under tightly controlled circumstances. [88]. In order to avoid habituation, randomized electrical stimuli are applied over a median nerve. Responses are recorded on the skin of the contralateral palm and sole as well as over the dorsum of the penis [90]. An absent response is considered pathological. While these tests have some degree of specificity, they tend to be insensitive.

Penile sympathetic skin responses are useful and may provide the only evidence for autonomic dysfunction in men with ED [91, 92]. A correlation has been demonstrated between SSR blocking in the foot and bladder neck dyssynergia in spinal cord injury [93]. One study reported that the use of perineal SSR in addition to that of the hand and foot was of diagnostic value for evaluating neurogenic bladder neck incompetence in spinal cord injured patients [94].

Quantitative Sensory Testing (QST) is used to evaluate small fiber function. Non-nociceptive cool stimuli are mediated by A-delta small myelinated fibers. Warm stimuli and nociceptive stimuli are mediated by C fibers. A-delta afferent fibers are evaluated using the cold perception test (CDT) whereas afferent C-fiber function is evaluated with heat thresholds. There are two methods to assess thermal thresholds; limits and levels. In the method of limits, the thermal stimulator (thermode) is applied to the skin and the temperature of the thermode increases until the subject presses a button indication that a warm sensation has been detected. This is the appearance threshold that can be influenced by reaction time. Variations of this algorithm have been described. Other algorithms utilizing the method of limits include the linear ramp algorithm with null stimuli and the Bekesy algorithm with null stimuli [95]. The method of levels overcomes the disadvantage of the inclusion of reaction time using predetermined levels of stimulus intensity and duration. QST is a psychophysical approach that requires an alert and cooperative patient. Therefore, this method cannot distinguish between feigned and true loss of sensation [96]. Age, gender, and site of stimulation influence thresholds results and must be incorporated into the normative data. Types of equipment, methodology, and testing algorithms may alter the results significantly with adverse effects on reproducibility [97]. As QST evaluates the integrity of the entire sensory neuraxis, from receptor to cortex, it is not a specific assessment of peripheral nerve function. Restated, dysfunction of the peripheral nerves or the central nervous system may give rise to abnormal results.

Besides its usefulness in the diagnosis of small fiber neuropathy, QST may have a role in the study of patients with PFD. Yarnitsky et al. reported that penile thermal thresholds are repeatable and may be used as a valid diagnostic tool to assess somatic small fiber function in patients with lower urinary tract disorders, [98]. Penile thermal thresholds have also been studied in premature ejaculation [99], in erectile dysfunction [100], and in patients who have undergone surgery for circumcision [101], correction of penile curvature [102] and transurethral resection of the prostate [103].

Urodynamic Tests

In patients with neurologic impairment and lower urinary tract symptoms, urodynamic testing may help to characterize the function of the bladder, the urethra, the pelvic floor muscles, and their coordination [104].

Uroflowmetry is a simple, noninvasive study of bladder emptying that measures the volume of urine released, the speed at which it is released, the duration of urinary release and the postvoid residual volume. Key measures include maximum and mean flow rates, voided volume, and flow time. The results are displayed as a graph. These studies are not specific but help document the typical flow pattern such that they provide a reasonable screen of voiding function when normal. Patients with neurologic impairment may have reduced flow either due to impaired detrusor contractility or because of outlet obstruction such as detrusor sphincter dyssynergia [5].

Cystometry is the measurement of the intravesical pressure during filling and/or emptying of the bladder. Additional information is provided by simultaneous recording of pelvic floor muscle contraction-relaxation patterns using surface or needle electrodes. Provocative measures such as coughing, straining or standing may be utilized to reproduce symptoms. Measures include the bladder volume at the first sensation of filling, normal desire to void, strong desire to void, the volume when uninhibited detrusor contractions first appear and if they are detected by the patient. Additional measures include the compliance and capacity of the bladder as well as whether or not incontinence occurs [5].

Stress urinary incontinence is diagnosed when urinary incontinence occurs with increased abdominal pressure in the absence of a detrusor contraction. In these cases, the Valsalva leak point pressure should be determined. The minimum pressure elevation sufficient to induce leakage is also a measure of continence. In contrast, if there is uninhibited detrusor activity present, the detrusor leak point pressure should be determined and the minimum detrusor pressure sufficient to induce leakage will be a measure of storage pressure in the urinary tract. In the absence of increased abdominal pressure or a detrusor contraction, leakage occurs when passive vesicular pressure exceeds outlet resistance.

Pressure Flow Studies are the simultaneous recording of detrusor pressure and urine flow during voiding. The addition of kinesiologic assessment of the pelvic floor with monitoring of EMG activity enhances interpretation, particularly in the presence of obstructive flow patterns [105]. Measures include the voided volume, maximum flow rate, and detrusor pressure at maximum flow. Determination of post-void residual volume, which helps to calculate the cystometric capacity, is especially helpful in neurological disease [104].

Patients with lower motor neuron dysfunction may also have impaired sensation with an elevated capacity and high compliance. The detrusor muscle may be underactive or acontractile such that there may be associated stress and/or "*overflow*" incontinence with an elevated residual [5, 106]. Patients with upper motor neuron dysfunction may also have impaired sensation but the capacity is often low such that compliance may be reduced. In such instances, neurogenic detrusor overactivity with incontinence is usually observed. The residual volume may be elevated from detrusor sphincter dyssynergia [107].

Functional testing of gastrointestinal tract may also provide information in patients with pelvic floor disorders. These studies have their own specific indications and methodology. However, a discussion of these studies is beyond the scope of this chapter.

Management of Peripheral Neuropathy in Pelvic Floor Dysfunction

Support and treatment of PFD include pharmacological, non-pharmacological and surgical approaches. In a patient with neurological disease, PFD is not likely to be an isolated issue. Therefore, optimal treatments approaches require an appropriate individualized assessment of pelvic organ dysfunction and neurological status. Treatment must also be appropriate for the patient's disability and cognitive functioning.

Non-pharmacological methods: The first-line management of neurogenic PFD is usually supportive and consists of non-pharmacological conservative measures. Non-pharmacological treatments may include education about normal bladder and bowel function as well as lifestyle modifications. These include timed or prompted urination and fluid management along with well established routines of regular bowel evacuation. Other interventions may include dietary manipulation, pelvic floor muscle training and peripheral neuromodulation by means of posterior tibial nerve stimulation.

Muscle training methods range from Kegel exercises to therapeutic electrical stimulation or biofeedback. Such treatments are directed at improving muscle function with respect to strength, endurance, coordination, and function. However, pelvic floor strengthening exercises should be avoided in interstitial cystitis/bladder pain syndrome [108].

Biofeedback can be used to teach patients to sustain, strengthen, direct, or eliminate a body action or reaction. Commonly used biofeedback techniques include digital (tactile), verbal, visual, electromyographic (visual or auditory), and manometric (simple or computerized) methods as well as vaginal retention sensation, (e.g. as provided by weighted vaginal cones) [109].

The aim of electrical stimulation within the pelvic floor region is to induce skeletal muscle training, remodel smooth muscle and connective tissues and to modulate bladder, bowel, or sexual function. It is indicated to control pelvic pain, to facilitate voiding, to restore continence, to control continence/defecation/constipation and to improve sexual function. [110]

Fluid management recommendations must be individualized in each case. By means of dietary manipulation, patients with reflex bowel function are encouraged to aim for a soft-formed stool consistency while those with flaccid bowel function the objective are should aim for firmer stools in order to avoid fecal incontinence.

Percutaneous tibial nerve stimulation is useful as a treatment for symptoms of urinary urgency, urinary frequency and urge incontinence in overactive bladder and interstitial cystitis [111]. It has also been used to treat fecal incontinence with good results. [112, 113]

Intermittent catheterization, as first suggested by Lapides, is well-tolerated for the management of neurogenic and non-neurogenic voiding dysfunction [114]. Indwelling catheterization should be recommended to patients who are unable or unwilling to self-catheterize or when containment devices are not suitable. Complications of indwelling catheters include infections, bladder spasms and urine leakage.

Other conservative methods that may be potentially useful in bowel dysfunction include abdominal massage, digital rectal stimulation, digital evacuation of feces, enemas, laxatives, antidiarrheal agents and transanal irrigation.

Medical therapy: Pharmacological approaches to neurogenic bladder dysfunction focus on controlling detrusor overactivity without interfering with bladder emptying. Systematic reviews and large meta-analyses of the most used antimuscharinic drugs have shown that these drugs provide a significant clinical benefit in the treatment of overactive bladder [115,116,117]. Intravesical injections of botulinum toxin may be an alternative therapy that may be considered in antimuscarinic resistant patients [118]. Injection of botulinum neurotoxin A in the urethral striated sphincter appears to be an effective therapy for the treatment of incomplete voiding after spinal cord injury.[119]

Oral phosphodiesterase 5 (PDE5) inhibitors are the first-line therapy in patients suffering from neurogenic ED. In certain cases, vacuum constriction devices may be considered as a first-line alternative. Second-line treatments include intracavernosal injections of alprostadil, a synthetic preparation of prostaglandin E1. Many neurological diseases cause or exacerbate ED. Men with an underlying neurological disorder frequently fail to respond to PDE5 inhibitors and other medical treatments. Female sexual dysfunction is a common problem in patients with neurological illnesses. At present, few effective treatments exist. Surgical treatments may be considered when non-pharmacological and pharmacological methods prove inadequate or intolerable. For men, this would include penile implants.

For bladder dysfunction, there are several different procedures which can be considered including sacral neurostimulation, reconstructive surgery, bladder outlet obstruction management and the treatment of stress urinary incontinence. Surgery for neurogenic bladder disorders is often performed in young people with a normal life expectancy such that the surgical benefits will be longstanding. As such, these surgical procedures not commonly performed in older patients or those with progressive neurological disorders.

Currently, the conservative approach remains the most common form of management in neurogenic bowel dysfunction. However, there are a small number of surgical interventions available to enhance the quality of life in these patients. Sacral neurostimulation may be used to treat both fecal incontinence and constipation. This procedure can only be performed when the sphincter and sacral nerves are intact, but it is not effective in complete spinal cord injury [120]

In conclusion, while many new treatments for PFD have been introduced in recent years, treatment failures still occur. For example, many men with ED reported a significant improvement in their quality of life with the introduction of phosphodiesterase type 5 (PDE5) inhibitors. However, there is a subset of patients that do not respond to these PDE5 inhibitors or in whom they are contraindicated [121, 122]. Similarly, a 29% reoperation rate for urinary incontinence and prolapse has been reported [123]. Treatment failures also occur with surgical procedures used to treat fecal disturbances or pudendal nerve entrapment. Failures have also occurred with sacral neurostimulation. A better understanding the pathophysiology of PFD will be essential to improve its management and for the development of new therapies.

References

[1] Sung VW, Hampton BS. Epidemiology of pelvic floor dysfunction. *Obstet Gynecol Clin North Am.* 2009; 36:421-43.

[2] Mayer EA, Naliboff BD, Craig AD. Neuroimaging of the brain-gut axis: from basic understanding to treatment of functional GI disorders. *Gastroenterology* 2006; 131:1925–42.

[3] Bannister LH, ed. Gray's anatomy. The anatomical basis of medicine and surgery (38th edition). New York: *Churchill Livingstone,* 1995.

[4] deGroat, W. C. and A. M. Booth Nervous Control of Urogenital System. *In The autonomic Nervous System.* Edited by C. A. Maggi. London. Harwood, 1993, vol 6, chap 13, p465-513

[5] Roberts MM. Neurophysiology in neurourology. *Muscle Nerve* 2008; 38:815–36.

[6] Nahm F, Freeman R. Sphincter electromyography and multiple system atrophy. *Muscle Nerve* 2003; 28:18-26.

[7] Swash M. The pelvic floor: functional concepts and neurocontrol. Pelvic Floor Disorders G.A. Santoro. A.P. Wieczorek C.I. Bartram Editors. *Springer Verlag* Italy 2010, p33-42.

[8] David B. Vodusek. Neural Control of Pelvic Floor Muscles. Pelvic Floor Re-education Principles and Practice. Kaven Baessler, Bernhard Schussler, Kathryn L. Burgio, Kate H.Moore, Peggy A. Norton, and Stuart L. Stanton (Eds). Second edition *Springer-Verlag* London 2008 p22-35

[9] Clare J. Fowler, Derek Griffiths, and William C. de Groat The neural control of micturition. *Nat Rev Neurosci.* 2008; 9: 453–66.

[10] Prateesh M. Trivedi and Derek J. Griffiths Neurological control of the bowel in health and disease In: Pelvic Organ Dysfunction in Neurological Disease Clinical Management and Rehabilitation Edited by Clare J. Fowler FRCP *Cambridge University Press* New York 2010. (Chapter 2)

[11] Clare J. Fowler, Jalesh N. Panicker and Rajesh B. C. Neurological control of sexual function in health and disease Kavia. Pelvic Organ Dysfunction in Neurological Disease. Clinical Management and Rehabilitation. Ed. Clare J. Fowler, Jalesh N. Panicker & Anton Emmanuel. *Cambridge University Press* 2010. Chapter 3

[12] Giuliano F. Neurophysiology of erection and ejaculation. *J Sex Med.* 2011 Oct; 8 Suppl 4:310-5.

[13] Jalesh N. Panicker, Vinay Kalsi and Marianne de Sèze. Approach and evaluation of neurogenic bladder dysfunction. Pelvic Organ Dysfunction in Neurological Disease. Clinical Management and Rehabilitation. Ed. Clare J. Fowler, Jalesh N. Panicker & Anton Emmanuel. *Cambridge University Press* 2010. Chapter 4

[14] Klaus Krogh. Approach and evaluation of neurogenic bowel dysfunction. Pelvic Organ Dysfunction in Neurological Disease. Clinical Management and Rehabilitation. ed. Clare J. Fowler, Jalesh N. Panicker & Anton Emmanuel. *Published by Cambridge University Press.* Cambridge 2010, (Chapter 8).

[15] Harris RD, Holtzman SR, Poppe AM. Clinical outcome in female patients with pelvic pain and normal pelvic US findings. Radiology 2000; 216: 440–43.

[16] Zermann DH, Ishigooka M, Doggweiler-Wiygul R, Schubert J, Schmidt RA. The male chronic pelvic pain syndrome. *World J Urol.* 2001; 19:173-9.

[17] NIH Consensus Conference. Impotence. NIH Consensus Development Panel on Impotence. *JAMA.* 1993 Jul 7; 270:83-90.

[18] Feldman HA, Goldstein I, Hatzichristou DG, Krane RJ, McKinlay JB. Impotence and its medical and psychosocial correlates: results of the Massachusetts Male Aging Study. *J Urol* 1994; 151: 54–61.

[19] Eardley I. Pathophysiology of erectile dysfunction. *Br J Diabetes Vasc Dis* 2002; 2:272-6

[20] Diseases of the Peripheral Nerves. In: Adams and Victor, Principles of Neurology by The McGraw-Hill Companies, Inc. Eighth Edition 2005 p111-1171

[21] Jalesh N. Panicker and Hadi Manji Neuromuscular disorders. Pelvic Organ Dysfunction in Neurological Disease. *Clinical Management and Rehabilitation.* Ed. Clare J. Fowler, Jalesh N. Panicker & Anton Emmanuel. Cambridge University Press 2010 Chapter 18

[22] Podnar S. Epidemiology of cauda equina and conus medularis lesions. *Muscle Nerve* 2007; 35:529–31.

[23] Jalloh I, Minhas P. Delays in the treatment of cauda equina syndrome due to its variable clinical features in patients presenting to the emergency department. *Emerg Med J* 2007; 24:33–4

[24] Lavy C, James A, Wilson-MacDonald J, Fairbank J. Cauda equina syndrome. *BMJ* 2009; 338: b936.

[25] Brindley GS. The Ferrier lecture, 1986. The actions of parasympathetic and sympathetic nerves in human micturition, erection and seminal emission, and their restoration in paraplegic patients by implanted electrical stimulators. *Proc R Soc Lond B Biol Sci.* 1988; 235(1279):111-20.

[26] Simon Podnar and Clare J. Fowler Pelvic organ dysfunction following cauda equina damage. Pelvic Organ Dysfunction in Neurological Disease. Clinical Management and Rehabilitation. Ed. Clare J. Fowler, Jalesh N. Panicker & Anton Emmanuel. *Cambridge University Press* 2010.

[27] Podnar S. Bowel dysfunction in patients with cauda equina lesions. *Eur J Neurol* 2006; 13:1112–7.

[28] Podnar S, Oblak C, Vodusek DB. Sexual function in men with cauda equina lesions: a clinical and electromyographic study. *J Neurol Neurosurg Psychiatry* 002; 73:715–20.

[29] Sipski ML, Alexander CJ, Rosen R. Sexual arousal and orgasm in women: effects of spinal cord injury. *Ann Neurol* 2001; 49:35–44.

[30] Brazis P, Masdeu J, Biller J. Cervical, Brachial and Lumbosacral Plexi Localization in Clinical Neurology, 5th Edition. *Lippincott Williams & Wilkins*. 2007. Chapter 3

[31] Feasby TE, Burton SR, Hahn AF. Obstetrical lumbosacral plexus injury. *Muscle Nerve* 1992; 15:937-40.

[32] Katirji B, Wilbourn AJ, Scarberry SL, et al. Intrapartum maternal lumbosacral plexopathy. *Muscle Nerve* 2002; 26:340-47

[33] Samer Sheikh Ismaela, Gerard Amarencoa, Béatrice Baylea, Jacques Kerdraon Postpartum lumbosacral plexopathy limited to autonomic and perineal manifestations: clinical and electrophysiological study of 19 patients. *J Neurol Neurosurg Psychiatry* 2000; 68:771-3

[34] Sultan AH, Kamm MA, Hudson CN. Pudendal nerve damage during labour: prospective study before and after childbirth. *BJOG* 1994;101:22–8

[35] Allen RE, Hosker GL, Smith AR, Warrell DW. Pelvic floor damage and childbirth: a neurophysiological study. *Br J Obstet Gynecol* 1990; 97:770–9.

[36] Gianfranco Minini, Silvia Zanelli, Patrizia Inselvini,Marcello Caria, Sara Grosso and Davide Quaresmini M. Mechanisms of Pelvic Floor Trauma During Vaginal Delivery. In Pelvic Floor Disorders. *Springer Verlag* Italy 2010.p137-142.

[37] Williams A et al. Risk scoring system for prediction of obstetric anal sphincter injury. *BJOG* 2005 112:1066–9

[38] Sartore A, Pregazzi R, Bortoli P, Grimaldi E, Ricci G, Guaschino S. Effects of epidural analgesia during labor on pelvic floor function after vaginal delivery. *Acta Obstet Gynecol Scand.* 200; 82:143-6.

[39] Amarenco G, Lanoe Y, Perrigot M, Goudal H. A new canal syndrome: compression of the pudendal nerve in Alcock's canal or perinal paralysis of cyclists]. *Presse Med.* 1987;16: 399.

[40] Antolak SJ Jr, Hough DM, Pawlina W, Spinner RJ Anatomical basis of chronic pelvic pain syndrome: the ischial spine and pudendal nerve entrapment. *Med Hypotheses.* 2002;59: 349-53

[41] Benson JT, McClellan .The effect of vaginal dissection on the pudendal nerve. *Obstet gynecol.* 1993; 82: 387-9

[42] Paulson JD, Baker J. De novo pudendal neuropathy after TOT-O surgery for stress urinary incontinence. *JSLS.* 2011; 15:326-30.

[43] Bondar A, Egan M, Jochum D, Amarenco G, Bouaziz H.. Case report: pudendal nerve injury after a sciatic nerve block by the posterior approach. *Anesth Analg.* 2010;111:573-5.

[44] Mazza L, Formento E, Fonda G. Anorectal and perineal pain: new pathophysiological hypothesis. *Tech Coloproctol* 2004; 8: 77-83

[45] Benson JT, Griffis K. Pudendal neuralgia, a severe pain syndrome. *Am J Obstet Gynecol* 2005; 192: 1663-8

[46] Labat JJ, Riant T, Robert R, Amarenco G, Lefaucheur JP, Rigaud J. Diagnostic criteria for pudendal neuralgia by pudendal nerve entrapment (Nantes criteria). *Neurourol Urodyn* 2008; 27: 306-10

[47] Chuang TY, Yu KJ, Penn IW, Chang YC, Lin PH, Tsai YA. Neurourological changes before and after radical hysterectomy in patients with cervical cancer. *Acta Obstet Gynecol Scand* 2003;82:954-9

[48] Pieterse QD, Maas CP, ter Kuile MM, et al. An observational longitudinal study to evaluate micturition, defecation, and sexual function after radical hysterectomy with pelvic lymphadenectomy for early-stage cervical cancer. *Int J Gynecol Cancer* 2006;16:1119–29

[49] Zippe CD, Raina R, Shah AD, et al. Female sexual dysfunction after radical cystectomy: a new outcome measure. *Urology* 2004; 63:1153-7.

[50] Lange MM, Marijnen CA, Maas CP, et al. Risk factors for sexual dysfunction after rectal cancer treatment. *Eur J Cancer.* 2009; 45:1578-88.

[51] Lange MM, van de Velde CJ.Urinary and sexual dysfunction after rectal cancer treatment. *Nat Rev Urol.* 2011; 8:51-7.

[52] Vinik A, Richardson D. Erectile dysfunction in diabetes. *Diabetes Rev* 1998; 6:16–33.

[53] Fatemi SS, Taghavi SM. Evaluation of sexual function in women with type 2 diabetes mellitus. *Diab Vasc Dis Res* 2009; 6:38–9.

[54] Fayyad AM, Hill SR, Jones G. Prevalence and risk factors for bothersome lower urinary tract symptoms in women with diabetes mellitus from hospital-based diabetes clinic. *Int Urogynecol J Pelvic Floor Dysfunct* 2009; 20:1339–44.

[55] Caruana BJ, Wald A, Hinds JP, Eidelman BH. Anorectal sensory and motor function in neurogenic fecal incontinence. Comparison between multiple sclerosis and diabetes mellitus. *Gastroenterology* 1991; 100:465–70.

[56] Ravaglia, S.; Marchione, E; Costa, A. et al.: "Erectile dysfunction as a sentinel symptom of cardiovascular autonomic neuropathy in heavy drinkers". *J. Peripher. Nerv. J Peripher Nerv Syst.* 2004; 9:209-14.

[57] Sakakibara R, Uchiyama T, Kuwabara S, Mori M, Ito T, Yamamoto T, Awa Y, Yamaguchi C, Yuki N, Vernino S, Kishi M, Shirai K. Prevalence and mechanism of bladder dysfunction in Guillain-Barré Syndrome. Neurourol. *Urodynam* 2009. 28:432-7.

[58] Sakakibara R, Hattori T, Kuwabara S, Yamanishi T, Yasuda K. Micturitional disturbance in patients with chronic inflammatory demyelinating polyneuropathy. *Neurology.* 1998 Apr; 50:1179-82

[59] Sakakibara R, Uchiyama T, Asahina M, et al. Micturition disturbance in acute idiopathic autonomic neuropathy. *J Neurol Neurosurg Psychiatry.* 2004;75:287-91

[60] Klein CM, Vernino S, Lennon VA, Sandroni P, Fealey RD, Benrud-Larson L, Sletten D, Low PA. The spectrum of autoimmune autonomic neuropathies. *Ann Neurol.* 2003; 53:752-8.

[61] McArthur JC, Brew BJ, Nath A. Neurological complications of HIV infection. *Lancet* Neurol. 2005; 4:543-55

[62] Planté-Bordeneuve V, Said G. Familial amyloid polyneuropathy. *Lancet Neurol.* 2011;10:1086-97.

[63] Weber AM, Abrams P, Brubaker L, Cundiff G, Davis G, Dmochowski RR et al. The Standardization of Terminology for Researchers in Female Pelvic Floor Disorders *Int Urogynecol J Pelvic Floor Dysfunct.* 2001; 12:178-86.

[64] Rosen RC, Riley A, Wagner G, et al. The international index of erectile function (IIEF): a international index of erectile function (IIEF): a multidimensional scale for assessment of erectile dysfunction. *Urology* 1997; 49:822–30.

[65] Rosen R, Brown C, Heiman J, et al. The Female Sexual Function Index (FSFI): a multidimensional self- report instrument for the assessment of female sexual function. *J Sex Marital Ther* 2000; 26:191–208.

[66] Uebersax JS, Wyman JF, Shumaker SA, McClish DK, Fantl JA. Short forms to assess life quality and symptom distress for urinary incontinence in women: the Incontinence Impact Questionnaire and the Urogenital Distress Inventory. Continence Program for Women Research Group. *Neurourol Urodyn* 1995; 14:131–9.

[67] The Measurement Committee of the American Urological Association. The American Urological Association symptom index for benign prostatic hyperplasia. *J Urol* 1992; 148:1549–57.

[68] Nandedkar SD, Barkhaus PE, Sanders DB, Stalberg EV. Analysis of amplitude and area of concentric needle EMG motor unit action potentials. *Electroencephalogr Clin Neurophysiol.* 1988; 69:561-7.

[69] Podnar S, Vodusek DB. Protocol for clinical neurophysiologic examination of the pelvic floor. *Neurourol Urodyn* 2001; 20:669–82.

[70] Kavia RB, Datta SN, DasGupta R, Elneil S, Fowler CJ. Urinary retention in women: its causes and management. *BJU Int* 2006; 97:281–7

[71] Vodusek DB.J Sphincter EMG in possible multiple system atrophy: to do or not to do? *Neurol Neurosurg Psychiatry.* 2001; 71:575-6.

[72] Smith AR, Hosker GL, Warrell DW. The role of partial denervation of the pelvic floor in the aetiology of genitourinary prolapse and stress incontinence of urine. A neurophysiological study. *Br J Obstet Gynaecol.* 1989; 96:24-8.

[73] Fowler CJ, Kirby RS, Harrison MJ. Decelerating burst and complex repetitive discharges in the striated muscle of the urethral sphincter, associated with urinary retention in women. *J Neurol Neurosurg Psychiatry.* 1985; 48:1004-9.

[74] Falck B, Stalberg E, Bischoff C. Sensory nerve conduction studies with surface electrodes. Methods in Clinical Neurophysiology. *Dantec* 1994; 5: 1–18

[75] Trojaborg W. Sensory nerve conduction: near nerve recording methods in clinical neurophysiology. *Dantec* 1992; 3: 41–4.

[76] Kerry H. Levin. Motor nerve conduction studies. In Peripheral Nerve Diseases Handbook of Clinical Neurophysiology, Vol. 7 J. Kimura (Ed.). *Elsevier* B.V. 2006.

[77] Tulio E. Bertorini. Sensory nerve conduction studies In Peripheral Nerve Diseases Handbook of Clinical Neurophysiology, Vol. 7 J. Kimura (Ed.) E*lsevier* B.V. 2006.

[78] Ochoa J, Mair WPG (1969). The normal sural nerve in man. I. Ultrastructure and numbers of fibers and cells. *Acta Neuropathol,* 13: 197-216.

[79] Kiff ES, Swash M. Normal proximal and delayed distal conduction in the pudendal nerves of patients with idiopathic (neurogenic) faecal incontinence. *J Neurol Neurosurg Psychiatry.* 1984; 47:820-3.

[80] Yeh M, Yamada T, Kimura K. Applications of SSEP recordings in the evaluation of the peripheral nervous system In Peripheral Nerve Diseases Handbook of Clinical Neurophysiology, Vol. 7 J. Kimura (Ed.) *Elsevier* B.V. 2006 pp. 443-466.

[81] Nuwer MR, Aminoff M, Desmedt J et al. IFCN recommended standards for short latency somatosensory evoked potentials. Report of an IFCN committee. International Federation of Clinical Neurophysiology. *Electroencephalogr Clin Neurophysiol* 1994; 9: 6–11.

[82] Cruccu G, Aminoff MJ, Curio G, Guerit JM, Kakigi R, Mauguiere F, Rossini PM, Treede RD, Garcia-Larrea L. Recommendations for the clinical use of somatosensory-evoked potentials. *Clin Neurophysiol.* 2008; 119:1705-19.

[83] Malaguti S, Spinelli M, Giardiello G, Lazzeri M, Van Den Hombergh U Neurophysiological evidence may predict the outcome of sacral neuromodulation. *J Urol.* 2003; 170(6 Pt 1):2323-6.

[84] Mazo EB, Sokolova AA, Krivoborodov GG, Shkolnikov ME, Moiseev PP. The role of somatosensory evoked potentials in prognosis of efficacy of tibial neuromodulation in patients with hyperactive urinary bladder. *Urologia.* 2005; 5: 49-52.

[85] Vodusek, DB, Janko, M and Lokar, J Direct and reflex responses in perineal muscles on electrical stimulation. *J. Neurol. Neurosurg. Psychiatry.* 1983; 46: 67–71.

[86] Ertekin C, Reel F. Bulbocavernosus réflex in normal men and in patients with neurogenic bladder and/or impotence. *J Neurol Sci* 1976; 28: 1–15

[87] Vodusek DB, Zidar J. Pudendal nerve involvement in patients with hereditary motor and sensory neuropathy. *Acta Neurol Scand* 1987; 76:457– 60.

[88] Claus D, Schondorf R. Sympathetic skin response. In, Recommendations for the Practice of Clinical Neurophysiology (EEG). (Suppl. 52). Amsterdam: *Elsevier,* 1999: 277–9.

[89] Shahani BT, Halperin JJ, Boulu P, Cohen J. Sympathetic skin response--a method of assessing unmyelinated axon dysfunction in peripheral neuropathies. *JNNP* 1984; 47:536-42.

[90] Ertekin C, Ertekin N, Mutlu S, Almis S, Akcam A, Zarola F, Bernardi G, Traversa R, La Pera G, Lavarone F Rossini PM. Skin potentials (SP) recorded from the extremities and genital regions in normal and impotent subjects. *Acta Neurol Scand.* 1987; 76:28-36.

[91] Daffertshofer M, Linden D, Syren M, Jünemann KP, Berlit P. Assessment of local sympathetic function in patients with erectile dysfunction. *Int J Impot Res.* 1994; 6:213-25.

[92] Valles-Antuña C, Fernandez-Gomez J, Escaf S, Fernandez-Gonzalez F. Sympathetic skin response in patients with erectile dysfunction. *BJU Int.* 2009; 104):1709-12.

[93] Schurch B, Curt A, Rossier AB The value of sympathetic skin response recordings in the assessment of the vesicourethral autonomic nervous dysfunction in spinal cord injured patients. *J Urol.* 1997; 157:2230-3.

[94] Rodic B, Curt A, Dietz V, Schurch B. Bladder neck incompetence in patients with spinal cord injury: significance of sympathetic skin response. *J Urol.* 2000; 163:1223-7.

[95] Dyck PJ, Karnes JL, Gillen DA, O'Brien PC, Zimmerman IR, Johnson DM. Comparison of algorithms of testing for use in automated evaluation of sensation. *Neurology* 1990; 40:1607–13.

[96] Freeman R, Chase KP, Risk MR. Quantitative sensory testing cannot differentiate simulated sensory loss from sensory neuropathy. *Neurology.* 2003; 60:465-70.

[97] Chong PS, Cros DP. Technology literature review: quantitative sensory testing. *Muscle Nerve.* 2004; 29: 734-47.

[98] Yarnitsky D, Sprecher E, Vardi Y. Penile thermal sensation. *J Urol.* 1996; 156 (2 Pt 1): 391-3.

[99] Salonia A, Saccà A, Briganti A, Del Carro U, Dehò F, Zanni G, et al. Quantitative sensory testing of peripheral thresholds in patients with lifelong premature ejaculation: a case-controlled study. *J Sex Med.* 2009; 6:1755-62.

[100] Bleustein CB, Arezzo JC, Eckholdt H, Melman A. The neuropathy of erectile dysfunction. *Int J Impot Res.* 2002; 14: 433-9.

[101] Bleustein CB, Fogarty JD, Eckholdt H, Arezzo JC, Melman A. Effect of neonatal circumcision on penile neurologic sensation. *Urology.* 2005; 65: 773-7.

[102] Rajmil O, Arrús J, Fernandez M, Sarquella J, Ruiz-Castañé E, Blasco A. Sensory changes after surgical correction of penile curvature. *Int J Impot Res.* 2009 Nov-Dec; 21: 366-71.

[103] Lefaucheur JP, Yiou R, Salomon L, Chopin DK, Abbou CC Assessment of penile small nerve fiber damage after transurethral resection of the prostate by measurement of penile thermal sensation. *J Urol.* 2000 Oct; 164:1416-9.

[104] Rivas DA, Chancellor MB. Neurogenic vesical dysfunction. *Urol Clin North Am* 1995; 22:579 –591.

[105] Abrams P, Cardozo L, Fall M, Griffiths D, Rosier P, Ulmsten U, et al. The standardisation of terminology of lower urinary tract function: report from the Standardisation Sub-committee of the International Continence Society. *Neurourol Urodyn* 2002; 21:167–78.

[106] Fowler CJ. Neurological disorders of micturition and their treatment. *Brain* 1999;122:1213–31.

[107] Weld KJ, Graney MJ, Dmochowski RR. Clinical significance of detrusor sphincter dyssynergia type in patients with posttraumatic spinal cord injury. *Urology* 2000; 56: 565–8.

[108] Hanno P, Burks DA, Clemens JQ, Dmochowski RR, Erickson D, FitzGerald MP et al. Diagnosis and treatment of interstitial cystitis/bladder pain syndrome. American Urological Association (AUA) Guideline. http://www.auanet.org/content/clinical-practice-guidelines/clinical-guidelines.cfm?sub=ic-bps] © 2011 by the American Urological Association

[109] Chiarelli PE, Moore KH. Techniques of Pelvic Floor Rehabilitation and Muscle Training: Exercise, Feedback and Biofeedback. Pelvic Floor Re-education Principles and Practice. Kaven Baessler, Bernhard Schussler, Kathryn L. Burgio, Kate H.Moore, Peggy A. Norton, and Stuart L. Stanton (Eds). Second edition *Springer-Verlag* London 2008p184-189

[110] Bower WF Techniques of Pelvic Floor Rehabilitation and Muscle Training: Electrical Stimulation. Pelvic Floor Re-education Principles and Practice. Kaven Baessler, Bernhard Schussler, Kathryn L. Burgio, Kate H.Moore, Peggy A. Norton, and Stuart L. Stanton (Eds). Second edition *Springer-Verlag* London 2008p190-195.

[111] Burton C, Sajja A, Latthe PM. Effectiveness of percutaneous posterior tibial nerve stimulation for overactive bladder: A systematic review and meta-analysis. *Neurourol Urodyn.* 2012 Nov; 31:1206-16.

[112] Hotouras A, Thaha MA, Boyle DJ, Allison ME, Currie A, Knowles CH, Chan CL. Short-term outcome following percutaneous tibial nerve stimulation for faecal incontinence: a single-centre prospective study. *Colorectal Dis.* 2012 Sep; 14:1101-5.

[113] Hotouras A, Thaha MA, Allison ME, Currie A, Scott SM, Chan CL. Percutaneous tibial nerve stimulation (PTNS) in females with faecal incontinence: the impact of sphincter morphology and rectal sensation on the clinical outcome. *Int J Colorectal Dis.* 2012 Jul;27:927-30.

[114] Lapides J, Diokno AC, Silber SJ, Lowe BS. Clean, intermittent self-catheterization in the treatment of urinary tract disease. *J Urol* 1972; 107:458–61.

[115] Chapple C, Khullar V, Gabriel Z, Dooley JA. The effects of antimuscarinic treatments in overactive bladder: a systematic review and meta-analysis. *Eur Urol* 2005; 48:5-26.

[116] Novara G, Galfano A, Secco S, D'Elia C, Cavalleri S, Ficarra V, Artibani W. A systematic review and meta-analysis of randomized controlled trials with antimuscarinic drugs for overactive bladder. *Eur Urol.* 2008. 54:740-63.

[117] Chapple CR, Khullar V, Gabriel Z, Muston D, Bitoun CE, Weinstein D. The effects of antimuscarinic treatments in overactive bladder: an update of a systematic review and meta-analysis Eur Urol. 2008. 54:543-62.

[118] Andersson KE, Chapple CR, Cardozo L, Cruz F, Hashim H, Michel MC, Tannenbaum C, Wein AJ. Pharmacological treatment of overactive bladder: report from the International Consultation on Incontinence. *Curr Opin Urol.* 2009 Jul; 19:380-94.

[119] Mehta S, Hill D, Foley N, Hsieh J, Ethans K, Potter P, Baverstock R, Teasell RW, Wolfe D; A meta-analysis of botulinum toxin sphincteric injections in the treatment of incomplete voiding after spinal cord injury. *Arch Phys Med Rehabil.* 2012 Apr; 93:597-603.

[120] Jarrett M, Mowatt G, Glazener C, et al. Systematic review of sacral nerve stimulation for faecal incontinence and constipation. *Br J Surg* 2004; 91:1559–69.

[121] Alwaal A, Al-Mannie R, Carrier S. Future prospects in the treatment of erectile dysfunction: focus on avanafil. *Drug Des Devel Ther.* 2011; 5:435-43.

[122] Angulo J, González-Corrochano R, Cuevas P, Fernández A, La Fuente JM, Rolo F, et al. Diabetes exacerbates the functional deficiency of NO/cGMP pathway associated with erectile dysfunction in human corpus cavernosum and penile arteries. *J Sex Med.* 2010 Feb; 7(2 Pt 1):758-68.

[123] Olsen AL, Smith VJ, Bergstrom JO, Colling JC, Clark AL Epidemiology of surgically managed pelvic organ prolapse and urinary incontinence. *Obstet Gynecol.* 1997; 89:501-6.

In: Contemporary Issues in Peripheral Neuropathy
Editor: Daniel L. Menkes
ISBN: 978-1-62948-681-9

Chapter XI

The Surgical Treatment of Peripheral Neuropathies: A Plastic Surgeon's Perspective

Sean Wolfort
Clinical Associate Professor of Surgery,
Florida State University,
University of Central Florida

Abstract

While many neuropathies are amenable to medical therapy, progressive compression neuropathies almost invariably require a surgical evaluation. Compression neuropathies are more likely to occur when there is a superimposed polyneuropathy as the affected nerve is less able to compensate for this process. It is important for the referring physician to understand the surgical approach to the treatment of compression neuropathies. This is best visualized by understanding the relevant "tunnels" commonly encountered with compression neuropathies. There are numerous similarities between the "tunnels" encountered in the upper extremity and those encountered in the lower extremity.

This chapter will address the surgical evaluation and treatment of the most commonly encountered upper and lower extremity entrapment neuropathies based on his extensive clinical experience. Although electrodiagnostic studies are helpful, this technique does not reliably identify each and every instance of a compression neuropathy. Therefore, a surgical referral is in order when the patient presents with symptoms of a compression neuropathy that is confirmed by specific physical examination signs.

Many of these patients with normal electrodiagnostic studies prove to have significant nerve compression at the time of their surgical intervention. The author reviews the surgical approach to these patients and concludes his chapter with a discussion of nerve repair techniques.

Introduction

Neurology is similar to other medical disciplines in that some conditions require surgical intervention given the inherent limitations of medical therapy. This is especially true for entrapment neuropathies as surgical intervention may eventually be required. Given the maxim that "sick nerves are liable to compression," many patients with an underlying polyneuropathy are at increased risk for a superimposed entrapment neuropathy. While most neurologists are able to identify the presence of an entrapment neuropathy, very few are aware of the surgical indications for a nerve release. Unlike other chapters in the textbook, the author will express his viewpoints even in the absence of "evidence- based medicine" to support them. This book chapter is based on extensive anecdotal experience as few surgical interventions have been assessed using Class I or Class II trials. That stated, this chapter will describe a surgical approach to entrapment neuropathies that is based on neuroanatomical concepts that focuses on the relevant "tunnels", through which nerves traverse. It is imperative that all physicians understand the salient anatomy of these anatomical tunnels such that the available surgical interventions can be visualized. From a surgical perspective, the evaluation of an entrapment neuropathy is relatively straightforward.

It should be stated that many surgeons view electrodiagnostic studies as specific but insensitive. Thus, a negative electrodiagnostic study neither excludes a diagnosis nor eliminates the option of a surgical intervention. The author is of the opinion that electrodiagnostic studies underestimate the true prevalence of entrapment neuropathies. Nerve conduction studies and needle electromyography [EMG/NCV] testing is insensitive, as reported by many studies attempting to correlate the EMG/NCVs with a true positive result and outcome following surgical releases [1]. One of the largest EMG/NCV studies reported a false negative rate of approximately 33% for carpal tunnel syndrome and 50% for cubital tunnel syndrome [2, 3]. As of the writing of this chapter, MRIs and CTs simply lack the resolution necessary to adequately evaluate for the presence of a compression neuropathy, even with larger nerves such as the sciatic. The author recalls numerous occasions when an imaging study was reported as normal and the nerve was found to be encased or even compressed by scar tissue. Until diagnostic tests with adequate sensitivity and specificity are developed, surgeons will continue to rely on their clinical judgment. The author routinely employs the use of other ancillary testing devices such as quantitative sensory testing. The Pressure-Specified Sensory Device has the advantages of being non-invasive, painless, simple, and inexpensive to perform [4]. When normative data are properly applied, the author has found this device to have a high degree of sensitivity. However, this machine is expensive (approximately $50,000). Moreover, many insurance plans do not reimburse testing with this device. Nonetheless, the author has found its results to be highly accurate and predictive of post-operative results.

The author will also caution the reader that not all clinical examination tests have a high degree of sensitivity and specificity as summarized in the text by Malanga and Nadler (5). For example, this text cites two studies in which the sensitivity of a Tinel's sign at the wrist was reported as 25% in one study and 44% in the other. Notably, these two studies estimated a specificity of over 90% [6]. Therefore, the results of these assessments should be interpreted with caution. Two studies in the aforementioned text determined that the sensitivity of a Tinel's sign at the wrist has a sensitivity of 25 and 44%. However, the specificity was approximately 95% in both studies [6]. When these techniques were compared with an electrophysiological examination as the "gold standard", one study found that the wrist flexion Phalen's test had a sensitivity of 71% and a specificity of 80% [7]. The author's experience is that several clinical tests that yield the same outcome prove most valuable. As such, the author hardly ever relies on a single test unless it has proven sensitivity and specificity. For example, the Durkan's carpal tunnel compression test has a higher sensitivity (87%) and specificity (90%) than either the Tinel's or Phalen's tests [8].

Once the diagnosis of compression of a peripheral nerve is established, the peripheral nerve surgeon must rely on the fundamentals of human anatomy. It should also be recalled that human anatomy is variable such that textbooks identify the "common" anatomical relationships. Individuals may have variations on this theme such that a surgeon should anticipate such anomalies. Furthermore, previous surgeries may result in new sites of entrapment due to the creation of new "tunnels", as may occur with an inguinal herniorrhaphy. Restated, the anatomy textbooks should serve as a rough guideline or 'road-map' rather than as "written in stone" topography. Notably, the "classic" anatomical illustrations are indicative of no more than forty percent of the general population as evidenced by cadaveric studies [9, 10]. Given the significant number of anatomical variants, a nerve release cannot be considered complete until all reasonable potential sites of compression have been addressed. This requires a comprehensive understanding of anomalous muscles, vascular 'leashes', and fibrous arches or arcades. This knowledge is important as the surgeon's goal is to perform a comprehensive yet minimally invasive operation that addresses all potential sites of compression. For example, the author notes that many electromyographers perform ulnar nerve inching studies to identify the specific compression site. This finding only identifies the most profound compression site and not each and every site of compression. A surgeon will perform an extensive ulnar nerve release in order to ensure that all potential sites of compression are addressed and not just the one detected by electrodiagnostic studies. As will be discussed later in this chapter, many nerve decompression surgeries are deemed "failures" because secondary compression sites were not considered in the first instance.

It is also this reconstructive surgeon's opinion that surgical principles that are useful in upper extremity entrapments are equally useful in the less frequently encountered lower extremity nerve entrapments. Much of what is described in this chapter should be attributed to the author's mentor, A. Lee Dellon, M.D., Ph.D. The author was able to translate much of what he learned from upper extremity neuropathies to those of the lower extremity. This chapter is focused on the treatment of entrapment neuropathies. As such, this chapter will not be discussing the surgical treatment of brachial plexopathies; a topic that has been addressed comprehensively in another textbook [11].

The author will now discuss his approach to the common entrapment neuropathies encountered in clinical practice. This will be approached in a slightly different manner than most chapters in that the upper extremity entrapment will be discussed followed by the analogous lower extremity entrapment. Embryology demonstrates that the lower extremity is similar to the upper extremity but that it is rotated 180 degrees. This approach will allow the reader to understand the surgical approach to these entrapment neuropathies. In this paradigm, the upper extremity entrapment will be discussed before its analogous lower extremity entrapment.

Carpal Tunnel Syndrome

Most patients with carpal tunnel syndrome due to median nerve compression at the wrist will present with some combination of symptoms that may include numbness, burning, paresthesias, and pain affecting the median innervated digits. Of these digits, the most reliable is that of the index finger's pulp due to overlapping sensory distributions in the other digits. If the small finger or the dorsum of the digit is involved, it cannot be due to carpal tunnel syndrome alone. Similarly, sensory loss over the back of the hand along the metacarpals cannot be due to carpal tunnel alone except if there is an unusual innervation pattern or an anastomosis [12, 13]. If the thenar eminence is involved with paresthesias, as supported by sensory testing and a comparison to the fellow hand, this simply cannot be ascribed to median nerve entrapment at the carpal tunnel alone. The palmar cutaneous branch of the median nerve originates from the median nerve proper approximately 5 cm proximal to the transverse carpal ligament such that there should not be sensory loss over the palm. If the lateral antebrachial cutaneous nerve contributes to the sensory innervation of the thenar eminence, it will never pass under the roof of the carpal tunnel. Given that electrodiagnostic studies may not be positive in the early stages of median nerve compression, a decision to proceed with surgical intervention is based on the clinical history and physical examination data. A positive Durkan's compression test with or without a Tinel's sign or positive Phalen's test, combined with a history of five out of seven nocturnal awakenings in a week and/or constant numbness for six weeks confirms the author's clinical diagnosis of carpal tunnel syndrome. If there is no evidence of weakness in the thenar eminence, conservative measures such as night splints, non-steroidal anti-inflammatory agents, and steroid injections should be attempted and proven inadequate before surgery is performed. However, surgery should be performed if these conservative measures fail even if nerve conduction studies are normal. Wasting of the abductor pollicis brevis muscle mandates surgical attention especially if noticed within the first year, when recovery may still be possible.

Once the need for a carpal tunnel release is established, the procedure is relatively straightforward. The author is of the opinion that instrumentation is unnecessary and complicates an otherwise simple procedure. The endoscopic approach should be avoided because of the variability of the origin of the recurrent motor branch of the median nerve. It may arise from the central volar surface of the median nerve proper and course through a fibrous and often thickened transverse carpal ligament and possibly proximal to the direct longitudinal path of the endoscopic blade releasing this ligament [14,15]. Moreover, a surgeon must expect to debulk the abundant degenerative tenosynovium from the 8 out of 9 flexors passing under the transverse carpal ligament. This is, especially the case in those patients with overuse syndromes or associated trigger digits where it is almost invariably present. The author has never observed the Flexor Pollicis Longus [FPL] to be encased in bulky tenosynovium except in those patients with rheumatoid arthritis. Bipolar electrocautery is mandatory for hemostasis in perineural procedures; a nearly impossible procedure when using an endoscopic approach. It is imperative to achieve complete hemostasis as a postoperative hematoma with the carpal tunnel release almost invariably leads to stiffness, pain, and a recurrence of paresthesias from the resultant fibrosis. There is some controversy regarding which layers to close after the carpal tunnel release. Some surgeons choose to close a released transverse carpal ligament to minimize scarring that might occur on the underside of the overlying dermis. The author is of the opinion that this is contrary to the goal of the release- increasing the volume of the tunnel. Dermal scarring is problematic in that it may stick to the underlying released nerve. Other surgeons may close the superficial palmar aponeurosis in an attempt to prevent dermal scarring, whereas some may only close the skin. The author then "stair-steps" the closure by joining the transverse carpal ligament to the superficial aponeurosis. This has the advantages of increasing the volume of the carpal tunnel while minimizing dermal scarring. Debulking of the tenosynovium is also recommended as it leads to an increased volume and transverse diameter of the carpal tunnel. Soft splints are used postoperatively as motion is encouraged within the confines of wound healing demands. This approach minimizes the adherence of scar tissue to the nerve. The important concept is that nerves were designed to move such that post-operative motion ought to be encouraged.

Tarsal Tunnel Syndrome

The lower extremity analogy to the carpal tunnel is the tarsal tunnel although there are fewer tendons passing through the tarsal tunnel by comparison. There are subdivisions within this tunnel such that case reports indicating a less than satisfactory result from tarsal tunnel releases may stem from the inadequate release of the subdivisions within this tunnel. This is why peripheral nerve surgeons often refer to the proper release as a "tarsal tunnel S" release. There are at least four subcomponent tunnels within the tarsal tunnel. The first is the flexor retinaculum roof, or lancinate ligament, which covers the posterior tibial neurovascular bundle, is the most proximal tunnel. The roof of this tunnel then blends with the abductor hallucis aponeurosis. A septum, often thickened, descends from the aponeurosis, and separates the medial from the lateral plantar nerve tunnels with their accompanying tendons underneath, the Flexor Digitorum Longus (FDL) and the Flexor Hallucis Longus (FHL), respectively.

It should be recalled from embryology that the foot is similar to the hand save for the fact that it is rotated 180 degrees. Thus, the lateral plantar nerve has a distribution similar to the ulnar nerve in that it innervates the lateral one and a half digits and the foot intrinsic muscles. There is also a similarity to the canal of Guyon. The fourth tunnel is smaller and directs the medial calcaneal branches to the sensory end organs in the skin. The author has observed a range from one to seven of these branches, with both high and low origins from the posterior tibial nerve proper to more distal jump-off points at the lateral and even medial plantar nerves.

In the author's practice, about half of the patients referred with lower extremity neuropathies are diabetic whereas approximately 40 percent have no known cause (idiopathic). The remaining 10 percent is comprised of miscellaneous causes including chemotherapy - induced neuropathy, HIV neuropathy, and uncommon causes such as environmental exposures.

In order to better understand lower extremity compression neuropathies, the author performed lateral tension testing in patients who presented with symptoms of a focal compression superimposed on a baseline neuropathy due to diabetes mellitus, HIV protease inhibitor use, and idiopathic neuropathies (Wolfort SF, unpublished data). A simple vessi-loop band was attached to a force pressure gauge and lateral tension was slowly applied to an

syndrome). Therefore, an entrapment of the median nerve in the forearm is analogous to an entrapment of the posterior tibial nerve at the soleal sling [17]. It is at this location that a fibrous arch derived from the two heads of the soleus muscle's origin might induce a significant degree of compression. The author recommends a similar surgical approach in which the nerve is freed from all potential sites of compression in this region.

Radial Tunnel Syndrome

The radial tunnel in the forearm is analogous to the fibular tunnel at the upper leg. The Arcade of Frohse, or the fibrous edge of the supinator muscle, may compress the radial nerve proper, proximal to the emergence of the motor branch innervating the extensor carpi radialis brevis (ECRB) and distal to the origin of the superficial radial nerve. This analogy should be remembered as a band of tissue under the peroneus longus muscle may compress the common fibular (peroneal) nerve distal to a lateral sural nerve branch.

Radial tunnel syndrome is especially difficult to diagnose as the chief complaint tends to be that of pain. The signs are not obvious in the absence of a posterior Interosseous Nerve (PIN) palsy presenting with weakness of finger and wrist extension. The area of lateral epicondylar tenderness often overlaps that of the radial tunnel territory. Thus, the key to this diagnosis is familiarity with the anatomy. Lateral epicondylar tenderness may be above and/or below the epicondyle at the origin of the wrist extensors. The variability of these origins explains the difficulty in targeting the tendinous inflammation. Several other clinical tests are useful. One is resisted dorsiflexion of the wrist, where the pain is near the epicondyle. The pain may be described as aching, severe, and burning. A middle finger resistance test to extension with resistance applied to the middle finger proximal phalanx dorsum tests the ECRB, as the insertion of this muscle is at the base of the middle finger metacarpal, and its fibrous edge compresses the posterior interosseous nerve. Resisted supination of the extended arm may produce pain at the radial tunnel as the fibrous arch of the supinator, the Arcade of Frohse, compresses the radial nerve proper as it plunges beneath this flat muscle. The forearm must be extended at the elbow to eliminate the powerful supinator effects of the biceps brachii muscle, thereby placing the load solely on the supinator itself. In an isolated radial tunnel syndrome there is no weakness and no sensory disturbance. Surgical release of the radial tunnel must include a debulking of any overly prominent ECRB, along with any fibrous edges, the supinator's Arcade of Frohse, and ligation of the commonly present vascular leash of Henry (the recurrent radial vessels). The author has observed these vessels in 80% of his radial tunnel cases.

Wartenberg's syndrome, or entrapment of the superficial radial nerve [SRN] between the muscle bellies of the brachioradialis and extensor carpi radialis longus [ECRL], may induce a sensory disturbance at the dorsal first web space of the hand from a "scissoring effect." It should be recalled that these nerve distributions can overlap, especially at the thumb, with digital nerve branches and a persistent lateral antebrachial cutaneous nerve that might confuse the examiner. This argues for using the volar pulp of the index finger as the most reliable area for sensory testing in a suspected median neuropathy at the wrist. While the precise mechanism by which two muscle bellies may compress the SRN over the radius has been debated, the author has often noted a nerve branch stuck to the underside of the muscle belly where there is a thickened fascia or epimysium. It appears shiny and white and is associated with adherence and resultant tethering.

The diagnosis of DeQuervain's stenosing tenosynovitis must be excluded when examining the patient for Wartenberg's syndrome. This is because of the proximity of the SRN, as it emerges from between the brachioradialis and ECRL, to the first extensor compartment. A Tinel's test of the SRN has an unknown sensitivity and specificity. However, when a positive Tinel's is noted and combined with a negative Finklestein's test, the likelihood of a Wartenberg's diagnosis is high. It should be stated that the Finklestein test, while useful, does not have a well defined sensitivity and specificity. The Finklestein's test is performed best by removing jewelry, having the patient hold the thumb loosely in the palm with a relaxed wrist and gently hyperpronating the wrist with a stabilized elbow. In a patient with DeQuervain's tenosynovitis, this test evokes significant pain. Also, a SRN tethered to the brachioradialis or ECRL will often elicit pain with this maneuver. Thus, the coexistence of DeQuervain's with Wartenberg's can easily be confirmed. It is also important not to stress the thumb carpometacarpal [CMC] joint during this maneuver as pain with an underlying grinding arthritic CMC can confuse the picture. The examiner must be specific about the pain's location and the quality as well as the presence of associated tenderness. There is no accurate analogue to Wartenberg's in the leg, although one could visualize a similar situation with the deep branch of the fibular (peroneal) nerve. Its terminal sensory branch provides cutaneous sensation to the web space between the first and second digits in the foot. It is susceptible to compression by the extensor hallucis brevis muscle. Often a fibrous edge at the musculotendinous junction will cause significant compression of the terminal sensory portion of this nerve. The superficial fibular (peroneal) nerve sensory branch is variable where it may travel in the septum between the lateral and anterior compartments, or directly travel into the anterior compartment, emerging through a small fascial window well above and medial to the lateral malleolus.

Common Fibular (Peroneal) Compression at the Fibular Tunnel

The most extreme presentation of a foot drop may occur from a compression of the common fibular (peroneal) nerve at the fibular tunnel. This is similar to a wrist drop due to compression of the radial nerve resulting in a PIN palsy. A more subtle presentation of common fibular nerve entrapment at the fibular tunnel might present as paresthesias in the distribution of both the superficial and deep fibular nerve cutaneous distributions. Common fibular nerve entrapment is often due to a fibrous band underneath the peroneus longus muscle, or by a fibrous edge of the lateral gastrocnemius muscle. If both superficial and deep distributions are compressed, then the entire dorsum of the foot may be affected by paresthesias. A more distal compression may affect one or the other nerves but not both never both unless there are two separate and distinct sites of compression. Another common compression site of the deep fibular nerve is on the foot dorsum itself just proximal to the first web space where the Extensor Hallucis Brevis muscle (EHB) can compress the terminal sensory branch of this nerve. Care must be taken not to damage the important dorsalis pedis artery when teasing apart adhesions at this site. The superficial fibular nerve cutaneous distribution is more expansive, and may lie in the septum between the anterior and posterior compartments. It also may emerge through a fenestration in the anterior compartment itself. These variations may set the stage for a traction injury from an ankle sprain near the sinus tarsi, where the superficial fibular nerve crosses the muscle belly of the EHB, and/or a motor branch of the deep fibular nerve. In some instances, both branches may be stretched and may result in persistent weakness in great toe extension. This diagnosis can be assessed by comparing the strength to the same muscle contralaterally. This diagnosis should also be suspected when the patient presents with pain with or without paresthesias in an otherwise uncomplicated sprain that should have healed. While this is a difficult and uncommon diagnosis, any persistent pain after an ankle inversion sprain where extreme inversion may cause an injury to those nerves near the sinus tarsi, should prompt the clinician to assess for a Tinel's sign at the sinus tarsi or EHB belly.

Saphenous Nerve

The saphenous nerve is hardly ever compressed. Nonetheless, a saphenous nerve compression ought to be considered when there are sensory symptoms affecting the medial leg and adjacent foot. It is the terminal sensory branch of the femoral nerve that accompanies the greater saphenous vein in its course. It can often be injured with vein stripping or harvesting for cardiac bypass grafts. This may present as discomfort on the top and medial portions of the ankle and foot. The lateral antebrachial or brachial cutaneous nerves similarly are subject to injury when harvesting or fistulizing the cephalic vein in the forearm or arm. The author often uses the saphenous nerve as an internal control for a patient with a baseline neuropathy when performing quantitative sensory testing, as it is rarely compressed except when it is involved with scar tissue. Similar statements may be rendered regarding the sural nerve, which is the lower extremity nerve that is usually assessed in routine electrodiagnostic studies given that it is more reliably obtained with cutaneous stimulation.

Interdigital Nerve Compression at the Foot

There is no analogue for a 'Morton's neuroma' in the hand, as the nerve arcade formed by the medial and lateral plantar nerves experience significant pressures that are not experienced in the upper extremity. The deep transverse metatarsal ligament exerts compression on the common digital nerve proximal to its branching into the proper digital nerves. This may result in a neuroma, which disturbs sensation in the web space and distal territories. Thus, the author recommends addressing this issue by relieving the compression by cutting or excising the ligament rather than the nerve itself. The author notes that nobody would advocate resecting or injecting the median nerve with alcohol at the carpal tunnel. However, these techniques are commonly employed in the foot with less than satisfactory results. In addition to a high failure rate, these techniques may result in a residual painful neuroma. The neuroma stump may then retract and become entangled with an adjacent ligament or scar tissue. When this situation occurs, the author opines that the only effective solution is to perform a microsurgical intrafascicular dissection for the purpose of sequestering the nerve ending in a "safe haven" such as in the belly of the quadratus plantae muscle or a bone window in the calcaneus (18).

Lateral Femoral Cutaneous Nerve Compression at the Anterior Pelvis

Meralgia paresthetica [MP] is an interesting and often overlooked compression of the lateral femoral cutaneous nerve (LFCN) of the thigh as it crosses over the anterosuperior iliac spine (ASIS). Five potential reported patterns have been described [19]. MP presents as numbness and burning pain along the anterolateral thigh area, which is reproduced by pressure or a Tinel's test at the bony landmark of compression, the ASIS. It is commonly encountered in military or police personnel who wear a holster too low. The author has also encountered it in patients who have undergone hip replacement surgery, especially revisions, seat belt injuries (including one in a commercial airline pilot), and even musicians. The author recalls one such case in a sedentary violist and cellist, where prolonged fixed positioning was required during practice and symphonic performances. The author has also observed this following tight hernia repairs, as a common course of the LFCN is through the inguinal ligament. Because the nerve may share a cutaneous branch with the genitofemoral nerve, which are more classically affected after a hernia repair, the correct diagnosis may not be readily apparent. Sensory nerve conduction studies or quantitative sensory testing in which the symptomatic limb is compared to the fellow limb is the recommended course of action.

Because the LFCN is a pure sensory nerve, the author recommends resection and implantation into the retroperitoneum. This is a relatively straightforward procedure to perform, as the resected nerve stump is simply 'dunked' into the pelvis. Violent coughing or straining with constipation may bring out the preoperative symptoms by increased intra-abdominal pressure.

Peripheral Nerve Injuries: Repair and Reconstruction

Over the last two decades there has been more interest regarding the optimal means by which a surgeon should repair a peripheral nerve injury. It should be recalled that the distal severed nerve end may direct the growth sprouting of a regenerated proximal nerve end to its native sensory or motor target. The author has experimented with alternative techniques that yield results similar to that of a surgical anastomosis with or without an autograft in neural regeneration. It cannot be overemphasized that any nerve repair that is placed under any tension is doomed to failure. Many new products touted as "nerve conduits" have appeared on the market given the limited availability of donor graft material. Many of these conduits have little evidence based medicine to support their use such that it would be difficult to make a specific recommendation. Nonetheless, the author is of the opinion that first principles of surgery need to be followed. The first concept is to determine what the goals of such conduits should be. The ideal conduit should not be recognized as foreign such that it would not provoke a strong inflammatory reaction. If it is chemically altered over time, it should be one that yields the least amount of scar tissue. It should also mimic the native surrounding environment of the nerve, preferably a soft bed of well-vascularized tissue that is pliable and protective as the nerve regenerates to join the distal end or target end organ. A nearly impermeable tube might significantly impair the nutrient lymphatico-vascular inflow and outflow in an already compromised neural junction, thus imposing great demands on the intraneural channels that have not yet been established. Moreover, gap length is inversely proportional to the clinical outcome. Therefore the conduit should allow for nerve regeneration to occur at the same pace as a simple tension-free anastomosis. Conduit outcomes should also be better than a long sural nerve graft. Given all these requirements, their use in mixed sensory and motor nerves is still in question [21]. Conduit tubes have included veins, polyglycolic acid [PGA], arteries, and hollowed out cadaveric nerves. Also, scaffolds that eliminate the antigenic stimuli yet provide the extracellular matrix framework to support a rapid regeneration have been designed, and skeletal muscles or fat has been stuffed in tubes [22].

Some of the more promising recent studies regarding conduits will be discussed. The use of bioabsorbable conduits such as PGA or a semi-permeable type I collagen conduit has demonstrated more favorable results when compared to direct repair for gaps $\leq$ 4mm and nerve grafts $\geq$ 8mm for sensory recovery in a trial addressing human digital nerves [23]. More recently, motor recovery in human brachial plexus nerve transfers using a type I collagen conduit demonstrated an equivalent clinical and EMG recovery to a direct anastomosis (24). The use of a polyglycolic bioabsorbable conduit has been shown to effectively bridge motor nerve gaps of up to 3 cm in humans [25]. Nonetheless, on any gap longer than 3 cm, the use of an autograft remains the gold standard. Processed nerve allografts offer an effective and safe alternative to autografts in achieving overall recovery of S3 or M4 and above in 86% of the nerve reconstructions in humans with sensory, motor, and mixed defects with gaps ranging from 0.5 to 5 cm [26]. Promising results in animal studies have favored the addition of co-cultured Schwann cells and adipose-derived or dental pulp-derived stem cells to nerve conduits in rat sciatic nerves with 15 mm gaps [27]. Another exciting advance in nerve regeneration comes from the logic applied to the area of tendon transfers, where one structure is sacrificed in order to repair another. As an example, consider a proximal ulnar nerve injury that has a poor prognosis in restoring intrinsic function in the hand. This is because the rate of regeneration is too slow to allow the regenerating nerve to reach the neuromuscular junctions of the distal muscles before the junction receptors disappear. This would be the case in even the most propitious circumstances in which the nerve is cleanly cut, minimal delay is seen in seeking attention or getting to the right caregiver, no infection and little collateral damage. In such an instance, the transfer of the terminal branch of the anterior interosseous nerve to the deep motor branch of the ulnar nerve will shorten recovery time with minimal donor morbidity. There are other such nerves that may be used in a similar manner that can even result in a potential M4 or M5 recovery [28].

In conclusion, a firm knowledge of the normal and variant anatomy is absolutely essential for any surgeon who will be addressing compression neuropathies. The importance of assessing for a superimposed compression neuropathy in a patient with a peripheral neuropathy cannot be overemphasized. Although nerve conduction studies and needle EMG can be helpful in establishing the correct diagnosis, especially when abnormal results are noted, nothing can replace a careful history and detailed physical examination. Thus, negative electrodiagnostic studies should not be interpreted as indicating the absence of a compression neuropathy. Surgical referral is recommended when conservative treatments have failed, even in those patients with normal electrodiagnostic studies. Surgical intervention must address the underlying anatomical issues while minimizing operative morbidity. Surgical release of nerve entrapments may lead to significant symptoms reduction and an improved quality of life. When nerves are not in continuity, surgical repairs are less than optimal. Although conduit technology is improving, their use is limited to very specific indications. Until conduit technology improves, nerve grafting and "nerve borrowing" techniques can lead to improved clinical outcomes in carefully selected patients.

References

[1] Lobar B. A neurologist's perspective: improved documentation of clinically suspect nerve compression by adding quantitative sensory testing when traditional NCV/EMG are normal. *J. Reconstr Microsurg* 1999; 15:616.

[2] AAEM Quality Assurance Committee. Literature review of the usefulness of nerve conduction studies and electromyography for the evaluation of patients with carpal tunnel syndrome. *Muscle Nerve 1993*; 16:1392-1414.

[3] Tomaino MM, Brach PJ, Vansickel DP. The rationale for and efficacy of surgical intervention for electrodiagnostic-negative cubital tunnel syndrome. *J. Hand Surg* 2001; 26: 1077-1081.

[4] Dellon AL. *Measuring peripheral nerve function: neurosensory testing versus electrodiagnostic testing, in Atlas of Hand Clinics: nerve repair and reconstruction*, D. Slutsky, ed., Philadelphia, PA: Elsevier Inc., Chapter 1, pp 1-31, 2005.

[5] Malanga GA and Nadler SF. *Musculoskeletal Physical examination: an evidence-based approach.* Philadelphia, PA: Elsevier Inc., 2006.

[6] Agesen T, Nadler ST, Wrightson J, Miller J. Physical examination of the elbow, wrist, and hand. In *Musculoskeletal Physical examination: an evidence-based approach*. eds. Malanga GA and Nadler ST. New York: Springer-Verlag., Ch. 5, p. 178. 2009.

[7] Gellman H, et al. Carpal tunnel syndrome: an evaluation of the provocative diagnostic tests. *J. Bone Joint Surg. Am.* 1986: 68:735-7.

[8] Durkan JA. A new diagnostic test for carpal tunnel syndrome. *J. Bone Joint Surg. Am.* 1991; 73:535-538.

[9] Brushart TM. The central course of primate digital nerve axons. *American Society for Surgery of the Hand*, Scientific Session, 1985.

[10] Terzis JK, Feeker BI, Sismour EN. A computerized study of the intraneural organization of the median nerve. *J. Hand Surg* 1984; 9:605.

[11] Leffert RD. *Brachial plexus injuries*. Churchill Livingstone, Inc., 1985.

[12] Learmonth JR. A variation in the distribution of the radial branch of the musculospiral nerve. *J. Anat* 1919; 53:371-372.

[13] Okwueze M, Cardwell NL, Wolfort SF, Nanney LB. Unexpected motor axons in the distal superficial radial and posterior interosseous nerves: a cadaver study. *Clinical Anatomy.* 2007; 20:790-794.

[14] Lanz V. Anatomic variations of the median nerve in the carpal tunnel. *J. Hand Surg.* 1977; 2:44-53.
[15] Bennett JB, Crouch CC. Compression syndrome of the recurrent branch of the median nerve. *J. Hand Surg.* 1982; 7:407-409.
[16] Stewart JD. *Focal peripheral neuropathies,* 4th edition. p.24, West Vancouver, BC: JBJ Publishing, 2010.
[17] Williams EH, Williams CG, Rosson GD, Dellon AL. Combined peroneal and proximal tibial nerve palsies. *Microsurgery.* 2009; 29: 259-264.
[18] Wolfort SF and Dellon AL. Treatment of recurrent neuroma of the interdigital nerve by implantation of the proximal nerve into muscle in the arch of the foot. *J. Foot & Ankle Surg.* 2001; 40:6, 404-410.
[19] Aszmann OC, Dellon ES, Dellon AL. Anatomical Course of the lateral femoral cutaneous nerve and its susceptibility to compression and injury. *J. of Plastic and Reconstructive Surgery* 1997; 100:600-604.
[20] Mackinnon SE and Dellon AL. *Surgery of the peripheral nerve.* New York: Thieme Medical Publishers, Inc., p. 179. 1988.
[21] Konofaos P, Ver Halen JP. Nerve repair by means of tubulization: past, present, future. *J. Reconstr. Microsurg.* 2013; 29:149-64.
[22] Papalia I, Raimondo S, Ronchi G, Magaudda L, Giacobini-Robecchi MG, Geuna S. Repairing nerve gaps by vein conduits filled with lipoaspirate derived entire adipose tissue hinders nerve regeneration. *Ann. Anat* 2013; 195(3): 225-230.
[23] Petrova ES. The use of stem cells to stimulate regeneration of damaged nerves. *Tsitologiia* 2012; 54(7):525-40.
[24] Mantovani C, Terenghi G, Shawcross SG. Isolation of adult stem cells and their differentiation to Schwann cells. *Methods of Mol Biol.* 2012; 916: 47-57.
[25] Weber RA, Breidenbach WC, Brown RE, Jabaley ME, Mass DP. A randomized prospective study of polyglycolic acid conduits for digital nerve reconstruction in humans. *Plast Reconstr. Surg.* 2000; 106:1036-1045.
[26] Wolfe SW, Strauss HL, Garg R, Feinberg J. Use of bioabsorbable nerve conduits as an adjunct to brachial plexus neurorrhaphy. *J. Hand Surg.* 2012; 37: 1980-5.
[27] Rosson GD, Williams EH, Dellon AL. Motor nerve regeneration across a conduit. *Microsurgery.* 2009; 29:107-14.
[28] Cho MS, Rinker BD, Weber RV, Chao JD, Ingari JV, Brooks D, Buncke GM. Functional outcome following nerve repair in the upper extremity using processed nerve allograft. *J. Hand Surg* 2012; 37:2340-9.
[29] Dai LG, Huang GS, Hsu SH. Sciatic nerve regeneration by co-cultured Schwann cells and stem cells on microporous nerve conduits. *Cell Transplant.* Nov 27, 2012. Accessed on 9/13/13 at http://www.ncbi.nlm.nih.gov/pubmed/23192007
[30] Mackinnon SE and Novak CB. Nerve transfers. *Hand Clinics* 2008, *24*:455-460.

Index

B

C

D

E

F

G

H

I

J

K

L

M

P

Q

R

S

T

U

V